South Asian Perspectives in Mental Health and Psychology

Series Editors

S. M. Yasir Arafat, Bangladesh Specialized Hospital, Dhaka, Bangladesh

Sujita Kumar Kar, Department of Psychiatry, King George's Medical University, Lucknow, Uttar Pradesh, India

This series of books is an endeavor to gather and present a comprehensive understanding of the various aspects of mental health that are relevant to people living in South Asia. The books aim to provide in-depth guidance and practical solutions to the mental health challenges that are unique to these areas. The content covers a wide range of topics, including but not limited to, climate change and its impact, prison mental health, perinatal mental health, social psychiatry, mental health and disorder among the elderly population, psychiatry education and training, suicide, SDGs and mental health, trauma, addiction, and social isolation. The books also emphasize the importance of early intervention and provide resources for seeking help. The ultimate goal of this series is to empower individuals and communities to take proactive steps toward enhancing their mental wellbeing. The proposed books will fill the existing unmet need in the region with huge populations in low and middle-income country (LMIC) settings.

South Asia, home to about 2 billion people, is a region of diverse cultures, languages, and religions. It caters to about 25% of the global population. This densely populated region faces a myriad of challenges, both natural and man-made. The frequent occurrence of natural disasters, such as earthquakes, floods, and landslides, threaten the lives and livelihoods of millions of people. War, terrorism, and political instability have caused significant disruptions to the region's socio-political fabric. Poverty, migration, and tropical infectious diseases remain major challenges that hinder progress towards sustainable development. Climate change exacerbates these challenges, causing widespread environmental degradation, food insecurity, and water scarcity. Despite these obstacles, South Asian people have shown remarkable resilience and strength in the face of adversity.

Mental health issues in the South Asian region significantly contribute to the global burden of mental illnesses. However, the region faces plenty of challenges such as high stigma, low mental health literacy, poor budgetary allocation, high out-of-pocket expense for mental health services, lack of adequate infrastructure, and limited human resources are significant barriers in mental healthcare. The majority of research on mental health issues is produced by the western countries which may not fit all in the South Asian culture, albeit evidence is needed to test. There is a paucity of research and evidence-based strategies that are region-specific. This series of books is an attempt to compile the important dimensions of mental health that will benefit the regional people.

Prerna Kukreti • Sujita Kumar Kar
S. M. Yasir Arafat
Editors

Women's Reproductive Mental Health in South Asia

Current Status, Challenges, and Ways Forward

Springer

Editors
Prerna Kukreti
Department of Psychiatry
Lady Hardinge Medical College
New Delhi, Delhi, India

Sujita Kumar Kar
Department of Psychiatry
King George's Medical University
Lucknow, Uttar Pradesh, India

S. M. Yasir Arafat
Department of Psychiatry
Bangladesh Specialized Hospital
Dhaka, Bangladesh

Department of Public and
Community Health
Faculty of Medicine and Health Sciences
Frontier University Garowe
Garowe, Somalia

ISSN 3059-3646 ISSN 3059-3522 (electronic)
South Asian Perspectives in Mental Health and Psychology
ISBN 978-981-96-9218-7 ISBN 978-981-96-9219-4 (eBook)
https://doi.org/10.1007/978-981-96-9219-4

This Springer imprint is published by the registered company Springer Nature Singapore Pte Ltd.
The registered company address is: 152 Beach Road, #21-01/04 Gateway East, Singapore 189721, Singapore

We dedicate this book to our beloved mothers
Shashi Kukreti
Urmila Kar
Amena Begum

Foreword

It is my great pleasure to write the foreword of the book—"Women's Reproductive Mental Health in South Asia: Current Status, Challenges, and Ways Forward," a publication authored by a dedicated group of scholars and emerging voices in the field. This book is a timely and much-needed contribution that explores the intricate and often overlooked intersection between reproductive health and mental well-being among women in South Asia.

South Asia consists of eight densely populated low- and middle-income countries (LMICs) that cater to about one-fourth of the global population. The region has multiple health challenges, such as low budgetary allocation, high out-of-pocket expenses, inadequate and inequitable human resources, and inadequate health literacy, and all these induced stress in mental health of the population. The region contains different characteristics compared to Western countries. The people of the region share similar cultural backgrounds and also face many social, economic, and health challenges that include male dominance and gender-based violence. In the case of mental health care, there are additional burdens and complexities due to enduring stigma. Additionally, there is a high treatment gap in the region, especially for mental disorders. Women's reproductive mental health is a trans-disciplinary issue where reproductive service providers play a significant role in the identification, referral, and collaboration for mental health sufferings.

Despite the necessity, there was no book considering the maternal mental health in the region, highlighting the strengths and weaknesses of their culture. This book certainly fills the gap, highlighting the various aspects of maternal mental health covered by both country-specific and topic-specific. The editors put their efforts into producing a well-crafted book based on available evidence and expertise. With remarkable depth and sensitivity, the authors have examined a range of pressing issues such as perinatal psychological disorders, domestic violence, substance abuse, suicidal tendencies, and the evolving role of forensic psychiatry in addressing mental health and legal challenges faced by women. Notably, the book also brings critical attention to gynecological and reproductive health conditions affecting adolescent girls and young women, including polycystic ovary syndrome, endometriosis, and adenomyosis and their significant psychological impacts. These conditions are not only medical concerns but are deeply tied to mental health, self-esteem, and quality of life, especially in cultural contexts where such topics remain stigmatized or inadequately addressed.

The insights offered in this book reflect the commitment, compassion, and academic rigor of its brilliant authors. Their interdisciplinary approach provides both a snapshot of current challenges and a visionary outlook on the future of women's mental health care in the region.

I commend these intelligent minds for initiating thoughtful discourse on such vital issues and hope this work will serve as a valuable resource for students, academics, practitioners, and policymakers dedicated to advancing women's health and mental well-being in the region and other LMIC settings.

I also hope the book will encourage enduring collaboration among reproductive and mental health services providers. As a region, for maternal mental health, we need to fight against stigma towards mental health among the patients as well as the service providers. I hope it will draw the attention of the local, regional, and international researchers to additional research in this neglected area.

Bangladesh Medical Research Council (BMRC) Sayeba Akhter
Dhaka, Bangladesh

Foreword

Why do we need a book on Reproductive Psychiatry specifically for South Asia? There are several reasons—the field of Reproductive Psychiatry is concerned with the complex interplay between mental health and the reproductive life of women, and it is a field garnering momentum across the globe. Yet in South Asia, where cultural, social, and structural barriers often dictate the boundaries of both psychiatric care and reproductive autonomy, the need for a nuanced, regionally grounded perspective has never been greater.

Gender inequality and the experience of violence are two important risk factors for poor mental health, including those related to one's reproductive health. If one looks at the Gender Gap Report published by the World Economic Forum in 2024, South Asia ranks seventh among all eight regions in the world, with a gender parity score of 63.7%. While the region has made some progress, it remains the region with one of the largest gender gaps, and it will take 149 years to close this gap if things don't change. South Asia also has the second-highest prevalence of intimate partner violence globally. Surveys indicate that between 11% and 64% of women have experienced physical and/or sexual violence by an intimate partner.

While there are commonalities, there is also wide variation within South Asia on several aspects. Let's look at a couple of examples. The first is period poverty and the impact it has on the mental health of girls and the second is related to laws and practices related to abortion.

Period poverty or the lack of access to menstrual products, education, and adequate sanitation remains a significant challenge across South Asia, adversely affecting the health, education, and dignity of millions of women and girls. Recent studies have found that water insecurity, stigma related to menstruation, and period poverty together are common reasons for psychological distress among young girls, leading to dropping out from school.

Abortion laws and practices in South Asia reflect a complex mix of cultural and religious influences, stigma, gender dynamics, and public health needs. While legal frameworks vary widely, actual access to safe abortion often depends on sociocultural and systemic factors rather than laws alone. Laws range from liberal (Nepal, India) to highly restrictive (Sri Lanka, Pakistan) while Bangladesh uses services like

Menstrual Regulation to support women with undesired pregnancies. However, legal does not always mean accessible. Several barriers exist including provider bias or refusal, lack of facilities in rural and remote areas, lack of awareness among women of legal rights and facilities, and consent requirements. Unwanted pregnancies are an important risk factor for poor mental health and access to safe abortion is essential.

Perinatal mental health however has received some attention in most South Asian countries with a fair amount of research done identifying the extent of the problem. There have also been several trials on psychological interventions including community-based interventions especially for perinatal mood and anxiety disorders.

However, given the high rates of suicide among women in the reproductive age group in South Asia there is a need for more data on suicidality in the perinatal period as well a need to develop confidential enquiries on maternal deaths related to psychiatric disorders and suicide. This will need collaboration between obstetric providers, mental health professionals, and policy makers and also capacity building for the same.

For all the above reasons, this book edited by Prerna Kukreti and Sujita Kumar Kar from India as well as S M Yasir Arafat from Bangladesh emerges at a pivotal time, when conversations about mental health are gradually overcoming long-standing stigmas, and when women's health is steadily but slowly beginning to receive the attention it deserves. By anchoring reproductive psychiatry within the socio-cultural realities of South Asia, the contributors to this volume offer not only clinical insight, but also an urgent call to recognize the unique intersections of biology, social determinants, and cultural issues that shape reproductive mental health in this context.

From perinatal mood disorders to the psychiatric implications of infertility, sexual health menstrual health, menopause, and gender-based violence, this text confronts topics often overlooked in mainstream psychiatric curricula. Importantly, it amplifies voices of authors from within the region on data and writings from South Asia with a representation from different countries. This gives us a glimpse of the wide variation in mental health services for women in the region and what needs to change.

Reproductive psychiatry is an upcoming specialty globally, and in countries such as Bhutan and Afghanistan where overall mental health services are still evolving, it may still be a luxury. The June 2025 issue of the journal World Psychiatry carries an authoritative review by Prof. Louise Howard and colleagues on women’s reproductive mental health, with emphasis on available evidence and future directions. In their powerful concluding statement they mention—“Reproductive health is foundational for women’s mental health and well-being.”

Violations of reproductive rights—including lack of access to reproductive health care, reproductive coercion, and a lack of gender-sensitive mental health care—can lead to enduring negative mental health outcomes.

They emphasize that psychiatrists should be advocates on behalf of their patients so that they can access reproductive health services. Psychiatrists should also educate themselves so that they acquire the knowledge and skills required to respond to their patients' reproductive health concerns.

In this context I congratulate the editors and authors for their commitment to bridge a critical gap in psychiatric knowledge and practice addressing the mental health of women.

NIMHANS
Bangalore, India

Prabha S. Chandra

Foreword

The eight countries of South Asia make about one quarter of the global population. The people of these countries share very similar religious cultural backgrounds and also face many social, economic, and health challenges that include gender inequality, gender-based violence, and high burden of mental ill health among its women. However, there is a considerable mental health treatment gap, and many areas of women's mental health are under-researched.

This book aims to look in to this gap by looking in to the epidemiology and burden of mental disorders during the perinatal period, psychological effects of contraception use, psychological issues related to menarche and menopause, domestic violence, substance abuse, and suicidal behavior during reproductive period as well as effects of various obstetric, gynecological, and surgical procedures including medical termination of pregnancy , hysterectomy, and mastectomy. In addition, it also highlights the current mental health services for women in the region and specific programs and policies utilized by each country. Finally the book also addresses challenges faced by the countries in region related to women's mental health and suggests ways forward.

The authors have produced valuable reading material for anyone who is interested in widening their knowledge in Women's Reproductive Mental Health in South Asia.

University of Kelaniya
Kelaniya, Sri Lanka

Aruni Hapangama

Alfred Hospital
Melbourne, VIC, Australia

Preface

South Asia, home to nearly a quarter of the world population, presents a unique context for understanding reproductive mental health. The region's women navigate a complex web of patriarchal norms, economic disparities, and limited access to healthcare, all of which profoundly influence their mental well-being during critical reproductive phases—menstruation, pregnancy, the perinatal period, and beyond. While strides have been made in maternal and reproductive health, mental health has often been sidelined, leaving a significant service gap that this book aims to highlight and address.

The intersection of women's reproductive health and mental well-being represents a profoundly complex and underexplored domain, particularly in the diverse and dynamic region of South Asia. The genesis of this book lies in the recognition of this critical oversight and the urgent need to bring women's reproductive mental health to the forefront of academic and clinical discourse. Its sixteen chapters offer a panoramic and nuanced exploration of the subject, blending empirical evidence, clinical insights, and sociocultural analysis. The volume begins with an overview of the disease burden and service gaps in reproductive psychiatry across South Asia, setting the stage for a series of country-specific chapters that delve into the unique contexts of Afghanistan, Bangladesh, Bhutan, India, Nepal, Pakistan, and Sri Lanka. Each of these chapters not only highlights the prevalence of mental health challenges but also underscores the influence of local cultural practices, healthcare systems, and socio-political realities on women's well-being.

Beyond these geographic perspectives, the book broadens its scope to address pressing public health concerns and marginalized experiences. Chapters on substance use and suicidal behavior in the perinatal period confront the alarming yet under-discussed risks faced by women, while discussions on domestic violence during pregnancy and the mental health of single mothers expose the intersecting vulnerabilities that exacerbate psychological distress. The reproductive mental health of marginalized women—those sidelined by caste, class, ethnicity, or displacement—receives dedicated attention, emphasizing the need for inclusive approaches to care. Equally compelling are the explorations of sexuality in the perinatal period and forensic issues in perinatal psychiatry, which tackle taboo subjects and legal complexities with sensitivity and rigor. Together, these contributions paint a holistic picture of the challenges and opportunities in this field.

This book, *Women's Reproductive Mental Health in South Asia: Current Status, Challenges, and Ways Forward* is not merely a documentation of challenges; it is a call to action. By synthesizing evidence, clinical insights, and policy recommendations, it aims to equip healthcare professionals, policymakers, researchers, and advocates with the knowledge and tools needed to advance reproductive mental health care in South Asia. It will also help the South Asian nations to learn from the neighboring countries and collaborate with them to strengthen the reproductive mental health facility for women. The collaborative effort of contributors from across the region underscores the importance of collective responsibility in tackling these issues while also recognizing the need for culturally sensitive and context-specific solutions.

We, the editors, are deeply grateful to Springer for providing a platform to amplify this critical conversation. We hope that this book serves as both a foundational resource and a catalyst for change, inspiring further research, dialogue, and intervention to ensure that the mental health of South Asian women is no longer an afterthought but a priority. As we move forward, we envision a future where every woman in this region, during her reproductive journey, can access the care and support she deserves, fostering resilience and well-being across generations.

Delhi, India — Prerna Kukreti
Uttar Pradesh, India — Sujita Kumar Kar
Dhaka, Bangladesh — S. M. Yasir Arafat

Contents

About the Editors

Prerna Kukreti is currently working as Professor of Psychiatry at Lady Hardinge Medical College (LHMC), New Delhi. She heads the women Mental Health Clinic and Perinatal Mental Health Unit at LHMC. She did her MBBS, MD Psychiatry from Maulana Azad Medical College, Delhi and WHO International diploma in mental health law and human rights from Indian Law Society, Pune. She is one of the lead investigators of the team developing the stepped care model, BIND-P (Brief Intervention for Depression in Pregnancy), for screening, providing brief intervention and referral for depression in perinatal period. She was convenor of Perinatal Psychiatry section of Indian Psychiatry Society (2023–24) and conducts workshops for nursing professionals, pediatricians, obstetricians, psychiatrists, mothers with high risk pregnancies for identification of maternal mental health conditions. Currently she is convenor of Biological Psychiatry section of Indian Psychiatry Society. She is Joint editor of Journal of Advanced Research in Psychology & Psychotherapy. She is reviewer of various national and international journals. She has authored book on "Forensic Psychiatry: Indian Perspective," 16 book chapters and 37 articles in in various national & international journals and made 50 presentations at various national and international conferences. Her research interests include women mental health, perinatal psychiatry, forensic psychiatry, community mental health, and neuropsychiatry.

Sujita Kumar Kar is currently working as an Additional Professor of Psychiatry at King George's Medical University, Lucknow, Uttar Pradesh, India. He is the editor-in-chief of Indian Journal of Health, Sexuality and Culture. He is also the editorial board member and reviewer of various national and international journals. He had written 88 book chapters and more than 540 articles in various national and international journals and made 70 presentations at various national and international conferences. He has been included in the global 2% researcher list released by Stanford University in 2021, 2022, 2023, 2024, and 2025. His research interests include brain stimulation, neuropsychiatry, and suicide prevention.

S. M. Yasir Arafat is currently working as an Associate Consultant of Psychiatry at Bangladesh Specialized Hospital, Dhaka, Bangladesh. He is affiliated with Dnet as an honorary Research Fellow and the Biomedical Research Foundation, Bangladesh, as Senior Research Fellow. He was affiliated with the University of Bristol, UK as Visiting Senior Research Associate (August 2021–2023). He completed an MD in Psychiatry, MPH in Health Economics, MBA in Marketing, and MBBS. Dr. Arafat has (co)authored more than 400 peer-reviewed articles and book chapters and (co)edited more than 15 books with Springer. He has been included in the global 2% researcher list in 2021, 2022, 2023, and 2025. He is acting as editorial member in more than 10 leading journals in mental health published by Elsevier, Wiley, Springer, and Taylor and Francis. His research focused on mental health, suicidal behavior, psychometrics, panic buying, and psycho-sexual disorders.

List of Figures

List of Tables

Chapter 1
Reproductive Psychiatry in South Asia: Disease Burden and Services Gap

Prerna Kukreti, Sujita Kumar Kar, and S. M. Yasir Arafat

1 Introduction

Mental health as a component of reproductive health has been unnoticed and marginalized. The lack of attention it has received is unfortunate, given the significant contributions of both mental health and reproductive health to the global burden of disease and disability (Fitch, 2024). The situation is further grave for women, where depression occurs approximately twice as often as in men. It is one of the most common mental health problems seen in women, and its rate is expected to increase further in the reproductive phase of life (Eloul et al., 2009).

The interplay of biological and socio-culturally determined factors is reasons that predispose women to develop mental illnesses. Specific phases of reproductive life, like the phase of the menstrual cycle, pregnancy, the postpartum period (Barnes, 2014), and menopause, accentuate these vulnerabilities, further increasing the risk ahead. However, the National Mental Health Survey of India, 2015–2016, found a lower lifetime and current prevalence of all psychiatric disorders in females than the males (Gautham et al., 2020). This might be due to the unusually high prevalence of

P. Kukreti (✉)
Department of Psychiatry, Lady Hardinge Medical College, New Delhi, Delhi, India

S. K. Kar
Department of Psychiatry, King George's Medical University, Lucknow, Uttar Pradesh, India

S. M. Y. Arafat
Department of Psychiatry, Bangladesh Specialized Hospital, Dhaka, Bangladesh

Department of Public and Community Health, Faculty of Medicine and Health Sciences, Frontier University Garowe, Garowe, Somalia

P. Kukreti et al. (eds.), *Women's Reproductive Mental Health in South Asia*, South Asian Perspectives in Mental Health and Psychology,
https://doi.org/10.1007/978-981-96-9219-4_1

substance use reported among males rather than females (Annajigowda et al., 2023; Gautham et al., 2020). The survey also reported that more than 82% of females with common mental illnesses were not on any psychiatric treatment, indicating a huge treatment gap (Annajigowda et al., 2023).

Women's mental well-being is by far more vulnerable during the years of young adulthood (between 20 and 40 years), associated with increased socio-cultural responsibilities, experience of reproductive processes including childbirth, child rearing, and so on. Motherhood has been particularly described as a pivotal transition in the life course of women, generating tumultuous waves of satisfaction, confidence, competence, a lack thereof, or a persisting sense of ambivalence. Misguided aspirations of achieving ever-increasing levels of societal expectations with regard to one's balancing role as wife, mother, daughter-in-law, and/or a working professional compound the levels of stress, impacting mental well-being in the short and long term (Barnes, 2014).

A widespread review to find the interaction between reproductive health and mental health is potentially a big task since each in itself is a large, specialized field of clinical as well as research venture. There are many places of intersection between mental health and reproductive health, premenstrual syndrome, the psychological issues related to pregnancy, postpartum period, childbirth including adverse maternal outcomes such as stillbirths and miscarriage, premarital pregnancies, the adverse mental health effects of sexual and physical violence, psychological issues related to surgical removal of reproductive organs, menopause, and infertility (Patel & Oomman, 1999).

Women's reproductive health in South Asia is shaped by a mixture of biological, sociocultural, and economic factors that significantly affect both physical and mental well-being. Challenges such as high fertility rates, limited access to reproductive healthcare, and deeply ingrained societal norms contribute to unique health issues for women in the region. Mental disorders, including antenatal and postpartum depression and anxiety, are prevalent yet often underdiagnosed and undertreated due to stigma and insufficient awareness (Mahendran et al., 2019).

2 Biological Aspects of Reproductive Health and Mental Health

Hormonal fluctuations throughout a woman's life profoundly affect mental health. Recent studies have highlighted the bidirectional relationship between depression and menstrual disorders. For instance, research indicates that individuals with depression are more likely to experience dysmenorrhea, suggesting that depression may be a primary cause rather than a consequence of menstrual pain. Additionally, gynecological conditions like polycystic ovary syndrome (PCOS) are more prevalent among South Asian women, which are further associated with increased risks of depression, anxiety, and body image disturbances (Kanagarajan et al., 2023).

3 Sociocultural and Psychological Factors

Cultural expectations regarding marriage, fertility, and motherhood impose significant psychological stress on South Asian women. Infertility, affecting approximately 10–15% of couples in the region, often leads to severe emotional distress exacerbated by societal stigma. Moreover, intimate partner violence (IPV) remains pervasive, with strong associations between IPV and increased risks of depression, post-traumatic stress disorder (PTSD), and suicidal tendencies among affected women (Srishti, 2023).

4 Common Psychiatric Disorders in Reproductive-Age Women

4.1 Perinatal Psychiatric Disorder

4.1.1 Antenatal and Postnatal Depression

As per a recent systematic review, the overall prevalence of antenatal depression was 24.3%. The lowest prevalence rates were seen in India (17.74%) and Sri Lanka (12.95%), while prevalence rates for Bangladesh were 20–25%. A review done in Bangladesh included 28 empirical studies published between 2007 and 2023, with sample sizes ranging from 100 to 39,434, and found that the *Edinburgh Postnatal Depression Scale (EPDS-B)* was used in 57% of studies and the prevalence of PPD ranged from 9% to 51.7% (Arafat & Rajkumar, 2024). The prevalence of mood disorders was present at 6.1%, and psychoses were noted at 4.5% for Bangladesh, 32.2% for Pakistan, and 50% for Nepal, much higher as compared to the global prevalence (Table 1.1). This variation in rates with respect to individual countries corresponds with their progress in terms of overall maternal health indicators. Rampant poverty in the region, coupled with factors such as food scarcity, inadequate housing for people, low socioeconomic status, high cost of living, financial instability, breakdown of traditional family structures into smaller families, and increased expenditure on healthcare, are all potential risk factors in this respect (Woody et al., 2017). Despite its prevalence, antenatal and postnatal depression often remain under-recognized due to cultural barriers and inadequate screening practices (Mahendran et al., 2019).

4.1.2 Postpartum Blues

Maternal Blues (MB), also known as *"postpartum blues," "third-day blues," "third-day syndrome," "baby blues," or "postnatal blues"* is a transient psychological condition with brief crying spells, irritability or emotional lability, weeping, insomnia, anxiety, loss of appetite, and poor concentration that occur in the first days after childbirth (Tosto et al., 2023). A recent systematic review and meta-analysis of 26

Table 1.1 Magnitude of antenatal and postnatal depression in South Asian countries

Country	Study	Assessing instrument	Reported prevalence
Bangladesh	Gausia et al. (2009)	EPDS	18% (postnatal)
Bangladesh	Alam et al. (2021)	EPDS	29.6% (postnatal)
India	Patel et al., (2002)	EPDS	23% (postnatal)
India	Mariam and Srinivasan (2009)	GHQ-28 & EPDS	20% (antenatal), 30% (postnatal)
India	Prabhu et al. (2022)	EPDS	19.8% (antenatal)
Nepal	Chalise et al. (2022)	EPDS	21.8% (antenatal)
Pakistan	Abdullah et al. (2024)	EPDS	28% (postnatal)
Pakistan	Rahman and Creed (2007)	ICD-10	25% (antenatal)

EPDS Edinburgh Postnatal Depression Scale, *ICD* International Classification of Diseases, *GHQ* General Health Questionnaire

studies reported a prevalence ranging from 13.7% to 76%, estimating an overall prevalence of 39% (95% confidence interval [32.3–45.6]; I^2 = 96.6%) (Rezaie-Keikhaie et al., 2020). The lowest prevalence was found in Malaysia at 3.5%, and the highest was 63.3% in Pakistan, while India had a prevalence of 58% (Tosto et al., 2023). These differences can be explained by the lack of mental healthcare integration into antenatal care, poor understanding and acceptance of mental health difficulties, and higher socioeconomic deprivation in LMICs (Insan et al., 2022).

Pathophysiology A sharp decline in progesterone, estradiol, and cortisol, coupled with rising prolactin, contributes to mood instability in maternal blues. Reduced *allopregnanolone* and GABA-A receptor density creates a withdrawal-like state, increasing anxiety and dysphoria. Dysregulation of the HPA axis, driven by decreased placental CRH, heightens stress responses. Serotonergic dysfunction, altered tryptophan metabolism, and increased monoamine oxidase activity impair mood regulation. Noradrenergic deficits, a sharp postpartum decline in β-endorphins, and low FT3/FT4 levels also contribute. MB is more common in women with early menarche, premenstrual dysphoric disorder, or passive coping styles, suggesting vulnerability to mood disorders (Payne & Maguire, 2019).

Assessment Scales used to measure MB include the Stein Maternity Blues Scale, Edinburgh Postnatal Depression Scale (EPDS), and Kennerley's Blues Questionnaire. Recently, the Maternal Blues Suryani (MBS) Scale was proposed for antepartum prediction (Tosto et al., 2023).

Management Given the unclear etiology, prevention strategies remain uncertain, but educating women during pregnancy helps prepare them for MB. Reassurance that symptoms are common and transient is crucial. Ensuring postpartum support, counseling, and emotional monitoring are key to differentiating MB from severe mood disorders. Higher-income countries often have better access to specialized mental healthcare and evidence-based treatments, while lower-income countries, including South Asian countries, face challenges in accessing these resources, relying more on community-based interventions and integration of mental healthcare within primary healthcare (Gajaria & Ravindran, 2018).

4.1.3 Postpartum Psychosis

Postpartum psychosis (PPP) is a rare but severe psychiatric emergency. Globally, its incidence ranges from 0.89 to 2.6 per 1000 births. In India, studies have reported an incidence rate of approximately 2.6 per 1000 births (Yang et al., 2023). Another narrative review from Bangladesh reported that 4.5% of mothers experienced psychoses during the postpartum period. Underreporting and limited mental health awareness may contribute to differences (Arafat & Rajkumar, 2024).

It manifests rapidly, posing risks to both mother and infant, with symptoms including delusions, hallucinations, mood instability, and cognitive impairment. PPP delusions evolve more quickly and are often directed at infants. Women with bipolar disorder are at higher risk, and PPP may be the first presentation of bipolar disorder. A history of affective psychosis or perinatal depression predicts recurrence. Symptoms typically emerge within 3–10 days postpartum, often after hospital discharge, making early detection challenging (Friedman et al., 2023).

Pathophysiology PPP peaks within the first two weeks postpartum, lasting weeks to months. While infanticide is rare (1–4.5% of cases), thoughts of harm—both self-directed and toward the infant—are frequent. Primiparity is the most consistent obstetric risk factor, and a recent psychiatric relapse increases the risk of recurrence. The pathophysiology involves genetic predisposition (polygenic risk for bipolar disorder), rapid estrogen decline, HPA axis dysregulation, thyroid dysfunction, and immune-related changes. Neuroimaging studies show altered connectivity in the prefrontal cortex, differentiating PPP from other psychoses (Friedman et al., 2023).

Assessment and Management PPP requires urgent intervention due to the risks of suicide, infanticide, and neglect. Hospitalization, psychoeducation, close monitoring, and pharmacologic treatment (lithium, antipsychotics, benzodiazepines) are key. Electroconvulsive therapy (ECT) has shown strong efficacy, with studies indicating better outcomes for PPP compared to other perinatal psychiatric conditions. Treatment approaches for PPP differ between Western countries and South Asian countries due to variations in healthcare infrastructure, resource availability, and cultural factors. Western countries often have specialized perinatal mental health services, including mother-baby units and multidisciplinary teams, providing comprehensive care. In contrast, South Asian countries lack such specialized services, relying more on general psychiatric care and community-based support. Additionally, cultural perceptions and stigma surrounding mental health may impact treatment-seeking behaviors and the type of care received (Kalra et al., 2022). PPP recovery and recurrence vary. Up to 50% of women with first-episode PPP only experience psychosis postpartum, while ~32% may develop affective or psychotic symptoms later. No clear risk factors predict recurrence, making long-term follow-up essential (Friedman et al., 2023).

4.2 Domestic Violence

Demographically, the highest rates of IPV are recorded in the South Asian continent, with prevalence rates between 33% and 51% among women aged 15–49 years. As per a recent study, the impact of domestic violence on South Asian women, particularly in India, Pakistan, Bangladesh, Bhutan, Nepal, Afghanistan, and Sri Lanka, remains a significant social issue influenced by social, economic, and cultural factors that may normalize violence experiences for women (Sardinha et al., 2022). Table 1.2 below summarizes studies on domestic violence (DV) and the mental health of women in South Asian countries. Research indicates that women in the South Asian region are less likely to report violence inflicted upon them due to associated stigma, shame, community isolation, and the importance placed on family reputation and social norms. It is important to note that statistics do not capture unreported cases, making it challenging to assess the impact of these barriers on reporting behaviors (Masih et al., 2024).

Domestic violence has severe consequences on women's reproductive health, affecting pregnancy outcomes, maternal well-being, and infant health. Physical violence during pregnancy poses significant risks, with reports of miscarriages due to physical assault or food deprivation by in-laws. Low infant birth weight was also

Table 1.2 Magnitude of mental health issues related to domestic violence in women of South Asian countries

Country	Study	Instruments used for the assessment	Findings
Bangladesh	Silverman et al. (2009)	Adapted WHO VAW Measure	DV prevalence of 53%; associated with child morbidity and maternal depression
India	Kumar et al. (2005)	SRQ-20	35% of women reported DV; strong association with poor mental health (depression, anxiety)
India	Chandra et al. (2009)	MINI & IES-R	Women reporting DV had higher rates of PTSD (33%) and depressive symptoms (42%)
Nepal	Bhatta and Assanangkornchai (2019)	WHO Structured Questionnaire	26.2% of pregnant women faced DV; higher rates of anxiety and stress reported
Pakistan	Ali and Gavino (2008)	WHO VAW Measure	70–90% of women experienced DV; linked to increased depression and anxiety symptoms
Pakistan	Alam and Nadeem (2023)	Rosenberg Self-Esteem Scale & Beck Scale	DV survivors showed low self-esteem and high suicidal ideation prevalence
Sri Lanka	Bandara et al. (2024)	SLDHS	Significant association between DV and household-level self-harm

SRQ Self-Reporting Questionnaire, *MINI* Mini-International Neuropsychiatric Interview, *IES-R* Impact of Event Scale-Revised, *WHO VAW* WHO Violence Against Women Instrument, *EPDS* Edinburgh Postnatal Depression Scale, SLDHS, Sri Lanka Demographic and Health Survey linked to maternal malnutrition caused by family abuse (Alhusen et al., 2015). Unwanted pregnancies and reproductive control were commonly reported, with some women denied contraception and forced into repeated pregnancies, leading to chronic malnutrition. Sexual coercion by husbands further exacerbated reproductive health risks, limiting women's ability to practice safe sex. Some victims resorted to induced abortions due to financial constraints, while others endured stillbirths under distressing conditions, often attributing them to marital abuse. The overarching impact of domestic violence highlights the urgent need for interventions to protect women's reproductive autonomy and health (Grace & Anderson, 2018).

4.3 Sexual Dysfunction

Sexual dysfunction in women is a prevalent issue in South Asia, with studies showing that the prevalence of sexual dysfunction in women ranges from 30% to 45%, with variations across different countries. Common types of dysfunction observed include low sexual desire, arousal disorder, orgasmic disorder, and dyspareunia (pain during intercourse). Cultural factors, such as societal expectations, restrictive norms around female sexuality, and stigma surrounding the discussion of sexual health, significantly impact the reporting and diagnosis of sexual dysfunction in these regions. In South Asia, these issues often remain underreported due to the fear of social stigma or marital implications. Specific regional insights highlight that in countries like India and Pakistan, women from rural areas report higher rates of sexual dysfunction compared to their urban counterparts, possibly due to lower levels of education, awareness, and access to healthcare services. While urban centers in countries like India, Bangladesh, and Pakistan have begun to provide counseling and specialized sexual health services, these resources are still limited and largely inaccessible in rural areas. Healthcare services aimed at addressing female sexual dysfunction are still developing, with only a few urban hospitals offering treatment options, including psychotherapy, sexual counseling, and medical interventions. In many cases, women continue to face challenges in seeking help due to the lack of open discussion about sexual health and a persistent cultural reluctance to address these concerns openly. Table 1.3 summarizes sexual dysfunction in women from South Asian countries.

Sexual function is a key component of reproductive health, yet it often declines during pregnancy due to hormonal, psychological, and physiological changes. Studies indicate that sexual activity significantly decreases across different trimesters, with 96% of women engaging in vaginal intercourse during the first trimester, which drops to 67% by the third trimester. The frequency of intercourse also declines, from 84.7% of women engaging in sexual activity one to four times per week before pregnancy to 70% in the first trimester, 61.3% in the second, and 32% in the third. Sexual dysfunction is highly prevalent, affecting 66.3% in the first trimester, 50.7% in the second, and 69.2% in the third trimester, with sexual desire disorder being the most frequently reported issue (Daescu et al., 2023).

Table 1.3 Female sexual dysfunction in South Asia: insights from population-based and clinical studies

Country	Study (Year & Population)	Instruments used	Prevalence	Salient findings
Bangladesh	Amin et al. (2022): Postmenopausal women (hospital-based, general sample)	FSFI	56.9%	Most affected domains: lubrication, arousal, desire; associated with age, education, and chronic illness.
India	Roy (2015): Comparative clinical vs community sample	FSFI	70.3% (clinical) vs. 43.3% (control)	Higher FSD rates in women on SSRIs and benzodiazepines; orgasm and arousal most impacted domains.
Nepal	Devkota et al. (2022): Women with depression (hospital-based, not general)	FSFI	58.8%	Depression severity significantly associated with lower FSFI scores; low desire and arousal predominant.
Pakistan	Noreen et al. (2024): Middle-aged and elderly women, community-attending	FSFI-derived structured tool	56.9%	Most women unaware of FSD as a treatable condition; low reporting due to cultural stigma and embarrassment.

FSD Female Sexual dysfunction, *FSFI* Female Sexual Function Index, *FSFI-derived tool* Structured questionnaire adapted from FSFI

The trajectory of sexual function varies across trimesters. In the first trimester, reduced libido is often attributed to fatigue, nausea, emotional instability, and anxiety, particularly concerning miscarriage. By the second trimester, some women report improvement in sexual desire which can be attributed to reduced nausea, increased vaginal lubrication, and psychological adaptation to pregnancy. However, in the third trimester, physical discomfort, weight gain, and fear of harming the baby often contribute to lower sexual activity. Studies show that 52% to 73% of women in the third trimester meet clinical criteria for sexual dysfunction, and only 11.2% report a positive attitude toward sexuality during pregnancy (Fernández-Carrasco et al., 2024).

Psychological and social factors further influence sexual health. Many pregnant women experience anxiety, emotional distress, and depressive symptoms related to sexual dysfunction. Common concerns include fear of harming the baby, worries about labor and delivery, increased responsibilities, reduced independence, and lack of partner support. Marital stress resulting from sexual dysfunction can lead to relationship dissatisfaction and even pregnancy complications. Despite the high prevalence of these issues, 68% of women report never discussing sexual concerns with their healthcare provider during pregnancy (Chauhan & Potdar, 2022).

Given its impact on emotional well-being, marital satisfaction, and overall quality of life, sexual health should be a routine part of prenatal care. Addressing these concerns through counseling and education can improve both maternal well-being and partner relationships, ultimately promoting healthier pregnancies and postpartum experiences (Daescu et al., 2023).

5 Psychological Impact of Gynecological Conditions

5.1 Polycystic Ovary Syndrome

It affects 6–10% of women in developed countries, while its prevalence is around 21.27% in Bangladesh, and in Indian women, it ranges from 3.7% to 22.5% (Kanagarajan et al., 2023). Women with PCOS face an increased risk of depression, anxiety, body image concerns, and disordered eating, largely due to symptoms such as weight gain, hirsutism, acne, and menstrual irregularities. The prevalence of specific psychiatric comorbidities in women with PCOS in India was found to be 5% for bipolar disorders, 1% for obsessive-compulsive disorder (OCD), 5% for social phobia, 4% for panic disorder, 34–57% for anxiety, and 28–64% for depression (Kanagarajan et al., 2023). Studies report depression prevalence rates of 40–50%, often associated with insulin resistance and metabolic dysfunction. Anxiety disorders, including generalized anxiety and binge eating disorder, are also more common. Negative self-perception, body dissatisfaction, and impaired sexual functioning further contribute to emotional distress. Given its psychological burden, PCOS management should integrate mental health screening and interventions. Cognitive-behavioral therapy (CBT), lifestyle modifications, and, when necessary, pharmacological treatments are essential for improving emotional well-being. A multidisciplinary approach addressing both physical and psychological aspects is crucial to enhancing the quality of life in women with PCOS (Kanagarajan et al., 2023).

5.2 PMS (Premenstrual Syndrome)

PMS significantly affects women's mental health, with symptoms including mood swings, anxiety, irritability, and depressive episodes, which follow a cyclic pattern. A severe form, premenstrual dysphoric disorder (PMDD), affects 3–8% of women worldwide, while the reported prevalence estimates of PMS in India have ranged from 14.3% to 74.4%, and for PMDD, it has varied widely between 3.7% and 65.7%. Psychological symptoms often coexist with physical discomfort, exacerbating emotional dysregulation and stress (Dutta & Sharma, 2021).

The etiology of PMS is multifactorial, involving hormonal fluctuations, psychosocial factors, and cognitive-emotional responses. Psychological interventions, particularly CBT, have shown moderate efficacy in reducing anxiety, depression, and functional impairment. Psychotherapeutic approaches emphasize coping strategies rather than symptom elimination, with mindfulness and acceptance-based interventions emerging as promising alternatives. While SSRIs remain a first-line treatment, high placebo rates and side effects limit their effectiveness. A multidisciplinary approach integrating pharmacotherapy, psychological therapies, and lifestyle modifications is essential for optimizing mental health outcomes in women experiencing PMS (Modzelewski et al., 2024).

5.3 Depression and Anxiety During the Menopausal Transition (MT)

The menopausal transition is a critical period of hormonal, psychological, and social change, often associated with an increased risk of depression and anxiety. Women in perimenopause are significantly more likely to experience depressive symptoms, particularly in the late transition phase. Psychological stressors, including prior depression, negative attitudes toward aging, role transitions, and health concerns, contribute to emotional distress. Data from the *Longitudinal Aging Study of India* showed a pooled prevalence of depression in postmenopausal women in India to be 21.76%.

Anxiety symptoms, such as excessive worry, panic, and cognitive difficulties, may also intensify during this period, often exacerbated by vasomotor symptoms like hot flashes. Subjective concerns about memory loss can further heighten distress. These psychological challenges can impair emotional regulation, self-esteem, and interpersonal functioning. Effective management includes cognitive-behavioral interventions, antidepressants (especially SSRIs/SNRIs for co-occurring vasomotor symptoms), and lifestyle modifications. Understanding the psychological impact of MT is crucial for tailoring mental health interventions to support women's emotional well-being during this transition (Santoro et al., 2015).

Table 1.4 highlights the significant mental health issues faced by postmenopausal women in South Asian countries. It shows that a substantial proportion of postmenopausal women experience high levels of depression, anxiety, and other psychological distress. Common mental health concerns, including mood disorders, insomnia, and emotional distress, have been found to be highly linked with menopausal symptoms like hot flashes, sleep disturbances, and social isolation. Research indicates that factors such as lower education, rural living conditions, lack of social support, and limited healthcare access have been found to be important determinants.

5.4 Female Genital Mutilation and Its Impact on Reproductive Mental Health

Female genital mutilation (FGM) is a deeply rooted cultural and religious practice that affects an estimated 200 million women worldwide, with four million girls at risk annually (Alradie-Mohamed et al., 2020). It is prevalent in 33 African countries

Table 1.4 Mental health issues around menopause in South Asian countries

Country	Author & Study	Tool used	Salient findings
Bangladesh	Bashar et al. (2017): Tangail women	MENQOL + BDI	Higher depression scores linked to concentration issues, fatigue, headaches
India	Basu and Aditya (2022): Postmenopausal women from LASI Wave-1 dataset (n = 18,475)	CIDI-SF (for depression)	Elevated risk of depression among postmenopausal women; associated with education, economic dependence, and marital status
Nepal	Baral & Kaphle (2023): Pokhara community women	MRS	51.4% poor QOL; education, activity, alcohol, treatment significant
Pakistan	Malik et al. (2021): Islamabad/ Rawalpindi women	MENQOL + HADS	Moderate depression; poor QoL among postmenopausal women
Sri Lanka	Rathnayake et al. (2019): Galle District women	MRS + SF-36	Depressive mood (43.4%), irritability (48.2%), mental exhaustion (53%)

MENQOL Menopause-Specific Quality of Life Questionnaire, *BDI* Beck Depression Inventory, *CIDI-SF* Composite International Diagnostic Interview—Short Form, *MRS* Menopause Rating Scale, *QOL* quality-of-life, *HADS* Hospital Anxiety and Depression Scale, *SF-36* 36-Item Short Form Health Survey, *MRS* Menopause Rating Scale, *LASI* Longitudinal Aging Study in India

and parts of Asia and the Middle East, where it is often performed as a rite of passage or for perceived religious and cultural purity. The World Health Organization (WHO) categorizes FGM into four types: Type I (clitoridectomy), Type II (excision), Type III (infibulation), and Type IV (other harmful procedures, including pricking, cauterization, and labia modification) (World Health Organization, 2025). Despite its widespread presence, national and international reproductive health policies rarely address its severe mental health consequences, leaving a critical gap in healthcare interventions for affected women. FGM is commonly practiced in parts of South Asia.

In India, FGM is primarily observed among the Bohra community, which numbers around one million. A 2018 study estimated that 75% of daughters in this community had undergone FGM (Khan et al., 2019). Additionally, some Sunni Muslim sects in Kerala are also reported to practice FGM, though data on its prevalence is limited.

Psychological and Reproductive Mental Health Consequences FGM has profound psychological and reproductive mental health consequences. Women who have undergone the procedure face increased risks of PTSD, depression, anxiety, and sexual dysfunction. The trauma associated with FGM is compounded by gendered power dynamics, socioeconomic restrictions, and cultural reinforcement of intimate partner violence. Many affected women report persistent fear, low self-esteem, and emotional distress, which can contribute to psychiatric disorders (Tammary & Manasi, 2023).

The psychological impact varies based on the severity of FGM. Infibulated women (Type III) often experience heightened psychological distress due to repeated trauma, particularly during menstruation, sexual intercourse, and childbirth. Studies have documented significant associations between FGM and memory disturbances, dissociation, and somatic disorders. While reconstructive surgery has been shown to improve sexual function and psychological well-being in some cases, the long-term emotional scars of FGM remain significant, underscoring the need for comprehensive mental health interventions (Bryant et al., 2014).

6 Mental Health Service Delivery Systems in South Asia for Women's Reproductive Psychiatry Issues

The mental health service delivery systems in South Asia have evolved considerably over the past years, with an emerging focus on maternal and reproductive psychiatry in recent years. This section explores mental health services in Bangladesh, India, Nepal, Pakistan, and Sri Lanka, highlighting country-specific systems, strengths, barriers, and the available services, including public health community outreach research projects like the *Thinking Healthy Program*, *Amma Manasu Asha*, and tele-mental health initiatives like *TeleManas*.

6.1 Bangladesh: Community-Based Approaches to Maternal Mental Health

Besides existing hospital-based mental health service delivery mechanisms, Bangladesh has made strides in addressing this issue through the involvement of community-based mental health workers by training them to identify signs of perinatal depression and provide basic counseling to affected women. Healthcare workers have also been trained to use screening tools like the EPDS for early detection of depression and anxiety and timely referral during pregnancy. The integration of mental health screening into routine antenatal care can emerge as a key strength for future programs (Dutta et al., 2024).

Tele-mental health services are still in the early stages of development in Bangladesh, and there are significant challenges in providing access to mental health care in rural areas (Hossain et al., 2025). Despite these efforts, mental health stigma remains a barrier to care, and there is still a long way to go in ensuring comprehensive maternal mental health services.

6.2 India: A Growing Focus on Maternal Mental Health

India has exhaustive mental health service delivery systems in the form of clinic-based services and community-based district mental health programs, but nothing exists in specific in programs or governmental service delivery systems to address women's mental health systems in specific. The country has a lot of centers running women's mental clinic and mother-baby unit but integration across departments is still lacking.

Innovative implementation research programs addressing women's mental health in specific have drawn attention toward reproductive psychiatry issues of relevance for women's health. Programs such as the Thinking Healthy Program, initially tested in Pakistan and India, have drawn attention toward the need for regularly screening pregnant women for depression and providing psychoeducation and have established that community health workers can offer brief psychological interventions (Vanobberghen et al., 2020). Another study conducted in different parts of India also established the feasibility of the development of a stepped-care model for use in antenatal care clinics, where nurses, after training, can play a key role in regular screening, providing brief intervention for mild cases and referral for high-risk cases of depression in pregnancy. The study revealed promising results in identifying and addressing perinatal depression through a structured, tiered approach, integrating healthcare workers, mental health professionals, and community support systems (Kukreti et al., 2022). Another key initiative in India has been *Amma Manasu*, where Auxiliary Nurse Midwives (ANMs) are trained to screen for depression and anxiety during pregnancy. This initiative has shown success in rural areas where access to mental health professionals is limited and can help in filling critical gaps in mental health services. Another study utilized these mental health principles and these stepped-care intervention models for addressing vaccine hesitancy during the COVID-19 pandemic among perinatal women (Ransing et al., 2022).

Additionally, TeleManas, a national tele-mental health initiative launched by the Indian government, aims to improve access to mental health services across the country, especially in underserved areas. Through this program, individuals can access mental health consultations over the phone, making it easier for pregnant and postpartum women in rural areas to get support (Sagar et al., 2022).

Despite these advances, a lack of integration between mental health services and maternal health programs and the stigma surrounding mental health issues continue to remain as one of the biggest challenges (Bhatia et al., 2021).

6.3 Nepal: Building Mental Health Capacity in Primary Care

Nepal is a country where maternal mental health has traditionally been under-addressed, but recent initiatives are helping to improve the situation. Postpartum depression affects a significant proportion of women in Nepal, but there is limited access to mental health professionals in rural areas. Community health workers are being trained to screen for mental health issues, and nurses in rural areas are increasingly being involved in maternal mental health care (Aryal et al., 2020).

In rural areas, where access to specialized care is minimal, community health workers play a vital role in identifying depression and providing support. Telemedicine initiatives are beginning to be used in Nepal to connect women with mental health professionals in urban centers, though these programs remain limited in scope.

6.4 Pakistan: Pioneering Maternal Mental Health Initiatives

Pakistan has made significant progress in addressing maternal mental health, particularly through its unique Thinking Healthy Program. As the program was first tested in Pakistan, it has played a pioneering role in shaping maternal mental health care in the region. The program trains community health workers to screen for perinatal depression, provide counseling, and refer women to mental health specialists if necessary (Rahman et al., 2019).

In Pakistan, Community health workers (CHWs) play a crucial role in identifying women at risk for depression and providing support in rural and remote areas. These workers are trained to use standardized screening tools like the Edinburgh Postnatal Depression Scale (EPDS) to detect perinatal depression early. Given the shortage of mental health professionals in rural areas, CHWs have become a vital resource for delivering essential mental health services at the community level.

However, challenges remain in Pakistan, including the limited availability of trained mental health professionals and the lack of specialized maternal mental health programs at the national level. While initiatives like *Tele-mental health* are beginning to emerge, there is still a significant gap in service delivery, especially in more remote regions (Choudhry et al., 2021).

6.5 Sri Lanka: Integrating Mental Health into Maternal Health Care

Sri Lanka's mental health services for women have made significant improvements over the years. The government has recognized maternal mental health as a key issue, and steps have been taken to integrate mental health services into maternal and child health care systems. Screening for postpartum depression and antenatal depression is regularly done in Sri Lankan health facilities and by healthcare providers. Nurses play a critical role in detecting depression and anxiety during pregnancy and the postpartum period, offering basic support, and referring women for further treatment if needed. This approach has proven effective, especially in rural and underserved areas where access to specialized care is limited (Agampodi et al., 2023).

Additionally, tele-mental health programs like *Tele-mental Health Sri Lanka* are beginning to provide remote support to women in rural areas, offering consultations via phone or video calls. These initiatives have helped bridge the gap in access to mental health services, particularly for women who may face cultural and logistical barriers to accessing traditional in-person care (Jayasinghe et al., 2016).

Despite these advances, Sri Lanka still faces challenges in scaling these programs to meet the needs of all women. There is a need for more widespread training of healthcare workers and increased investment in mental health services for reproductive health (Agampodi & Agampodi, 2023).

7 Disease Burden and Service Gaps Across South Asian Countries

Despite efforts to enhance maternal and reproductive healthcare, mental health services remain inadequately integrated into primary care in South Asia. Table 1.5 summarizes disease burden and service gaps across South Asian countries. Common

Table 1.5 Disease burden and services available in South Asian countries

Country	Disease burden	Screening programs	Service delivery programs	Tele-mental health	Barriers
Bangladesh (Arafat & Rajkumar, 2024)	19% depression during pregnancy	Antenatal screening utilizing community health workers in implementation research mode	No specific national program	Emerging Telehealth	Stigma, rural access
India (Kukreti et al., 2022)	15–20% depression in pregnancy, 22% PPD	*Thinking Healthy Program*, Amma Manasu in implementation research mode	No specific national program Tele Manas Amma Manasu program in a few states	Tele Manas	Stigma, rural access, poor integration with ANC clinics
Nepal (Aryal and Pant 2020)	High rates of postpartum depression	CHW screenings in implementation research mode	No specific national program	Limited telemedicine	Lack of specialized care in rural areas
Pakistan (Rahman et al., 2025)	High perinatal depression, 15–20% PPD	*Thinking Healthy Program*	CHWs being utilized for depression screening, community-based care	Emerging telehealth	Shortage of mental health professionals
Sri Lanka (Agampodi & Agampodi, 2023)	10–15% PPD	Routine screening at health facilities by nurses	Tele-mental health services	Tele-mental health	Limited rural outreach

CHW, Community health worker, *ANC*, Antenatal care

barriers include a shortage of trained mental health professionals, pervasive stigma, and economic constraints hindering women's access to psychiatric. The lack of specific women-friendly mental health facilities further deters women from seeking timely interventions. Comprehensive reforms, integrating mental health screenings, awareness campaigns, and gender-sensitive approaches, are essential to bridge these gaps in reproductive mental health care.

8 Conclusion

The intricate relationship between reproductive and mental health in South Asia presents a pressing concern that demands a multidisciplinary approach. Tackling biological, sociocultural, and systemic barriers is essential for improving women's health outcomes. South Asian countries have been making significant strides in addressing mental health issues related to women's reproductive health. However, there remain substantial gaps in service delivery, especially in rural and underserved regions. The integration of mental health care into maternal and newborn health services involving community health workers holds great promise. Future research should focus on region-specific interventions to bridge the existing gap between reproductive and psychiatric care.

References

Abdullah, M., Ijaz, S., & Asad, S. (2024). Postpartum depression-an exploratory mixed method study for developing an indigenous tool. *BMC Pregnancy and Childbirth, 24*, 49. https://doi.org/10.1186/s12884-023-06192-2

Agampodi, T., & Agampodi, S. (2023). Perinatal mental health in Sri Lanka: Current status, programmes, gaps, and recommendations. *The Ceylon Medical Journal,* 68(Supplement 1), 53–57. https://doi.org/10.4038/cmj.v68iSI1.9792

Agampodi, T., Amarasinghe, G., Wickramasinghe, A., Wickramasinghe, N., Warnasekara, J., Jayasinghe, I., Hettiarachchi, A., Nimesha, D., Dilshani, T., Senadheera, S., & Agampodi, S. (2023). Incorporating early pregnancy mental health screening and management into routine maternal care: Experience from the Rajarata Pregnancy Cohort (RaPCo), Sri Lanka. *BMJ Global Health, 8*, e012852. https://doi.org/10.1136/bmjgh-2023-012852

Alam, M. M., Haque, T., Uddin, K. M. R., Ahmed, S., Islam, M. M., & Hawlader, M. D. H. (2021). The prevalence and determinants of postpartum depression (PPD) symptomatology among facility delivered mothers of Dhaka city. *Asian Journal of Psychiatry, 62*, 102673. https://doi.org/10.1016/j.ajp.2021.102673

Alam, N., & Nadeem, M. (2023). Self-esteem and suicidal ideation among victims of violence women Southern Punjab. *Journal of Social Sciences Review, 3*(1), 1. https://doi.org/10.54183/jssr.v3i1.205

Alhusen, J. L., Ray, E., Sharps, P., & Bullock, L. (2015). Intimate partner violence during pregnancy: Maternal and neonatal outcomes. *Journal of Women's Health, 24*(1), 100–106. https://doi.org/10.1089/jwh.2014.4872

Ali, P. A., & Gavino, M. I. B. (2008). Violence against women in Pakistan: A framework for analysis. *The Journal of the Pakistan Medical Association, 58*(4), 198–203.

Alradie-Mohamed, A., Kabir, R., & Arafat, S. M. Y. (2020). Decision-making process in female genital mutilation: A systematic review. *International Journal of Environmental Research and Public Health, 17*(10), 3362. https://doi.org/10.3390/ijerph17103362

Amin, M. A., Mozid, N.-E., Ahmed, S. B., Sharmin, S., Monju, I. H., Jhumur, S. S., & Hawlader, M. D. H. (2022). Status of female sexual dysfunction among postmenopausal women in Bangladesh: A cross-sectional study in a tertiary hospital. *BMC Women's Health, 22*(1), 401. https://doi.org/10.1186/s12905-022-01991-9

Annajigowda, H. H., Nirisha, L. P., Ganjekar, S., Rao, G. N., Gururaj, G., Varghese, M., Benegal, V., & Group, N. N. C. (2023). Common mental disorders among women in reproductive age group: An analysis of national mental health survey, India 2016. *Indian Journal of Psychiatry, 65*(12), 1238. https://doi.org/10.4103/indianjpsychiatry.indianjpsychiatry_832_23

Arafat, S. M. Y., & Rajkumar, R. P. (2024). Mental disorders during pregnancy and postpartum in Bangladesh: A narrative review. *Health Science Reports, 7*(9), e70027. https://doi.org/10.1002/hsr2.70027

Aryal, S., & Pant, S. B. (2020). Maternal mental health in Nepal and its prioritization during COVID-19 pandemic: Missing the obvious. *Asian Journal of Psychiatry, 54*, 102281. https://doi.org/10.1016/j.ajp.2020.102281

Baral, S., & Kaphle, H. P. (2023). Health-related quality of life among menopausal women: A cross-sectional study from Pokhara, Nepal. *PLoS One, 18*(1), e0280632. https://doi.org/10.1371/journal.pone.0280632

Bandara, P., Page, A., Rajapakse, T., & Knipe, D. (2024). Intimate partner violence, suicide and self-harm in Sri Lanka: Analysis of national data. *PloS One, 19*(3), e0298413. https://doi.org/10.1371/journal.pone.0298413

Barnes, D. L. (Ed.). (2014). *Women's reproductive mental health across the lifespan* (pp. xxvii, 333). Springer International Publishing/Springer Nature. https://doi.org/10.1007/978-3-319-05116-1

Bashar, M. I., Ahmed, K., Uddin, M. S., Ahmed, F., Emran, A. A., & Chakraborty, A. (2017). Depression and quality of life among postmenopausal women in Tangail, Bangladesh: A cross-sectional study. *Journal of Menopausal Medicine, 23*(3), 172–181. https://doi.org/10.6118/jmm.2017.23.3.172

Basu, S., & Aditya, S. (2022). Menopause and depression: Evidence from the longitudinal aging study in India (LASI). *Asian Journal of Psychiatry, 76*, 103174. https://doi.org/10.1016/j.ajp.2022.103174

Bhatta, N., & Assanangkornchai, S. (2019). Patterns of domestic violence against women during pregnancy and the postpartum period in Kathmandu, Nepal. *Asia-Pacific psychiatry: Official Journal of the Pacific Rim College of Psychiatrists, 11*(1), e12342. https://doi.org/10.1111/appy.12342

Bhatia, M., Dwivedi, L. K., Banerjee, K., Bansal, A., Ranjan, M., & Dixit, P. (2021). Pro-poor policies and improvements in maternal health outcomes in India. *BMC Pregnancy and Childbirth, 21*(1), 389. https://doi.org/10.1186/s12884-021-03839-w

Bryant, C., Kleinstäuber, M., & Judd, F. (2014). Aspects of mental health care in the gynecological setting. *Women's Health, 10*(3), 237–254. https://doi.org/10.2217/WHE.14.16

Chalise, A., Shrestha, G., Paudel, S., & Poudyal, A. K. (2022). Antenatal depression and its associated factors among women of Godawari Municipality, Lalitpur, Nepal: A cross-sectional study. *BMJ Open, 12*(11), e063513. https://doi.org/10.1136/bmjopen-2022-063513

Chandra, P. S., Satyanarayana, V. A., & Carey, M. P. (2009). Women reporting intimate partner violence in India: Associations with PTSD and depressive symptoms. *Archives of Women's Mental Health, 12*(4), 203–209. https://doi.org/10.1007/s00737-009-0065-6

Chauhan, A., & Potdar, J. (2022). Maternal mental health during pregnancy: A critical review. *Cureus, 14*(10), e30656. https://doi.org/10.7759/cureus.30656

Choudhry, F. R., Khan, N., & Munawar, K. (2021). Barriers and facilitators to mental health care: A systematic review in Pakistan. *International Journal of Mental Health*. Advance online publication. https://doi.org/10.1080/00207411.2021.1941563

Daescu, A.-M. C., Navolan, D.-B., Dehelean, L., Frandes, M., Gaitoane, A.-I., Daescu, A., Daniluc, R.-I., & Stoian, D. (2023). The paradox of sexual dysfunction observed during pregnancy. *Healthcare, 11*(13), 1914. https://doi.org/10.3390/healthcare11131914

Devkota, L., Pant, S. B., Ojha, S. P., & Chapagai, M. (2022). Prevalence of sexual dysfunction in women with depressive disorder at a tertiary hospital in Nepal. *Journal of Psychosexual Health, 4*(2), 123–128. https://doi.org/10.1177/26318318221080751

Dutta, A., & Sharma, A. (2021). Prevalence of premenstrual syndrome and premenstrual dysphoric disorder in India: A systematic review and meta-analysis. *Health Promotion Perspectives, 11*(2), 161–170. https://doi.org/10.34172/hpp.2021.20

Dutta, G. K., Ahmed, H. U., Talukder, M. Q., Bhattacharyya, D. S., Reza, M. S., Rahman, M. M., Majumdar, R., Tofail, F., Perry, H. B., & Biswas, T. K. (2024). Effectiveness of a package of community-based mental healthcare services to address perinatal mental disorders in Bangladesh: A cluster-randomized controlled trial. *Asian Journal of Psychiatry, 102*, Article 104290. https://doi.org/10.1016/j.ajp.2024.104290

Eloul, L., Ambusaidi, A., & Al-Adawi, S. (2009). Silent epidemic of depression in women in the Middle East and North Africa Region. *Sultan Qaboos University Medical Journal, 9*(1), 5–15.

Fernández-Carrasco, F. J., Batugg-Chaves, C., Ruger-Navarrete, A., Riesco-González, F. J., Palomo-Gómez, R., Gómez-Salgado, J., Rodriguez Diaz, L., Vázquez-Lara, M. D., Fagundo-Rivera, J., & Vázquez-Lara, J. M. (2024). Influence of pregnancy on sexual desire in pregnant women and their partners: Systematic review. *Public Health Reviews, 44*, 1606308. https://doi.org/10.3389/phrs.2023.1606308

Fitch, M. I. (2024). Editorial: Reproductive health and mental health in LMICs: Adolescent health. *Frontiers in Reproductive Health, 6*, 1383170. https://doi.org/10.3389/frph.2024.1383170

Friedman, S. H., Reed, E., & Ross, N. E. (2023). Postpartum psychosis. *Current Psychiatry Reports, 25*(2), 65–72. https://doi.org/10.1007/s11920-022-01406-4

Gajaria, A., & Ravindran, A. V. (2018). Interventions for perinatal depression in low and middle-income countries: A systematic review. *Asian Journal of Psychiatry, 37*, 112–120. https://doi.org/10.1016/j.ajp.2018.08.014

Gausia, K., Fisher, C., Ali, M., & Oosthuizen, J. (2009). Magnitude and contributory factors of postnatal depression: A community-based cohort study from a rural subdistrict of Bangladesh. *Psychological Medicine, 39*(6), 999–1007. https://doi.org/10.1017/S0033291708004455

Gautham, M. S., Gururaj, G., Varghese, M., Benegal, V., Rao, G. N., Kokane, A., Chavan, B. S., Dalal, P. K., Ram, D., Pathak, K., Lenin Singh, R. K., Singh, L. K., Sharma, P., Saha, P. K., Ramasubramanian, C., Mehta, R. Y., Shibukumar, T. M., Deuri, S. P., Krishnatreya, M., et al. (2020). The National Mental Health Survey of India (2016): Prevalence, socio-demographic correlates and treatment gap of mental morbidity. *International Journal of Social Psychiatry, 66*(4), 361–372. https://doi.org/10.1177/0020764020907941

Grace, K. T., & Anderson, J. C. (2018). Reproductive coercion: A systematic review. *Trauma, Violence & Abuse, 19*(4), 371–390. https://doi.org/10.1177/1524838016663935

Hossain, A. T., Rahman, M. H., Manna, R. M., Akter, E., Islam, S. M. H., Hossain, M. A., Ara, T., Usmani, N. G., Chandra, P., Khan, M. A., Rahman, S. M. M., Ahmed, H. U., Mozumder, M. K., Juthi, J. M., Shahrin, F., Shams, S. A., Afroze, F., Banu, M. J., Ameen, S., Jabeen, S., … Rahman, A. E. (2025). Enhancing Access to Mental Health Services for Antepartum and Postpartum Women Through Telemental Health Services at Wellbeing Centers in Selected Health Facilities in Bangladesh: Implementation Research. *JMIR pediatrics and parenting, 8*, e65912. https://doi.org/10.2196/65912

Insan, N., Weke, A., Forrest, S., & Rankin, J. (2022). Social determinants of antenatal depression and anxiety among women in South Asia: A systematic review & meta-analysis. *PLoS One, 17*(2), e0263760. https://doi.org/10.1371/journal.pone.0263760

Jayasinghe, D., Crowder, R. M., & Wills, G. (2016). Model for the adoption of telemedicine in Sri Lanka. *SAGE Open, 6*(3). https://doi.org/10.1177/2158244016668565

Kalra, H., Tran, T., Romero, L., Chandra, P., & Fisher, J. (2022). Burden of severe maternal peripartum mental disorders in low- and middle-income countries: A systematic review. *Archives of Women's Mental Health, 25*(2), 267–275. https://doi.org/10.1007/s00737-021-01201-9

Kanagarajan, S. S., Varshney, P., Ganjekar, S., Muralidhar, A., & Desai, G. (2023). Psychiatric comorbidities among Indian Women with polycystic ovary syndrome: A scoping review. *Journal of Psychiatry Spectrum, 2*(1), 7. https://doi.org/10.4103/jopsys.jopsys_30_22

Khan, A., Shekhani, S. S., Jafarey, A. (2019). Demystifying the practice of khafd in the Dawoodi Bohra community: A commentary on the WeSpeakOut report from India. *Indian Journal of Medical Ethics, 4*(1), 65–70. https://doi.org/10.20529/IJME.2018.075

Kukreti, P., Ransing, R., Raghuveer, P., Mahdevaiah, M., Deshpande, S. N., Kataria, D., Puri, M., Vallamkonda, O. R., Rana, S., Pemde, H. K., Yadav, R., Nain, S., Prasad, S., & Garg, B. (2022). Stepped care model for developing pathways of screening, referral, and brief intervention for depression in pregnancy: A mixed-method study from development phase. *Indian Journal of Social Psychiatry, 38*(1), 12–20. https://doi.org/10.4103/ijsp.ijsp_372_21

Kumar, S., Jeyaseelan, L., Suresh, S., & Ahuja, R. C. (2005). Domestic violence and its mental health correlates in Indian women. *The British Journal of Psychiatry, 187*, 62–67. https://doi.org/10.1192/bjp.187.1.62

Mahendran, R., Puthussery, S., & Amalan, M. (2019). Prevalence of antenatal depression in South Asia: A systematic review and meta-analysis. *Journal of Epidemiology and Community Health, 73*(8), 768–777. https://doi.org/10.1136/jech-2018-211819

Malik, M., Mahjabeen, M., Rana, S., Hussain, A., & Hashmi, A. (2021). Quality of life and depression among postmenopausal women in Pakistan. *Archives of Pharmacy Practice, 12*(3), 29–33. https://doi.org/10.51847/MAPShK83EB

Mariam, K. A., & Srinivasan, K. (2009). Antenatal psychological distress and postnatal depression: A prospective study from an urban clinic. *Asian Journal of Psychiatry, 2*(2), 71–73. https://doi.org/10.1016/j.ajp.2009.04.002

Masih, M., Wagstaff, C., & Kaur-Aujla, H. (2024). The global psychological and physical effects of domestic abuse and violence on South Asian women: A qualitative systematic review. *Frontiers in Global Women's Health, 5*, 1365883. https://doi.org/10.3389/fgwh.2024.1365883

Modzelewski, S., Oracz, A., Żukow, X., Iłendo, K., Śledzikowka, Z., & Waszkiewicz, N. (2024). Premenstrual syndrome: New insights into etiology and review of treatment methods. *Frontiers in Psychiatry, 15*. https://doi.org/10.3389/fpsyt.2024.1363875

Noreen, K., Ayyaz, F., Meraj, L., Khalid, T., Malik, J., & Randhawa, M. A. (2024). Estimation of knowledge, attitude and prevalence of female sex dysfunction in elderly Pakistani women. *Journal of Rawalpindi Medical College, 28*(3), 426–432. https://doi.org/10.37939/jrmc.v28i3.2540

Patel, V., & Oomman, N. (1999). Mental health matters too: Gynaecological symptoms and depression in South Asia. *Reproductive Health Matters, 7*(14), 30–38.

Patel, V., Rodrigues, M., & DeSouza, N. (2002). Gender, poverty, and postnatal depression: A study of mothers in Goa, India. *The American Journal of Psychiatry, 159*(1), 43–47. https://doi.org/10.1176/appi.ajp.159.1.43

Payne, J. L., & Maguire, J. (2019). Pathophysiological mechanisms implicated in postpartum depression. *Frontiers in Neuroendocrinology, 52*, 165–180. https://doi.org/10.1016/j.yfrne.2018.12.001

Prabhu, S., Guruvare, S., George, L. S., Nayak, B. S., & Mayya, S. (2022). Prevalence and associated risk factors of antenatal depression among pregnant women attending tertiary care hospitals in South India. *Depression Research and Treatment, 2022*, 9127358. https://doi.org/10.1155/2022/9127358

Rahman, A., & Creed, F. (2007). Outcome of prenatal depression and risk factors associated with persistence in the first postnatal year: Prospective study from Rawalpindi, Pakistan. *Journal of Affective Disorders, 100*(1–3), 115–121. https://doi.org/10.1016/j.jad.2006.10.004

Rahman, A., Akhtar, P., Hamdani, S. U., Atif, N., Nazir, H., Uddin, I., Nisar, A., Huma, Z., Maselko, J., Sikander, S., & Zafar, S. (2019). Using technology to scale-up training and supervision of community health workers in the psychosocial management of perinatal depression: A non-inferiority, randomized controlled trial. *Global Mental Health, 6*, e8. https://doi.org/10.1017/gmh.2019.7

Rahman, A., Malik, A., Nazir, H., Hamdani, S. U., Atif, N., Huma, Z. E., Maselko, J., Sikander, S., Zafar, S., & Patel, V. (2025). Technology-assisted cognitive-behavioral therapy for perinatal depression delivered by lived-experience peers: A cluster-randomized noninferiority trial. *Nature Medicine, 31*(10), 2196–2203. https://doi.org/10.1038/s41591-025-03655-1

Ransing, R., Kukreti, P., Raghuveer, P., Puri, M., Paranjape, A. D., Patil, S., Hegde, P., Padma, K., Kumar, P., Kishore, J., & Deshpande, S. N. (2022). A brief psycho-social intervention for COVID-19 vaccine hesitancy among perinatal women in lowand middle-income countries: Need of the hour. *Asian Journal of Psychiatry, 67*, 102929. https://doi.org/10.1016/j.ajp.2021.102929

Rathnayake, N., et al. (2019). Prevalence and severity of menopausal symptoms and the quality of life in middle-aged women: A study from Sri Lanka. *Nursing Research and Practice, 2019*, 2081507. https://doi.org/10.1155/2019/2081507

Rezaie-Keikhaie, K., Arbabshastan, M. E., Rafiemanesh, H., Amirshahi, M., Ostadkelayeh, S. M., & Arbabisarjou, A. (2020). Systematic review and meta-analysis of the prevalence of the maternity blues in the postpartum period. *Journal of Obstetric, Gynecologic, and Neonatal Nursing, 49*(2), 127–136. https://doi.org/10.1016/j.jogn.2020.01.001

Roy, P. (2015). Female sexual dysfunction: A comparative study in drug-treated populations. *Indian Journal of Psychiatry, 57*(1), 30–34. https://doi.org/10.4103/0019-5545.148509

Sagar, R., & Singh, S. (2022). National Tele-Mental Health Program in India: A step towards mental health care for all?. *Indian Journal of Psychiatry, 64*(2), 117–119. https://doi.org/10.4103/indianjpsychiatry.indianjpsychiatry_145_22

Santoro, N., Epperson, C. N., & Mathews, S. B. (2015). Menopausal symptoms and their management. *Endocrinology and Metabolism Clinics of North America, 44*(3), 497–515. https://doi.org/10.1016/j.ecl.2015.05.001

Sardinha, L., Maheu-Giroux, M., Stöckl, H., Meyer, S. R., & García-Moreno, C. (2022). Global, regional, and national prevalence estimates of physical or sexual, or both, intimate partner violence against women in 2018. *Lancet (London, England), 399*(10327), 803–813. https://doi.org/10.1016/S0140-6736(21)02664-7

Silverman, J. G., Decker, M. R., Gupta, J., Kapur, N., Raj, A., & Naved, R. T. (2009). Maternal experiences of intimate partner violence and child morbidity in Bangladesh: Evidence from a national Bangladeshi sample. *Archives of Pediatrics & Adolescent Medicine, 163*(8), 700–705. https://doi.org/10.1001/archpediatrics.2009.115

Srishti, D. (2023). Infertility and patriarchy in India: Causes and Consequences. *International Journal of Health Sciences and Research, 13*, 353. https://doi.org/10.52403/ijhsr.20230748

Tammary, E., & Manasi, K. (2023). Mental and sexual health outcomes associated with FGM/C in Africa: A systematic narrative synthesis. *eClinicalMedicine, 56*. https://doi.org/10.1016/j.eclinm.2022.101813

Tosto, V., Ceccobelli, M., Lucarini, E., Tortorella, A., Gerli, S., Parazzini, F., & Favilli, A. (2023). Maternity blues: A narrative review. *Journal of Personalized Medicine, 13*(1), 154. https://doi.org/10.3390/jpm13010154

Vanobberghen, F., Weiss, H. A., Fuhr, D. C., Sikander, S., Afonso, E., Ahmad, I., Atif, N., Bibi, A., Bibi, T., Bilal, S., De Sa, A., D'Souza, E., Joshi, A., Korgaonkar, P., Krishna, R., Lazarus, A., Liaqat, R., Sharif, M., Weobong, B., Zaidi, A., … Rahman, A. (2020). Effectiveness of the thinking healthy programme for perinatal depression delivered through peers: Pooled analysis of two randomized controlled trials in India and Pakistan. *Journal of Affective Disorders, 265*, 660–668. https://doi.org/10.1016/j.jad.2019.11.110

World Health Organization. (2025, January 31). Female genital mutilation [Fact sheet]. https://www.who.int/news-room/factsheets/detail/female-genital-mutilation

Woody, C. A., Ferrari, A. J., Siskind, D. J., Whiteford, H. A., & Harris, M. G. (2017). A systematic review and meta-regression of the prevalence and incidence of perinatal depression. *Journal of Affective Disorders, 219*, 86–92. https://doi.org/10.1016/j.jad.2017.05.003

Yang, J. M. K., Vaiphei, K., Siliya, M., Mkandawire, T., Dolman, C., Heron, J., Wilson, S., Yaresheemi, S., Kitney, D., Bailey, L., Apsey, C., Liwimbi, O., Stewart, R., Thippeswamy, H., Jones, I., Chorwe-Sungani, G., Chandra, P., & Di Florio, A. (2023). Postpartum psychosis: A public involvement perspective across three continents. *Archives of Women's Mental Health, 26*(6), 831–837. https://doi.org/10.1007/s00737-023-01347-8

Chapter 2
Women's Reproductive Mental Health in Afghanistan

Isha Batra and Gunja Sengupta

1 Introduction

Afghanistan is a landlocked country located in South Asia. As per the data published by the National Statistics and Information Authority (NSIA) of Afghanistan, the total population of 2023–2024 was 39.5 million, with a female population of 17.1 million, and a sex ratio of 104 males per 100 females (National Statistics and Information Authority (NSIA), 2024). The female reproductive population statistics are not available in this report. Food and Agriculture Organization (FAO) data (2019) shows 3.8 million women of reproductive age suffer from anemia, the proportion of which is 42.6%, according to World Bank data (UNdata, 2019; World Bank Gender Data Portal, 2019). We can get a rough indirect estimate of the numbers from these data.

It is a country that has suffered multiple, often simultaneous, humanitarian crises over the years. The worst-impacted population appears to be that of women. The Taliban, since its takeover in 2021, has passed multiple directives that have curbed the rights and autonomy of women. There is a lack of access to education, public spaces, healthcare, reproductive rights, and mental health services. There is also, consequently, a lack of data on many domains of reproductive mental health (UN Women, 2024a, b). The regulations and restrictions on women have been seen to have mental health repercussions. A report from early 2022 found that women make up 75% of those who visit Herat's psychiatric hospital, with an increase of 7% in the number of mentally ill women receiving psychological treatment over the past year (Schwartz et al., 2023).

However, even in the face of these restrictions and challenges, many have found a way to conduct some research in this area. This chapter presents the summary of

I. Batra · G. Sengupta (✉)
Department of Psychiatry, ABVIMS & Dr RML Hospital, New Delhi, India

P. Kukreti et al. (eds.), *Women's Reproductive Mental Health in South Asia*, South Asian Perspectives in Mental Health and Psychology,
https://doi.org/10.1007/978-981-96-9219-4_2

the available research and data that has been published on women's mental health in Afghanistan, with a focus on the reproductive period.

2 Perinatal Mental Health Issues

2.1 Context and Prevalence

The perinatal period is a critical period for women's mental health. Mental disorders during this period, including depression, anxiety, and postpartum psychosis, represent a significant public health concern globally. The World Health Organization (WHO) estimates that approximately 15.6% of pregnant women and 19.8% of postpartum women experience a mental disorder, primarily depression, in developing countries (WHO, 2025). In Afghanistan, precise epidemiological data on perinatal mental health are scarce due to systemic barriers to healthcare access and limited research infrastructure, but studies suggest an alarmingly high prevalence.

A feasibility study conducted in two Afghan health facilities reported a screening prevalence of postnatal depression as high as 61% among women who had given birth in the past 12 months, based on the *Patient Health Questionnaire-9 (PHQ-9)* with a cut-off score of 12 (Tomlinson et al., 2020). This figure is strikingly higher than global estimates, which suggest that approximately 10–15% of women in high-income countries and 15–20% in low- and middle-income countries experience perinatal depression (WHO, 2025). Another report highlighted that the prevalence of depression among pregnant women was as high as 80.4%, which is notably higher than the national average for major depressive episodes, reported to be 11.7% (Kovess-Masfety et al., 2021; Sarem et al., 2024). Furthermore, a cross-sectional study conducted among pregnant women in Herat province suggested that the overall prevalence of depression, anxiety, and stress as measured by Depression, Anxiety and Stress Scale (DASS-42) was 42.8%, 40.0%, and 59.5%, respectively (Niazi et al., 2023).

2.2 Risk Factors

The high incidence of perinatal mental illnesses in Afghanistan is mediated by a number of risk factors, such as *socioeconomic challenges* like high rates of unemployment, poverty, and lack of access to healthcare (World Health Organization, 2025); *conflict and displacement* (Chin et al., 2022; Yin et al., 2021); *cultural and social norms* like gender-based violence, early marriage, limited autonomy, abusive relationships, or forced marriages (Gelaye et al., 2016); *lack of mental health support* (Tomlinson et al., 2020); and *previous history of mental illness* (Kovess-Masfety et al., 2021) (especially depression or anxiety disorders).

2.3 *Impact*

The burden of perinatal mental health disorders in Afghanistan extends beyond individual suffering to impact families and communities. Untreated prenatal mental illnesses can have serious repercussions that impact both maternal and child outcomes. Untreated maternal depression and anxiety are linked with various adverse outcomes, including reduced breastfeeding initiation, impaired mother-infant bonding, and increased risks of infant malnutrition and developmental delays (Field, 2009). Women with untreated mental health conditions, particularly postpartum depression and psychosis, may be at risk of suicide and harm to the infant. These effects are especially catastrophic in situations where there is minimal psychiatric support.

Many Afghan women may not seek treatment because of the associated stigma with mental illnesses, which can cause them to become isolated and worsen their condition. This lack of social support can further increase psychological distress and perpetuate the cycle of mental illness (Najafizada et al., 2017).

3 Mental Health During Menarche and Menopause

The onset of menarche or menopause can be a challenging time for Afghan women, often accompanied by psychological stress due to cultural taboos and a lack of education about menstruation.

3.1 *Menarche and Mental Health*

Menarche, the onset of menstruation, marks a significant developmental milestone for girls. The experience of menarche is particularly difficult in Afghanistan, a nation defined by prolonged conflict, gender inequality, and inadequate access to healthcare.

3.1.1 Traumatic First Experiences

Most Afghan girls face menstruation unprepared, describing their first period as "terrifying" and "shameful" due to societal taboos. Families often avoid discussions, leaving girls to interpret menstruation as punishment or injury. According to a UNICEF survey in Afghan schools, 50% of girls who are menstruating for the first time are unaware of it, 38% of girls skip school when they are menstruating, and 12% do not utilize sanitary goods like soap, sanitary napkins, and clean water. According to their beliefs, 70% of these girls do not take a bath during their periods (UNICEF, 2018; Odey et al., 2022). A study on menstrual hygiene management in

Afghan schools reported that 70% of girls felt embarrassed or anxious about their first period, with many lacking prior knowledge due to limited sexual and reproductive health education (UNICEF, 2019; Odey et al., 2022).

3.1.2 Lack of Education and Support

No formal menstrual health education exists in schools or communities in Afghanistan. Knowledge about puberty and menstruation is minimal, with only 30% of Afghan girls receiving any formal education on reproductive health, according to a 2018 WaterAid study (WaterAid & UNICEF, 2018).

3.1.3 Cultural Stigma and Isolation

Menstruation is heavily stigmatized, with practices such as seclusion during periods (e.g., exclusion from religious activities or household tasks). Menstruation is perceived as “impure,” limiting girls’ mobility and social engagement. The UNICEF report on menstrual health in Afghanistan noted that 29% of girls missed school during menstruation, often due to shame or lack of sanitation facilities, contributing to social withdrawal and depressive symptoms (UNICEF, 2018).

3.1.4 Increased Vulnerability to Mental Health Issues

The onset of menarche often leads to fluctuations in hormone levels, which can contribute to emotional disturbances such as mood swings, irritability, and anxiety. For many Afghan girls, these natural hormonal changes may coincide with psychological distress due to societal expectations around puberty and menstruation, combined with a lack of access to mental health education, leading to depression and anxiety (Neyazi et al., 2023).

3.2 Menopause and Mental Health

Menopause marks the end of reproductive years and is a significant life transition in a woman’s life, accompanied by physical, hormonal, and psychological changes. Studies have shown that women’s attitudes toward menopause have a significant impact on their acceptance and management of the problems of this period. Middle-aged women who have more knowledge and awareness about menopause are more likely to manage menopause better, as compared to those with a negative attitude toward it (Kwak et al., 2014). A study conducted on the level of knowledge and attitude of Afghan women regarding the phenomenon of menopause depicted that 64% of women had a negative attitude toward menopause (Hakim, 2024).

4 Psychological Issues Associated with Reproductive Interventions

4.1 Contraception Use

The use of contraceptives by Afghan women reflects a complex interplay of reproductive autonomy, cultural norms, healthcare access, and mental health outcomes. Contraceptive use in Afghanistan remains low despite high awareness, with a national prevalence of 21.8%. Regional variations exist, with Herat province having the highest prevalence at 49.4% and Paktika the lowest at 2% (Rasooly et al., 2015). Urban areas usually depict higher usage rates (36.4%) than rural settings (18.4%) (Shafiqullah et al., 2018).

Women's decision to use contraception is frequently influenced by familial pressure, religious beliefs, and male partner approval, adding layers of psychological complexity to its adoption. Factors associated with higher contraceptive use include higher education, urban background, greater wealth, larger family size, and exposure to antenatal care (Osmani et al., 2015; Rasooly et al., 2015). Barriers to contraceptive use include lack of education, conservative beliefs, and spousal disapproval (Masudi & Alami, 2023; Todd et al., 2008). There was no published data found on the psychological impact of contraception in Afghanistan.

4.2 Medical Termination of Pregnancy

Medical termination of pregnancy (MTP), the deliberate ending of a pregnancy through medical means, is a deeply sensitive and complex issue in Afghanistan, shaped by legal restrictions, cultural norms, and limited access to healthcare.

4.2.1 Legal Status and Access to MTP

Abortion is illegal in Afghanistan except to save a woman's life, as per the Afghan Penal Code (Government of the Republic of Afghanistan, 1976), (United Nations, 2001). Nevertheless, unsafe abortions still happen, frequently as a result of unwanted pregnancies, which account for 24% of births, according to the 2015 Afghanistan Demographic and Health Survey (Central Statistics Organization (CSO) Afghanistan et al., 2017). Although exact data on abortion incidence in Afghanistan are lacking, the abortion rate in the South Central Asia region was 46 abortions per 1000 women aged 15–49 years old from 2015 to 2019; over half of abortions in the area were unsafe (Bearak et al., 2020).

Additionally, due to social, economic, and geographical constraints, Afghan women have limited access to abortion-related health facilities. A study conducted on Afghan women suggested that 73.7% of women did not have good knowledge about the legal conditions under which abortion is allowed in Afghanistan. Good knowledge of abortion among participants was significantly associated with their ethnicity, educational level, father's knowledge level, mother's knowledge level, and economic status (Saeed et al., 2022).

4.2.2 Psychological Outcomes and Prevalence

Qualitative insights suggest that Afghan women face intense emotional distress post-MTP. Feelings of shame, guilt, and fear of discovery are common, driven by cultural and religious condemnation of abortion as a sin or moral failing. The secrecy needed to obtain an abortion—often without spousal or familial knowledge—can lead to isolation and chronic stress, while the physical risks of unsafe methods may trigger trauma responses (Perera et al., 2021).

5 Suicide and Substance Use

5.1 Suicide

As per the National Mental Health Survey 2022, women experience significantly higher rates of both suicidal thoughts and attempts compared to men, although the incidence of suicide planning is similar between the genders. In total, 9.1% of women have reported experiencing suicidal thoughts at some point in their lives. Approximately 4.8% of women have reported having made a suicide plan during their lifetime, and 4.6% have reported attempting suicide. All the above proportions are higher than those of their male counterparts. This disparity may be attributed to the prevalent violence against women in the country. Furthermore, women are more likely than men to report suicidal behaviors, with the most pronounced difference observed in lifetime suicide attempts (Sabawoon et al., 2022; Paiman, 2024). As per a report from UN Women, a survey conducted in March 2023 depicted that 48% of respondents indicated knowing at least one woman who had suffered from anxiety or depression, and, alarmingly, 8% of respondents indicated knowing a woman who had attempted suicide, yet none were receiving treatment for this (UN Women, 2024a). One report suggests that up to 80% of people who died by suicide in Afghanistan were women (Tharwani et al., 2022).

Common methods include self-immolation (setting oneself on fire), hanging, drug overdose, and consuming chemicals like detergents. Self-immolation is particularly prevalent among young women aged 14–19 (Tharwani et al., 2022).

Traumatic event exposures, particularly sexual violence, and psychiatric disorders such as depression, anxiety, and PTSD are strongly associated with increased risk of suicidal behavior (Sabawoon et al., 2022). Domestic violence, family conflicts, forced marriages, and cultural practices are major contributors to the high suicide rates among Afghan women (Tharwani et al., 2022). Lack of access to mental health services further exacerbates the problem. Despite high rates of depression among those attempting suicide, treatment for mental health issues is lacking (Paiman et al., 2019). In Afghanistan's Islamic context, suicide is considered forbidden, leading many families to conceal suicide attempts. No suicide surveillance systems are in place. The data collected on incidences of burns and organophosphate poisonings do not delineate whether it was related to a suicide attempt. The lack of awareness and stigma together further compound the problem (Paiman, 2024). The situation has worsened since the Taliban's return to power, with restrictive policies and systemic oppression disproportionately affecting women (Sabawoon et al., 2022).

5.2 Substance Use Disorders

Afghanistan is among the leading producers of opium and other illicit drugs. The easy availability of drugs and the presence of conflict and instability resulted in a high prevalence of drug use in all the population subgroups, including women and children. In a nationwide survey conducted in 2015 on 3723 women aged 15 and above, the prevalence of drug use was reported to be 9.5%, the most common being opioids (6.7%). Notably, the prevalence was significantly higher in rural areas at 11.2% compared to urban areas, which stood at 4.3% (SGI Global, 2015; Singh et al., 2024). A survey conducted in 2009 found that the prevalence of injecting drug use among women was 0.07% (UNODC, 2009). Women who use drugs are more likely to be widowed or divorced, less educated, and over twice as likely to be unemployed compared to their non-drug-using counterparts. 78% of women who consume opium have given it to their children or other family members. The most common method of consumption is ingestion, perceived as more socially acceptable and often associated with medical use. Over half (52.2%) were first introduced to drugs by a close family member, often a husband, and nearly half are unemployed. Women are seen as bearers of family honor, maintained through seclusion and chastity, with men controlling their interactions. While upholding family honor can sometimes protect against drug use, when women are introduced to drugs by male members of the family, seeking help becomes more challenging. Women are integral to agricultural production, including opium cultivation, though they seldom manage the marketing, which is typically handled by male relatives (Momand & Jones, 2020).

Women face unique challenges, as substance dependence among them is rising but remains underreported due to cultural barriers (WHO EMRO, 2024b; Singh et al., 2024). While treatment services have expanded in urban areas, rural areas still lack evidence-based, culturally appropriate prevention and treatment programs (Momand & Jones, 2020).

A study comparing treatment outcomes between men and women in drug treatment centers in Afghanistan showed that women have better outcomes of treatment than men. But women are usually able to utilize only home-based services due to lack of access (Schweinhart et al., 2022).

Despite challenges, some organizations in Afghanistan are advancing harm reduction and community-based rehab for substance use disorders (SUDs). More accessible, evidence-based treatments adapted to low-resource settings are needed. The Ministry of Counter Narcotics leads drug demand reduction through policies like the National Drug Treatment Guidelines, National Guidelines for Drug Education and Harm Reduction Strategy (Singh et al., 2024).

6 Psychosocial and Cultural Indices

6.1 Gender-Based Violence (GBV)

Most of the research on GBV in this section is on intimate partner violence. However, in the context of Afghanistan, manifestations of gender-based violence against women may encompass domestic violence inflicted by spouses and/or mothers-in-law, honor-related killings, forced marriages, sexual assault by strangers, mutilation, and involuntary engagement in (Mannell et al., 2021).

A survey in 2018, conducted by the Central Statistical Organisation in Kabul, showed that 50.8% of women had a lifetime history of physical and/or sexual IPV and 46.1% of women had a history of IPV in the last year. The numbers varied with provinces, the maximum proportion of women with a history of IPV reaching up to 92% in some provinces (UN Women, 2024a). A United Nations Population Fund study revealed that 87% of Afghan women have suffered from at least one type of violence, with 62% enduring multiple types of abuse over their lifetime. These numbers are much higher than the prevalence of IPV worldwide (30%) and in the WHO Southeast Asia region (33%) (WHO, 2024).

6.2 Risk and Protective Factors

A variety of IPV risk and protective factors were found in Afghan studies. A review (Wachter et al., 2024) summarized the risk and protective factors of IPV identified in the literature from Afghanistan, which are as follows:

- Individual factors: Older age (except sexual violence), employment, exposure to trauma and violence (sexual violence), disability, and acceptance of violence have been seen to increase the likelihood of IPV, while higher education for self and husband has been associated with a lower likelihood of IPV.
- Interpersonal and household level factors: Early age of marriage, unequal educational status, polygamous marriages, longer marriages, contraceptive (especially female contraceptive) use, conflict about contraceptive use, having more children

associated, violence by in-laws, and food insecurity have been seen to be associated with a higher likelihood of IPV. Decision-making in the household has a complex relationship with IPV. More participation in decision-making is associated with a lower likelihood of IPV. However, sole decisions regarding big purchases increased the risk of IPV.
- Societal level factors: Living in a rural area, acceptance of IPV in the province, and armed conflict have been seen to be associated with increased risk of IPV.

6.3 Outcomes of GBV

Physical and Mental Health of Women A study on the associated factors and consequences of IPV showed that diminished life satisfaction was correlated with female individuals undergoing one or more instances of emotional IPV. Those who indicated experiencing one or more episodes of physical IPV alongside one or more episodes of emotional IPV exhibited heightened depressive symptoms, PTSD symptoms, reduced life satisfaction, deteriorated overall health, amplified suicidal ideation, and an escalated degree of disability. Furthermore, women who experienced two or more episodes of both physical and emotional IPV reported exacerbated depressive symptoms, PTSD symptoms, lowered life satisfaction, worsened general health, increased suicidal ideation, and an intensified severity of disability (Gibbs et al., 2018). Women with a history of physical or sexual violence were more likely to have pregnancy complications (Rahman et al., 2021).

Stigma There are multiple sources of stigma that a woman faces in the context of IPV and its after-effects. A qualitative study on survivors of IPV and the stigma they face after IPV showed that the stigma was experienced from natal family, husband and in-laws, friends and community, authorities, and the survivors themselves (self-stigma). IPV was seen as a private family matter, and speaking up against violence or considering divorce was seen to be against the honor of the family. Survivors reported that authorities, including healthcare workers and law enforcement, either did not take their claims seriously or maintained silence (Mukerji et al., 2023).

Intergenerational Impact A study focused on Afghan women revealed that they reported observing instances of physical abuse directed at their mothers and articulated how such experiences manifested in violent behaviors toward their children during periods of emotional distress (Ndungu et al., 2021). Within the demographic of children and adolescents, studies have indicated that family violence, to a greater extent than violence associated with warfare, serves as a significant catalyst for mental health issues, including but not limited to depression and anxiety. Moreover, within educational settings, instances of violence among children have been correlated with exposure to domestic violence occurring in the home environment (Alemi et al., 2023).

6.3.1 Interventions on GBV

The interventions on GBV are multi-faceted. The first is prevention, that focuses on strengthening policy and targeting gender norms in society. The second are interventions for survivors of violence. Trauma-focused therapies are the mainstay of treatment of women impacted by violence. There is a dearth of literature in this area, as women do not have access to these interventions. A study on a group counselling intervention, based on developing networks of support, psychoeducation, social skills, and stress management, on female survivors of GBV in Kabul showed improvement in general health or social life. (Manneschmidt & Griese, 2009) Narrative storytelling was another method tried on women in safe houses as a mental health support intervention and it was found that there were many stories of trauma waiting to be told and that storytelling under specifically formulated conditions was perceived as a positive experience for a sense of identity, learning, and challenging societal norms. (Mannell et al., 2018).

6.4 Gender Inequality

Afghanistan is a country that is among the last in rank worldwide for indices of gender equality. The table below shows the rankings in gender equality indicators. Afghanistan ranks last on the World Economic Forum's Global Gender Gap Index (2022) (World Economic Forum, 2022). All measurable indicators of gender equality have had a setback since the new regulations targeted women's autonomy and rights and made them largely homebound. Around 80% of girls don't go to school. More than 100,000 girls have been banned from university. Only 6% of women have internet access (UN Women, 2024a, b).

This jarring state of inequality has had mental health repercussions in terms of anxiety, fear, and hopelessness (Alemi et al., 2023). Most of the women patients treated in psychiatric hospitals are those who were formerly employed or pursuing education and are being treated for depression and anxiety (Schwartz et al., 2023).

7 Mental Health Services for Women: Availability and Utilization

The NSIA data on health indices does not include reproductive mental health indices; thus, the data presented here is from a review adapted from the Health Resources and Services Availability Monitoring System (HeRAMS) data from WHO. There are 4760 health facilities in Afghanistan with 42,691 health staff, of whom 41.5% are women. About 20% of specialists and 33.05% of nurses are women, while

99.41% of midwives are women and only 8.29% of technicians and pharmacists are women (Hegazy et al., 2025).

7.1 Mental Health Services Availability

According to the review, the availability of mental health services (in general) across different regions remains under 50%. The southeastern and eastern areas have the highest availability, whereas the central highland and northern regions have the lowest. The central highland region is affected by a lack of staff, which is the only barrier reported. On the other hand, the northern regions face challenges in shortages of funding, medical supplies, personnel, and training, all of which are significant hurdles to service availability. Likewise, psychological first aid is most accessible in the southern region at 47.6% and least accessible in the southeastern region at 8.5%. Inpatient care for mental disorders is not widespread, with the Eastern, Southern, and Northeastern regions showing availability between 16% and 18%, while the Central Highland region has a mere 4.3% availability rate (Hegazy et al., 2025).

Specifically in terms of women's mental health, the provision of mental health services in Afghanistan, which was already challenging, has been severely hindered by the administration's limitations on civil society, a shortage of trained mental health professionals within the public health sector, reductions in funding, and minimal investment in mental health initiatives, including those addressing drug and substance abuse. Additionally, the stigma associated with seeking services further complicates the difficulties faced by women in accessing healthcare (Ezadi et al., 2021; UN Women, 2024a, b).

7.2 Service Utilization

A survey in 2022 showed that just 10% of Afghan women surveyed reported that the health services accessible to them were sufficient to meet their basic health needs. Women encounter extra economic challenges and limitations on their movement and access to public space. In certain regions of Afghanistan, mahram (compulsory accompanying male person) rules are enforced for both female healthcare workers during their shifts and female patients for the entirety of their time at medical facilities, even within the operating room. This also precludes women from reporting GBV, availing contraception, and reporting mental health problems. The extra cost of mahram rules also limits access to healthcare facilities (UN Women, 2024a, b).

In a survey, women reported that either clinics providing mental health services have shut down or there are only a few staff members left who are trained in mental health (Safi & Rivas, 2023). There are only two psychiatric hospitals in the country (Schwartz et al., 2023).

An anonymous survey was conducted among doctors in Afghanistan. Based on the criteria of access, none of the respondents indicated that services for gender-based violence were accessible (Endler et al., 2023).

7.3 Liaison Between Reproductive Health and Mental Health Services

The strategies planned by the erstwhile government had included plans to liaise reproductive and mental health services (see point no. 5 in the Programs and Policies section below). However, the implementation has likely not happened with the barriers due to the change in administration. There is no data available on any such liaison service.

7.4 International Agencies

There are international agencies that have programs listed for women's mental health in Afghanistan. The United Nations, via UN Women, United Nations High Commissioner for Refugees (UNHCR), and other UN agencies, have services for women. In the mental health domain, the services mainly focus on GBV reduction and psychosocial support for women (UN Women, 2024a). WHO and UN Women have recently launched an initiative to target substance use in women (WHO EMRO, 2024a) HealthNet TPO, in collaboration with UNHCR, provides counseling services (Gluck, 2024). After 2021, there were challenges of withdrawal of funding as well as a ban on women working in NGOs (Schwartz et al., 2023; UN Women, 2024a, b).

8 Programs and Policies

After the end of the first Taliban rule, the elected government had taken steps to improve women's rights and access to services. The positive consequences of these were seen in the reduction in the maternal mortality rate and in the increase in the number of girls receiving education (UN Women, 2024b).

1. Afghanistan's National Action Plan (NAP) on United Nations Security Council Resolution (UNSCR) 1325 Women, Peace and Security: It was formulated and officially came into force in 2015 to implement the provisions of the UNSCR 1325 and to tackle the issues women encountered following the war and humanitarian conflict in Afghanistan. Included in its aims were prevention and protection

of women from discrimination and violence and providing psychosocial and healthcare support for survivors of GBV (Ministry of Foreign Affairs, 2015).

2. Law on the Elimination of Violence Against Women (EVAW), 2009: The implementation of the EVAW Law led to the designation of specialized EVAW prosecutors in various government sectors, the appointment of female judges and defense attorneys, as well as the creation of Family Response Units in each of Afghanistan's 34 provinces. However, the implementation was challenging due to the lack of knowledge and access of women to the provisions set by this law (UNAMA & OHCHR, 2011).
3. National Reproductive, Maternal, Newborn, Child, & Adolescent Strategy (RMNCAH), 2017–2021: It had a section on mental health and aimed to optimize mental health and psychosocial support services (MHPSS) for women for mental health problems related to pregnancy, violence, and conflict. The strategy aimed at optimizing the screening of maternal mental health and training of health personnel like obstetricians, physicians, and midwives for screening and psychosocial support (Ministry of Public Health, 2017).
4. National Strategy for Mental Health, 2019–2023: Among the strategy approaches, there is a section titled Mental health for pregnant and post-partum women and survivors of gender-based violence, complementing the aims of RMNCAH. It includes forming a program for maternal mental health in liaison with departments like obstetrics and ensuring training of health personnel in the community in screening and MHPSS. It also included a plan for ensuring the availability of mental health services for GBV survivors and widening its ambit in women protection centers, shelters, prisons, family protection centers, etc. (Ministry of Public Health, 2018).

However, after the new administration took over since 2021, all these policies have come to a halt, and women's rights have been replaced with a decrees and regulations, The former Ministry of Women's Affairs building being taken over by the Ministry for the Propagation of Virtue and the Prevention of Vice, which oversees the morality based decrees, symbolically represents this (UN Women, 2024a, b).

9 Research Gap

There exists a very stark deficit of current data regarding women's health in Afghanistan due to underreporting, restrictions, lack of access, and barriers to research. Most work that has been published comes internationally or are analyses of old data. There is barely any current epidemiological data available. Though the HeRAMS data lists the availability of reproductive services and mental health services, the data on the utilization of these services is either unavailable or sometimes contradictory.

10 Country-Specific Challenges

The challenges in assessing, optimizing, and providing services for reproductive mental health in Afghanistan are at a very basic level. Owing to the lack of access of women to public spaces and mahram rules, women are not able to access health-care services, and even if they do, they are not able to disclose sensitive or personal details, which is essential for assessment of reproductive mental health. Strict regulations and the implementation of gender norms result in the requirement of female healthcare workers for a therapeutic relationship. Though the ban on women's employment excludes healthcare workers, they are often not able to work to their optimum capacity due to the mahram rules that apply to them. Lack of access for girls to education also prevents the development of a future female workforce in healthcare. The policy measures for mental health for women in the reproductive population also largely stand incapacitated, thus preventing the development of health systems for them (UN Women, 2024a, b).

11 Way Forward

Increased awareness and research are one way forward. Social reforms may be practically difficult in the current setting. The recommendations given by women in Afghanistan are what matter in this regard. Women have appreciated the availability of counselling services provided by the UNHCR with the help of Afghan women, and the demand for it has greatly increased since its inception. A study on the experiences of displaced populations in Afghanistan revealed that the population wants accessible, affordable MHPSS services that are sensitive to their culture (Gluck, 2024). Due to stigma in society regarding mental health conditions, the people of Afghanistan found it difficult to utilize MHPSS services and also recommended integrating MHPSS with other services to reduce stigma. The women of Afghanistan faced a lack of accessibility to public spaces and recommended gender-specific mobile services providing door-to-door care or providing services from the community mosque (IOM Afghanistan, 2023).

12 Conclusion

Afghanistan is a country that has had ongoing wars and humanitarian crises for more than four decades. The pre-existing societal gender norms and stigma around mental health problems have been intensified manifold. This is a fertile ground for mental health problems for women during the reproductive period, which is already a vulnerable period for the onset and exacerbation of mental illnesses. Barely any epidemiological data is available on the magnitude of the problem. Till the country attains a state of sustainable stability, any possible effort of healthcare systems, including those of international agencies, in providing accessible MHPSS services to women would be a welcome step forward.

References

Alemi, Q., Panter-Brick, C., Oriya, S., Ahmady, M., Alimi, A. Q., Faiz, H., Hakim, N., Sami Hashemi, S. A., Manaly, M. A., Naseri, R., Parwiz, K., Sadat, S. J., Sharifi, M. Z., Shinwari, Z., Ahmadi, S. J., Amin, R., Azimi, S., Hewad, A., Musavi, Z., Ventevogel, P. (2023). Afghan mental health and psychosocial well-being: Thematic review of four decades of research and interventions. *BJPsych Open*, 9(4), e125. https://doi.org/10.1192/BJO.2023.502

Bearak, J., Popinchalk, A., Ganatra, B., Moller, A. B., Tunçalp, Ö., Beavin, C., Kwok, L., & Alkema, L. (2020). Unintended pregnancy and abortion by income, region, and the legal status of abortion: Estimates from a comprehensive model for 1990–2019. *The Lancet Global Health, 8*(9), e1152–e1161. https://doi.org/10.1016/s2214-109x(20)30315-6

Central Statistics Organization (CSO) Afghanistan, Ministry of Public Health (MoPH) Afghanistan, & ICF. (2017). *Afghanistan Demographic and Health Survey 2015.* https://www.rhsupplies.org/uploads/tx_rhscpublications/Afghanistan_-_2017.pdf

Chin, K., Wendt, A., Bennett, I. M., & Bhat, A. (2022). Suicide and maternal mortality. *Current Psychiatry Reports, 24*(4), 239–275. https://doi.org/10.1007/s11920-022-01334-3

Endler, M., Hassan, L., Gemzell-Danielsson, K., Babak, S., Sohail, R., & FIGO Committee on Women Facing Crisis. (2023). "I hope to all the world they don't forget women of Afghanistan": An interrupted survey among doctors in Afghanistan. *International Journal of Gynecology & Obstetrics, 163*(2), 402–408. https://doi.org/10.1002/ijgo.14979

Ezadi, Z., Mohammadi, N., Sarwari, R., & Jafari, S. M. (2021). Afghan women and access to health care in the past 25 years. *EClinicalMedicine, 43*, 101235. https://doi.org/10.1016/j.eclinm.2021.101235

Field, T. (2009). Postpartum depression effects on early interactions, parenting, and safety practices: A review. *Infant Behavior & Development, 33*(1), 1–6. https://doi.org/10.1016/j.infbeh.2009.10.005

Gelaye, B., Rondon, M. B., Araya, R., & Williams, M. A. (2016). Epidemiology of maternal depression, risk factors, and child outcomes in low-income and middle-income countries. *The Lancet Psychiatry*, 3(10), 973–982. doi:https://doi.org/10.1016/s2215-0366(16)30284-x

Gibbs, A., Corboz, J., & Jewkes, R. (2018). Factors associated with recent intimate partner violence experience amongst currently married women in Afghanistan and health impacts of IPV: A cross sectional study. *BMC Public Health, 18*(1), 593. https://doi.org/10.1186/S12889-018-5507-5/TABLES/4

Gluck, C. (2024, October 10). *Counselling offers Afghan women a safe space to share their mental health struggles. UNHCR Afghanistan.* Retrieved April 8, 2025, from https://www.unhcr.org/af/news/stories/counselling-offers-afghan-women-safe-space-share-their-mental-health-struggles

Government of the Republic of Afghanistan (1976). *Penal Code.* Retrieved on August 05, 2025, from https://antislaverylaw.ac.uk/wp-content/uploads/2019/08/Afghanistan-Penal-Code.pdf

Hakim Hekmati, P. D. A. (2024). Investigating the relationship between attitudes towards menopause and sexual function in menopausal women in war-torn Afghanistan. *Journal for Research in Applied Sciences and Biotechnology, 3*(6), 81–87. https://doi.org/10.55544/jrasb.3.6.11

Hegazy, N., El Deeb, S., Salem, M. R., Shaguy, J. A., Mohammed, R. N., Khawari, A., Tanoli, J., & Abouzeid, A. (2025). The availability and distribution of health services and resources across different regions in Afghanistan. *Frontiers in Public Health, 12*, 1371104. https://doi.org/10.3389/fpubh.2024.1371104

IOM Afghanistan. (2023). *Displacement trends and challenges in Afghanistan since August 2021*. https://afghanistan.iom.int/sites/g/files/tmzbdl1071/files/inline-files/Digital_RADA%20research%20papers_mental%20health.pdf

Kovess-Masfety, V., Keyes, K., Karam, E., Sabawoon, A., & Sarwari, B. A. (2021). A national survey on depressive and anxiety disorders in Afghanistan: A highly traumatized population. *BMC Psychiatry*, 21(1), 314. doi:https://doi.org/10.1186/s12888-021-03273-4

Kwak, E. K., Park, H. S., & Kang, N. M. (2014). Menopause knowledge, attitude, symptom and management among midlife employed women. *Journal of Menopausal Medicine, 20*(3), 118–125. https://doi.org/10.6118/jmm.2014.20.3.118

Mannell, J., Ahmad, L., & Ahmad, A. (2018). Narrative storytelling as mental health support for women experiencing gender-based violence in Afghanistan. *Social Science & Medicine, 1982*(214), 91–98. https://doi.org/10.1016/j.socscimed.2018.08.011

Mannell, J., Grewal, G., Ahmad, L., & Ahmad, A. (2021). A qualitative study of women's lived experiences of conflict and domestic violence in Afghanistan. Violence Against Women, 27(11), 1862–1878. https://doi.org/10.1177/1077801220935191

Manneschmidt S. & Griese K. (2009). Evaluating psychosocial group counselling with afghan women: Is this a useful intervention? Torture, 19(1), 41–50.

Masudi, M., & Alami, S. N. (2023). A review of contraceptive prevalence rates in Afghanistan. *Jami Scientific Research Quarterly Journal, 8*(2), 15–28. https://doi.org/10.61438/jsrqj.v8i2.24

Ministry of Foreign Affairs. (2015). *Afghanistan's National Action Plan on UNSCR 1325 women, peace and security*. Retrieved April 8, 2025, from http://pwnap1.tetra.in/wp-content/uploads/2020/10/NAP-Afghanistan.pdf

Ministry of Public Health. (2017). *National Reproductive, Maternal, Newborn, Child and Adolescent Health (RMNCAH) Strategy 2017–2021*. Retrieved April 8, 2025, from https://platform.who.int/docs/default-source/mca-documents/policy-documents/plan-strategy/afg-cc-10-03-plan-strategy-2017-eng-national-rmncah-strategy-2017-2021.pdf

Ministry of Public Health. (2018). *National Strategy for Mental Health 2019–2023*. Retrieved April 8, 2025, from https://moph.gov.af/sites/default/files/2019-09/Mental%20Health%20Staregy%202019-2023.pdf

Momand, A. S., & Jones, H. E. (2020). Drug use among women and children in Afghanistan: The complexities of an important public health issue. *HSOA Journal of Addiction & Addictive Disorders, 7*(1), 033. https://doi.org/10.24966/aad-7276/100033

Mukerji, R., Saboor, L., Paphitis, S., Devakumar, D., & Mannell, J. (2023). How does domestic violence stigma manifest in women's lives in Afghanistan? A study of survivors' lived experiences of help-seeking across three provinces. *Global Public Health, 18*(1). https://doi.org/10.1080/17441692.2023.2212035

Najafizada, S. A. M., Bourgeault, I. L., & Labonté, R. (2017). Social determinants of maternal health in Afghanistan: A review. *Central Asian Journal of Global Health, 6*(1), 240. https://doi.org/10.5195/cajgh.2017.240

National Statistics and Information Authority (NSIA). (2024). *Key Indicators 2023–24*. https://nsia.gov.af:8443/wp-content/uploads/2025/03/Key-Indicators-1402_2.pdf

Ndungu, J., Jewkes, R., Ngcobo-Sithole, M., Chirwa, E., & Gibbs, A. (2021). Afghan women's use of violence against their children and associations with IPV, adverse childhood experiences and poverty: A cross-sectional and structural equation modelling analysis. *International Journal of Environmental Research and Public Health, 18*(15), 7923. https://doi.org/10.3390/IJERPH18157923

Neyazi, A., Padhi, B. K., Mohammadi, A. Q., Ahmadi, M., Erfan, A., Bashiri, B., Neyazi, M., Ishaqzada, M., Noormohammadi, M., & Griffiths, M. D. (2023). Depression, anxiety and quality of life of Afghan women living in urban areas under the Taliban government: A cross-sectional study. BMJ Open, 13(8), e071939. https://doi.org/10.1136/bmjopen-2023-071939.

Niazi, A. R., Alekozay, M., Osmani, K., & Najm, A. F. (2023). Prevalence and associated factors of depression, anxiety, and stress among pregnant women in Herat, Afghanistan: A cross-sectional study. *Health Science Reports, 6*(8), e1490. https://doi.org/10.1002/hsr2.1490

Odey, G. O., Adegbite, M., Razaqi, N., Faizi, G., Afzali, H., Ahmadi, M., Frough, Z., Bhattacharya, S., & Lucero-Prisno, D. E., III. (2022). Knowledge and practice of menstrual hygiene among adolescent girls in secondary schools of Herat, Afghanistan. *Razi International Medical Journal, 2*(1), 1–9. https://doi.org/10.56101/rimj.v2i1.20

Osmani, A. K., Reyer, J. A., Osmani, A. R., & Hamajima, N. (2015). Factors influencing contraceptive use among women in Afghanistan: Secondary analysis of Afghanistan Health Survey 2012. *Nagoya Journal of Medical Science, 77*(4), 551–561.

Paiman, M. A. (2024). Suicidal behavior in Afghanistan. In S. M. Y. Arafat, M. Rezaeian, & M. M. Khan (Eds.), *Suicidal behavior in Muslim majority countries*. Springer. https://doi.org/10.1007/978-981-97-2519-9_2

Paiman, M. A., Khan, M., Ali, T., Asad, N., & Azam, I. (2019). Psychosocial factors of deliberate self-harm in Afghanistan: A hospital based, matched case-control study. *Eastern Mediterranean Health Journal, 25*(11), 798–805. https://doi.org/10.26719/emhj.19.021

Perera, S. M., Achakzai, H., Giuffrida, M. M., Kulkarni, M. J., Nagle, D. C., Wali, M. K., & Casey, S. E. (2021). Barriers to seeking post-abortion care in Paktika Province, Afghanistan: A qualitative study of clients and community members. *BMC Women's Health, 21*(1), 1–11. https://doi.org/10.1186/s12905-021-01529-5

Rahman, M., Saha, P., Anwar, N., & Hossain, A. (2021). He hurts her womb: Physical-sexual violence and pregnancy complications among women in Afghanistan. *Health Promotion Perspectives, 11*(4), 485–491. https://doi.org/10.34172/hpp.2021.61

Rasooly, M. H., Ali, M. M., Brown, N. J. W., & Noormal, B. (2015). Uptake and predictors of contraceptive use in Afghan women. *BMC Women's Health, 15*(1), 1–7. https://doi.org/10.1186/s12905-015-0173-6

Sabawoon, A., Keyes, K. M., Karam, E., & Kovess-Masfety, V. (2022). Associations between traumatic event experiences, psychiatric disorders, and suicidal behavior in the general population of Afghanistan: Findings from Afghan National Mental Health Survey. *Injury Epidemiology, 9*(1), 31. https://doi.org/10.1186/S40621-022-00403-8

Saeed, S., Jain, S., Emma, N., Afzali, H., Razaqi, N., Ahmadi, M., Yousufi, M., Bhattacharya, S., & Lucero-Prisno, D. E., III. (2022). Knowledge and attitude towards abortion among women in Afghanistan. *Razi International Medical Journal, 2*(2), 52–62. https://doi.org/10.56101/rimj.v2i2.58

Safi, M., & Rivas, A.-M. (2023). *The mental health crisis among Afghan women and girls*. ODI Policy brief. London: ODI. Retrieved April 8, 2025, from https://media.odi.org/documents/The_mental_health_crisis_among_Afghan_women_and_girls_mh6O2uX.pdf

Sarem, S., Neyazi, A., Mohammadi, A. Q., Neyazi, M., Ahamdi, M., Razaqi, N., Wali, S., Timilsina, S., Faizi, H., & Griffiths, M. D. (2024). Antenatal depression among pregnant mothers in Afghanistan: A cross-sectional study. *BMC Pregnancy and Childbirth, 24*(1), 342. https://doi.org/10.1186/s12884-024-06548-2

Schwartz, L., Lane, H., & Hassanpoor, Z. (2023). Overview and understanding of mental health and psychosocial support in Afghanistan. *International Health, 15*(5), 601–607. https://doi.org/10.1093/inthealth/ihad055

Schweinhart, A., Shamblen, S., Shepherd, C., Courser, M. W., Young, L., Morales, B., & Redpath, B. (2022). Gender differences in patient outcomes following drug abuse treatment in Afghanistan: Results from a new evaluation. *Journal of Substance Abuse Treatment, 134*, 108475. https://doi.org/10.1016/j.jsat.2021.108475

SGI-GLOBAL. (2015). *Afghanistan National Drug Use Survey 2015*. Retrieved April 8, 2025, from https://colombo-plan.org/wp-content/uploads/2020/03/Afghanistan-National-Drug-Use-Survey-2015-compressed.pdf

Shafiqullah, H., Morita, A., Nakamura, K., & Seino, K. (2018). The family planning conundrum in Afghanistan. *Health Promotion International, 33*(2), 311–317. https://doi.org/10.1093/HEAPRO/DAW081

Singh, A., Joshi, M., & Parmar, A. (2024). Substance use disorder among women and children in South Asia. In S. M. Y. Arafat & S. K. Kar (Eds.), *Current perspectives on substance use disorders in South Asia*. Springer. https://doi.org/10.1007/978-981-97-6619-2_14

Tharwani, Z. H., Essar, M. Y., Farahat, R. A., & Shah, J. (2022). The urgency of suicide prevention in Afghanistan: Challenges and recommendations. *The Lancet Regional Health – Southeast Asia, 8*, 100082. https://doi.org/10.1016/j.lansea.2022.100082

Todd, C. S., Isley, M. M., Ahmadzai, M., Azfar, P., Atiqzai, F., Smith, J. M., Ghazanfar, S. A., Strathdee, S. A., & Miller, S. (2008). Cross-sectional analysis of factors associated with prior contraceptive use among hospitalized obstetric patients in Kabul, Afghanistan. *Contraception*, 78(3), 249–256. https://doi.org/10.1016/j.contraception.2008.05.005

Tomlinson, M., Chaudhery, D., Ahmadzai, H., Rodríguez Gómez, S., Rodríguez Gómez, C., van Heyningen, T., & Chopra, M. (2020). Identifying and treating maternal mental health difficulties in Afghanistan: A feasibility study. *International Journal of Mental Health Systems*, 14(1), 1–8. https://doi.org/10.1186/s13033-020-00407-1

UN data. (2019). *Number of women of reproductive age (15–49 years) affected by anemia (million)*. Retrieved April 8, 2025, from https://data.un.org/Data.aspx?q=women+of+reproductive+age&d=FAO&f=itemCode%3a210430#FAO

UN Women. (2024a). *Afghanistan gender country profile 2024*. https://www.unwomen.org/sites/default/files/2024-06/Gender-country-profile-Afghanistan-en.pdf

UN Women. (2024b, August 12). *FAQs: Afghan women three years after the Taliban takeover*. Retrieved April 8, 2025, from https://www.unwomen.org/en/articles/faqs/faqs-afghan-women-three-years-after-the-taliban-takeover

UNAMA, & OHCHR. (2011). *A long way to go: Implementation of the elimination of violence against women law in Afghanistan*. https://unama.unmissions.org/sites/default/files/november_23_unama-ohchr-joint-report-on-implementation-of-evaw-law_eng_1.pdf

UNICEF. (2018). *Let us break the taboos and silence*. Retrieved April 8, 2025, from https://www.unicef.org/afghanistan/stories/let-us-break-taboos-and-silence

UNICEF. (2019). *Celebration of menstruation hygiene management day in Afghanistan*. Retrieved April 8, 2025, from https://www.unicef.org/afghanistan/press-releases/celebration-menstruation-hygiene-management-day-afghanistan

United Nations. (2001). *Abortion policies: A global review*. https://www.un.org/development/desa/pd/sites/www.un.org.development.desa.pd/files/files/documents/2021/Nov/undesa_pd_2001_abortion-policies-a-global-review-volume-i-afghanistan-to-france.pdf

UNODC. (2009). *Drug use in Afghanistan: 2009 Survey Executive summary*. https://www.unodc.org/documents/data-and-analysis/Studies/Afghan-Drug-Survey-2009-Executive-Summary-web.pdf

Wachter, K., Baccam, Z., Burgess, T., & Alemi, Q. (2024). A scoping review of the intimate partner violence literature among afghans across contexts. *Trauma, Violence, and Abuse*. https://doi.org/10.1177/15248380241271419

WaterAid & UNICEF. (2018). *Menstrual hygiene management in schools in South Asia*. https://washmatters.wateraid.org/sites/g/files/jkxoof256/files/menstrual-hygiene-management-snapshot%2D%2D-afghanistan.pdf

WHO. (2024, March 25). *Violence against women*. Retrieved April 8, 2025, from https://www.who.int/news-room/fact-sheets/detail/violence-against-women

WHO. (2025). *Mental health, brain health and substance use*. Retrieved April 8, 2025, from https://www.who.int/teams/mental-health-and-substance-use/promotion-prevention/maternal-mental-health

WHO EMRO. (2024a, July 17). *WHO and UN Women launch joint initiative to support women and children with substance use disorders in Afghanistan*. Retrieved April 8, 2025, from https://www.emro.who.int/afg/afghanistan-news/who-and-un-women-launch-joint-initiative-to-support-women-and-children-with-substance-use-disorders-in-afghanistan.html

WHO EMRO. (2024b, July 23). *WHO strengthens public health response to substance use in Afghanistan*. Retrieved April 8, 2025, from https://www.emro.who.int/afg/afghanistan-news/who-strengthens-public-health-response-to-substance-use-in-afghanistan.html

World Bank Gender Data Portal. (2019). *Prevalence of anemia among women of reproductive age (% of women ages 15–49)*. Retrieved April 8, 2025, fromhttps://genderdata.worldbank.org/en/indicator/sh-anm-allw-zs?year=2019

World Economic Forum. (2022). *Global gender gap report 2022*. https://www3.weforum.org/docs/WEF_GGGR_2022.pdf

Yin, X., Sun, N., Jiang, N., Xu, X., Gan, Y., Zhang, J., Qiu, L., Yang, C., Shi, X., Chang, J., & Gong, Y. (2021). Prevalence and associated factors of antenatal depression: Systematic reviews and meta-analyses. *Clinical Psychology Review, 83*, 101932. https://doi.org/10.1016/j.cpr.2020.101932

Chapter 3
Women's Reproductive Mental Health in Bangladesh

S. M. Yasir Arafat, Chandrima Mourin, and Fahmida Sharmin Joty

1 Introduction

The South Asian lower-middle-income category nation of Bangladesh is home to more than 170 million people, has an area of 147,570 km^2, and has more than 3,000,000 births annually (Arafat & Rajkumar, 2024; Bangladesh Bureau of Statistics, 2024; Countrymeters, 2024; World Bank, 2024). Among the population, 50.5% are females with a male-to-female ratio of 1.02, and 56.2% of females are aged between 15 and 44 years (Arafat & Rajkumar, 2024; Bangladesh Bureau of Statistics, 2024; Countrymeters, 2024). According to national statistics, maternal morbidity and death have decreased, and healthcare utilization has improved over the past 20 years, indicating a significant improvement in the quality of maternal healthcare in Bangladesh (Arifeen et al., 2014). Nevertheless, maternal mental health is frequently overlooked, particularly in environments with limited resources (Rahman et al., 2008). Due in large part to a lack of funding and targeted planning, this has not been linked to a commensurate increase in maternal mental health services (Insan et al., 2022). In its *National Mental Health Strategic Plan for 2020–2030*, the Government of Bangladesh has included two recommendations about maternal mental health in light of the evidence reviewed above: training

S. M. Y. Arafat (✉)
Department of Psychiatry, Bangladesh Specialized Hospital, Dhaka, Bangladesh

Department of Public and Community Health, Faculty of Medicine and Health Sciences, Frontier University Garowe, Garowe, Somalia

C. Mourin
Department of Clinical Psychology, University of Dhaka, Dhaka, Bangladesh

F. S. Joty
Department of Gynaecology and Obstetrics, Bangladesh Medical College, Dhaka, Bangladesh

P. Kukreti et al. (eds.), *Women's Reproductive Mental Health in South Asia*, South Asian Perspectives in Mental Health and Psychology,
https://doi.org/10.1007/978-981-96-9219-4_3

healthcare workers in maternal mental health literacy and integrating depression screening into maternal health (Government of The People's Republic of Bangladesh, 2022). There has been a recent focus highlighting the burden and consequences of maternal mental health in Bangladesh. This chapter highlights the epidemiological burden of psychiatric disorders among women during reproductive period, the current services status, enduring challenges and ways forward in Bangladesh.

2 Epidemiology and Burden of Psychiatric Disorders During Women's Reproductive Period

The prevalence of psychiatric disorders is higher among females than males, as revealed by two previous national mental health surveys (Alam et al., 2024; Firoz et al., 2006). It was 21.5% (male 15.7%) in the 2019 survey (Alam et al., 2024) and 19% (male 12.9%) in the previous survey (Firoz et al., 2006). The rate was lower (16–22%) among females in the reproductive age group (18–49 years) than the older age group (>25%) in Bangladesh (Alam et al., 2024). One hospital-based study with 197 prenatal women (135 antepartum, 62 postpartum) assessed the prevalence of psychiatric disorders determined by the *Structured Clinical Interview for DSM-IV Axis-I Disorders – Clinician Version* (SCID-CV) in Dhaka between 2012 and 2013 (Parveen et al., 2015). It found the prevalence was 14.2%. Among them, affective disorder was found in 6.1%, psychoses were present in 4.5%, and other disorders were found in 3.6%. As a single disorder, major depressive disorder was noted as the most common (3.6%) (Parveen et al., 2015).

One study determined the common mental disorders (CMD) among 264 mothers with children under five years (Khan & Flora, 2017). It found that about 46% of mothers were indicative of having CMD. Mothers with a higher age, lower educational attainment and social status, food insecurity, and under-nutrition were noted as risk factors (Khan & Flora, 2017). Bangladeshi women may be more susceptible to depression and anxiety due to factors such as unintended pregnancies, intimate partner violence (IPV), traditional views on gender preference for children, and family strife (Insan et al., 2022). Additionally, Bangladesh is susceptible to flooding and other natural disasters, which could raise the risk of mental health issues among mothers (Futterman et al., 2023). The COVID-19 pandemic's psychological and financial effects have also made mothers in the nation more susceptible to worry and depression (Nishat et al., 2023).

2.1 Psychiatric Disorders in the Antenatal Period

A study conducted in Chandpur in 2005 evaluated depression by the *Bangla Edinburgh Postnatal Depression Scale* (EPDS-B) among 361 pregnant women during the antenatal period at 34 to 35 weeks. Thirty-three percent of pregnant women had depression. Depression risk variables included a history of physical abuse, an unsupportive family (husband or mother-in-law), and expectations of a male child from family members (Gausia et al., 2009). A study conducted in Mymensingh evaluated 720 women from the third trimester to 6–8 months postpartum. It showed that throughout the prenatal period, the prevalence of anxiety and depression was 29% and 18%, respectively (Nasreen et al., 2011). Women's literacy was found to be protective against the development of depression and anxiety, while negative spousal connections, aggressive sexual encounters, and physical abuse by the spouse were identified as risk factors (Nasreen et al., 2011). A study in Chattogram, including 435 pregnant women evaluated how depression symptoms changed throughout the course of the antepartum period in each trimester. About 58% of women had depression in at least one trimester, with the prevalence being higher in the first trimester (35.4%) and progressively declining in the third (third trimester 30.1% and second trimester 33.7%). Throughout the entire prenatal period, roughly 13% experienced depression symptoms (Begum & Biswas, 2020).

Another study conducted in Nilphamari determined depression and sleep problems in 481 expectant mothers. About 39% of women experienced sleep issues, while 9% of women suffered from depression. Sleep problems were linked to depressive symptoms. Compared to women who did not lose their children, those who did so during the postpartum period were more likely to experience depression (Shaun et al., 2022).

2.2 Postpartum Depression

Studies assessing postpartum depression (PPD) found a wide range of prevalence in various settings measured by different tools like EPDS-B, *Self-Report Questionnaire* (SRQ-20), and SCID-CV (Table 3.1). The majority (10 out of 12) of the studies used EPDS-B, which is a screening tool for measuring depression. The rate ranged between 9% and 60.6%. Studies using EPDS-B found a range between 11% in Mymensingh (Edhborg et al., 2011) and 60.6% in the hospital samples (Al-Mamun et al., 2024). One study assessed PPD among 461 fathers living in different parts of the country by EPDS-B (Yesmin et al., 2023). It found that about 35% of fathers had moderate depressive symptoms and about 17% had severe symptoms of depression.

Several risk factors for PPD have been identified by studies, including age, parental age, pregnancy after 30 years of age, first baby, working mothers with job problems, physical comorbidities like hypertension, neonatal problems, poor family support, loss of a previous baby, having a loan to meet the delivery expenses, mood

Table 3.1 Postpartum depression in Bangladesh (Adapted from Arafat & Rajkumar, 2024)

SN	Study	Study place	Method	Sample source	Sample size	Measuring instrument	Data collection place	Prevalence (%)
1	Alam et al. (2021)	Urban	Cross-sectional	Community	291	EPDS-B	Dhaka	29.6
2	Azad et al. (2019)	Urban	Cross-sectional	Slum	376	EPDS-B	Dhaka	39.4
3	Al-Mamun et al. (2024)	Urban	Cross-sectional	Hospital	259	EPDS-B	Dhaka	60.6
4	Edhborg et al. (2011)	Rural	Cohort	Community	672	EPDS-B	Mymensingh	11
5	Gausia et al. (2007)	Urban	Cross-sectional	EPI center	100	SCID	Dhaka	9
6	Hamadani et al. (2012)	Rural	Longitudinal	Community	488	EPDS-B	Chandpur	17
7	Hossain et al. (2020)	Rural	Cross-sectional	Community	591	SRQ-20	Sirajganj	51.7
8	Islam et al. (2017)	Rural	Cross-sectional	Community	426	EPDS-B	Chandpur	35.2
9	Kabir et al. (2014)	Rural	Longitudinal	Community	660	EPDS-B	Mymensingh	32
10	Sharmin et al. (2019)	Urban	Cohort	Community	287	EPDS-B	Dhaka	25.7
11	Tasnim et al. (2021a)	Urban	Cross-sectional	Primary health centers	497	EPDS-B	Rajshahi	34
12	Tasnim et al. (2023)	Urban	Cross-sectional	Primary health center	497	EPDS-B	Rajshahi	34
13	Valdes et al. (2021)	Urban	Cross-sectional	Community	235	EPDS-B	Dhaka	24.3

EPDS-B Bangla Edinburgh Postnatal Depression Scale, *SCID* Structured Clinical Interview for DSM-IV Axis-I Disorders, *SRQ* Self -Report Questionnaire symptoms during the antenatal period, intimate partner violence, bad marital relationship, recent adverse events in life, perceived stress, and unplanned pregnancy (Arafat & Rajkumar, 2024).

2.3 Abortion and Mental Health in Bangladesh

One study of 240 women with spontaneous abortion assessed depressive and anxiety symptoms by *Generalized Anxiety Disorder* (GAD-7) and *Patient Health Questionnaire* (PHQ-9) (Koly et al., 2023). It found more than two-thirds of the respondents (77.5%) and more than half of the women (58.7%) had anxiety symptoms within 18 months of a spontaneous abortion. A higher educational status and being employed were noted as protective factors, and attaining post-abortion health services was associated with the reduction of symptoms (Koly et al., 2023).

2.4 Tubal Ligation and Mental Health in Bangladesh

One study was conducted among 100 ligated females in 1991, assessing the psychiatric morbidity after the ligation (Khanam et al., 1996). The mean age was 29.23 (SD = 3.91) years living in urban poor socioeconomic conditions. It found that 73% of the considerable amount of psychological symptoms. About 60% of the cases had pure psychological symptoms and about 40% had both physical and mental symptoms (Khanam et al., 1996).

2.5 Hysterectomy and Mastectomy, and Mental Health

One case-control study with 365 women after three to six months of planned hysterectomy in Sylhet in 2012 found that mental illness was more common among women after hysterectomy (38.3% vs. 28.1%), where depression (26.5%) was the most common diagnosis (Roy et al., 2015). Diagnoses were assigned according to the *Diagnostic and Statistical Manual of Mental Disorders, Fourth Edition, Text Revision* (DSM-IV-TR) for Axis I disorders. An earlier study found about 73% of women after hysterectomy had psychological symptoms (Khanam et al., 2000). Another study with 54 women after 3–6 months of hysterectomy found the prevalence of psychiatric morbidity at 38.8%, where depression and anxiety disorders were prominent (Habib et al., 2011).

Mastectomy deteriorates the emotional health of women, which is not an exception in Bangladesh. One study assessed the quality of life among 151 women before and after mastectomy between 2012 and 2013 in Dhaka. It found a reduction in physical and emotional well-being along with cognitive function after the operation (Rahman et al., 2014).

2.6 *Infertility and Mental Health*

Infertility has been associated with poor mental health status when compared to fertile women in Bangladesh (Saha et al., 2015). A high rate of anxiety (62.5%) and depression (89.3%) has been noted among patients with infertility attending hospitals (Alam et al., 2018; Chowdury et al., 2019). One study assessed the mental health status of 375 infertile women who were taking treatment for infertility (Hasan et al., 2023). It found the corresponding prevalence rates for stress, anxiety, and depression were 48.7%, 55.0%, and 59.7%. Infertile homemakers had about 3 times the odds of depression compared to government service holders; the chances of depression were 1.8 times higher for infertile women who had abortions (Hasan et al., 2023). One study assessed depression (woman 54.4%, man 38.4%), anxiety (woman 53.6%, man 26.8%), and stress (woman 30.4%, man 21.4%) among both partners of 112 couples with infertility (Irfan et al., 2018). It found that women were more affected than their male partners.

2.7 *Domestic Violence and Mental Health*

Bangladesh is a male-dominated country where females have a minimal role in partner choice, and they are blamed for trivial failures in the family (Hossain et al., 2022; Islam et al., 2018). However, the association between violence and psychiatric illness varies depending on the nature of the disorder and types of violence (Islam et al., 2018). Sometimes, violence may be a consequence of psychiatric morbidity (Islam et al., 2018). Several studies assessed the relationship between IPV and mental disorders (Tran et al., 2020; De & Murshid, 2018; Ziaei et al., 2016; Tasnim et al., 2021b; Esie et al., 2019; Islam et al., 2017; Ellsberg et al., 2008; Khan, 2015; Bakchi et al., 2018; Kabir et al., 2014). IPV was found to increase the risk of mental disorders more than two times (Tran et al., 2020; De & Murshid, 2018). It is associated with depression, CMD, emotional distress, and suicidal behavior. Nevertheless, the association has been affected by the attribution of violence by women (De & Murshid, 2018). The prevalence of domestic violence was 57% in a lifetime and emotional distress was 35% during pregnancy. Along with all forms of violence, emotional violence and behavior control were more related to emotional distress (Ziaei et al., 2016; Tasnim et al., 2021b; Esie et al., 2019). The prevalence was 77.2% in a year in a rural setting and depression was about 17% (Esie et al., 2019). The recent COVID-19 pandemic made the situation worse, as it has been reported to increase the rate of IPV during the pandemic in Bangladesh (Mahmood et al., 2022; Rashid Soron et al., 2021; Nishat et al., 2023).

2.8 Menopause and Mental Health

Every menopausal symptom affects a woman's quality of life (QoL). Evidence indicates that Asian women have greater menopausal suffering than women in North America and Europe, albeit the effects may differ from person to person and from place to place. According to estimates, during their menopausal transition, over two-thirds of middle-aged women in Bangladesh experienced stress, irritability, insomnia, mental tiredness, and difficulty concentrating (Ahmed et al., 2016; Rahman et al., 2011; Tasnim et al., 2016).

Furthermore, unusual symptoms are common in menopausal women, and in Bangladesh, they may be more severe (Ahmed et al., 2016; Rahman et al., 2011). A cross-sectional survey conducted in Bangladesh found that the majority of women in the country began to experience depression before menopause, which eventually led to headaches, excessive weariness, and impaired concentration in daily life (Bashar et al., 2017).

One study assessed depression among 326 women at 41–60 years of age to compare the rates among pre-, peri-, and post-menopausal stages (Alam et al., 2020). It found depression was higher among peri- (34.2%) and post-menopausal (33.2%) groups than pre-menopausal (26.8%) women.

3 Substance Abuse and Suicidal Behavior During the Reproductive Period

3.1 Substance Abuse

We did not find any study assessing substance abuse among females during pregnancy in Bangladesh. We know a little about the estimates, risk factors, interventions, and prevention of substance abuse among females of reproductive age in Bangladesh. One study assessed substance abuse among 296 female university students (22 ± 1.98 years) in Dhaka (Akhter, 2012). It found the prevalence of substance abuse was 17%; cannabis and phensidyl were the most common (44%) substances, followed by benzodiazepines (32%). One qualitative study assessed the risk factors for substance abuse among twelve female drug abusers (12–30 years of age) admitted to different rehabilitation centers in Dhaka (Mahbub & Rahman, 2023). It found that adverse life events, peer pressure, curiosity and novelty-seeking behavior, easy availability, and social stigma work as precipitating and perpetuating factors for substance abuse among females. One study assessed substance abuse among 360 "Dalit Married Adolescent Girls" (Haque et al., 2022). It found that the prevalence of drug addiction was 11.3%. Personal smoking, spousal smoking, and habits of using highly risky substances were associated with drug addiction (Haque et al., 2022). Gender-based violence was attributed to the risky behaviors among women who inject drugs, revealed in a qualitative study (Irfan et al., 2021). Another qualitative study found that social influence, problems within the family, lack of awareness about the bad impact of drugs, easy availability, stress, and curiosity were the attributing factors for substance abuse among females in Bangladesh.

3.2 *Suicidal Behavior*

One study among 361 pregnant mothers in Chandpur assessed thoughts of self-harm by the Bangla version of the *Edinburgh Postnatal Depression Scale (EPDS-B)*. It found that 4.7% of the mothers with depression had ideas of self-harm during the pregnancy (Gausia et al., 2009). Another study among 426 mothers during the six months after birth assessed the rate of suicidal thoughts in Chandpur district. The rate was 30.8% postpartum (Islam et al., 2020). One study assessed suicide attempts among the 940 pregnant mothers at an adolescent age. It found that 6.5% of the participants had suicide attempts during the last year (Li et al., 2021).

4 Current Status of Services and Care Seeking

Bangladesh has a well-structured health system that extends from the center to the primary care level for maternal and child health at the local to the national level (Dutta et al., 2022). Bangladesh has made substantial progress in maternal and child health due to this well-designed service structure at primary, secondary, and tertiary care levels. However, there is still inequitable and inadequate access to maternal mental health treatments. The number of mental health professionals is insufficient, as well as the national budget for mental health services is less than 0.05% of the total national budget allocated for mental health (Arafat et al., 2024). Bangladesh needs to integrate mental health support and services into existing health services for physical health.

Considering all these, maternal mental health is committed to being promoted by the Bangladesh government in the *National Mental Health Strategic Plan 2020–2030*. This strategy places a strong emphasis on incorporating mental health services into primary healthcare, including training healthcare professionals to increase mental health literacy and integrating depression screening into maternal health services (Government of The People's Republic of Bangladesh, 2022). There is no specialized center for maternal mental health care. The country still lacks special courses and trainings in perinatal mental health. Also, there is no placement of psychiatry residents to gynecology and gynecology residents to psychiatry during the post-graduation training period and curriculum.

The treatment gap for maternal mental health is high (Dutta et al., 2022; Koly et al., 2022). Most of the women do not receive mental health support during the perinatal period. Poor mental health literacy, high stigma toward mental health services, and unavailability of mental health services were the major barriers (Koly et al., 2022).

5 Liaison Between Maternal and Mental Health Services Providers

There has been discussion of efforts to incorporate mental health into basic healthcare in Bangladesh, with a focus on the necessity of identifying and treating mental illnesses in primary care settings (Arafat et al., 2018; Government of The People's Republic of Bangladesh, 2022). The collaboration between maternal and mental health service providers is still very limited in the context of Bangladesh. Specialized mental hospitals are centralized in cities, and in rural areas, mental health professionals are rarely found. A study carried out within a rural sub-region in Bangladesh indicates that two-thirds of women never sought mental health care during the perinatal period. This was mainly because the women and their families were unaware of the programs and providers that were available. In addition, community-level service providers are not properly trained and do not have suitable guidelines to provide primary support as well as referral to the appropriate place (Dutta et al., 2022). The scenario is a bit different in urban areas. Most women in urban areas get treatment from a gynecologist during the perinatal period, where the gynecologists can refer them to psychiatrists if they find any mental health issues in the patient. However, the referral rate is substantially low from reproductive health services providers to mental health providers, as this referral is not a common practice; most of the time, physical health is prioritized, and the mental health part is ignored.

6 Challenges for Women's Reproductive Mental Health Care

The current state of mental healthcare in Bangladesh has several challenges: an inadequate number of mental health facilities, a shortage of mental health practitioners, an unequal distribution of financial resources, poorly managed mental health policies, and stigma (Arafat et al., 2024; Williams et al., 2018). This small number of mental health professionals is not enough to provide maternal mental health care to a huge number of the population, as mental health services are not integrated into the primary care level, and there is no available post for mental health services in the primary and secondary care levels of services in the country. There is no epidemiological catchment area or functioning referral system. Additionally, there is an enduring stigma regarding psychotropics that hinders mental health care seeking as well as referral. Community mental health workers do not have specific training in maternal mental health, so they cannot help with the required action in time of need. The recent policy taken by the government is a small step to improve the condition of maternal mental health by detecting the problems and providing appropriate training to the professionals (Government of The People's Republic of Bangladesh, 2022).

7 Available Research and Gaps

Maternal reproductive health is a widely studied area in Bangladesh. As a result, reproductive health has been improved and infant mortality rate has been significantly reduced. However, little is known about reproductive mental health. The prevalence and factors contributing to reproductive mental health difficulties were not studied thoroughly. Moreover, most of the studies are centralized in urban areas, especially among the people from privileged societies. Studies about services and service users of maternal mental health have not been found yet. In addition, no longitudinal or cross-sectional studies about reproductive mental health were found. These issues have to be addressed, and studies have to be conducted in broader aspects (Arafat & Rajkumar, 2024).

8 Ways Ahead

A multidimensional strategy is needed to address maternal mental health services, including introducing awareness campaigns, integrating maternal mental health into primary healthcare, identifying common mental health disorders, and developing policies for community-level service providers. Telemedicine services can help in the initial stages of the development of the disorders. Furthermore, a collaboration of the government with NGOs can make the services more accessible for people from every corner of the country.

9 Conclusions

Along with the reduction of maternal physical morbidity and mortality, maternal mental health care warrants attention in Bangladesh. Although there are variations in the prevalence of psychiatric disorders in women of reproductive age depending on methods, time, and places of the study, the rates are higher compared to males. It needs the collaboration of policymakers, local communities, healthcare providers, educators, and civil society to reduce the unmet needs for mental health services in Bangladesh.

References

Ahmed, K., Jahan, P., Nadia, I., Ahmed, F., & Abdullah-Al-Emran. (2016). Assessment of menopausal symptoms among early and late menopausal midlife Bangladeshi women and their impact on the quality of life. *Journal of Menopausal Medicine, 22*(1), 39–46. https://doi.org/10.6118/jmm.2016.22.1.39

Akhter, J. (2012). Prevalence of substance abuse among female residential students of Dhaka University. *ASA University Review, 6*(1), 115–127.

Alam, M. J., Rahman, M. M., & Afsana, N. E. (2018). Psychological impacts of infertility among married women attending in a tertiary hospital, Dhaka. *Anwer Khan Modern Medical College Journal, 9*(1), 10–14. https://doi.org/10.3329/akmmcj.v9i1.35817

Alam, M. M., Ahmed, S., Dipti, R. K., Siddiquee, R. E., & Hawlader, M. D. H. (2020). The prevalence and associated factors of depression during pre-, peri-, and post-menopausal period among the middle-aged women of Dhaka city. *Asian Journal of Psychiatry, 54*, 102312. https://doi.org/10.1016/j.ajp.2020.102312

Alam, M. M., Haque, T., Uddin, K. M. R., Ahmed, S., Islam, M. M., & Hawlader, M. D. H. (2021). The prevalence and determinants of postpartum depression (PPD) symptomatology among facility delivered mothers of Dhaka city. *Asian Journal of Psychiatry, 62*, 102673. https://doi.org/10.1016/j.ajp.2021.102673

Alam, M. F., Ahmed, H. U., Alam, M. T., Sarkar, M., Khan, N. M., Uddin, M. J., & Sarkar, A. A. (2024). Community prevalence of psychiatric disorders: Findings from a nationwide survey in Bangladesh. *Asian Journal of Psychiatry, 92*, 103897. https://doi.org/10.1016/j.ajp.2023.103897

Al-Mamun, F., Sultana, M. S., Momo, M. A., Malakar, J., Bahar, S. B., Uddin, I., Murshida, M., Akter, M. M., Begum, M. M., Nodi, T. S., Al Habib, A., Kaggwa, M. M., Roy, N., & Mamun, M. A. (2024). Exploring the burden of postpartum depression in urban Bangladesh: Prevalence and its associations with pregnancy-related factors from a cross-sectional study. *Health Science Reports, 7*(4), e2035. https://doi.org/10.1002/hsr2.2035

Arafat, S. M. Y., & Rajkumar, R. P. (2024). Mental disorders during pregnancy and postpartum in Bangladesh: A narrative review. *Health Science Reports, 7*(9), e70027. https://doi.org/10.1002/hsr2.70027

Arafat, S. M. Y., Roy, S., & Huq, N. (2018). Integrating mental health into primary health care in Bangladesh: Problems and prospects. *Mental Health and Addiction Research, 3*(2). https://doi.org/10.15761/MHAR.1000158

Arafat, S. M. Y., Giasuddin, N. A., & Mazumder, A. H. (2024). Access to mental health care in Bangladesh—Current status, potential challenges, and ways out. In S. M. Y. Arafat & S. K. Kar (Eds.), *Access to mental health care in South Asia* (pp. 29–55). Springer Singapore. https://doi.org/10.1007/978-981-99-9153-2_3

Arifeen, S. E., Hill, K., Ahsan, K. Z., Jamil, K., Nahar, Q., & Streatfield, P. K. (2014). Maternal mortality in Bangladesh: A countdown to 2015 country case study. *The Lancet, 384*(9951), 1366–1374. https://doi.org/10.1016/s0140-6736(14)60955-7

Azad, R., Fahmi, R., Shrestha, S., Joshi, H., Hasan, M., Khan, A. N. S., Chowdhury, M. A. K., Arifeen, S. E., & Billah, S. M. (2019). Prevalence and risk factors of postpartum depression within one year after birth in urban slums of Dhaka, Bangladesh. *PloS One, 14*(5), e0215735. https://doi.org/10.1371/journal.pone.0215735

Bakchi, J., Kundu, S., Ghosh, S., & Akter, S. (2018). Intimate partner violence in Bangladesh: A scoping review. *Bangladesh Journal of Bioethics, 9*(3), 15–27.

Bangladesh Bureau of Statistics. (2024). *Population & Housing Census 2022*. https://bbs.gov.bd/site/page/47856ad0-7e1c-4aab-bd78-892733bc06eb/Population-&-Housing (accessed on 02 December, 2024).

Bashar, M., Ahmed, K., Uddin, M. S., Ahmed, F., Emran, A. A., & Chakraborty, A. (2017). Depression and quality of life among postmenopausal women in Bangladesh: A cross-sectional study. *Journal of Menopausal Medicine, 23*(3), 172–181. https://doi.org/10.6118/jmm.2017.23.3.172

Begum, M. R., & Biswas, S. C. (2020). Changes in depressive symptoms during the antenatal period: A Cohort study from Bangladesh. *Indian Journal of Psychological Medicine, 42*(6), 519–524. https://doi.org/10.1177/0253717620954337

Chowdury, T. S., Chowdhury, T. A., Begum, S. A., Begum, Y., & Amatullah, M. (2019). Depressive morbidity among female partner of infertile couple in a tertiary care setup in Bangladesh: Depressive morbidity in infertile female partner. *Bangladesh Medical Research Council Bulletin, 45*(2), 93–98. https://doi.org/10.3329/bmrcb.v45i2.42537

Countrymeter. (2024). *Bangladesh population.* https://countrymeters.info/en/Bangladesh (accessed on 02 December, 2024).

De, P. K., & Murshid, N. S. (2018). Associations of intimate partner violence with screening for mental health disorders among women in urban Bangladesh. *International Journal of Public Health, 63*(8), 913–921. https://doi.org/10.1007/s00038-018-1139-x

Dutta, G. K., Sarker, B. K., Ahmed, H. U., Bhattacharyya, D. S., Rahman, M. M., Majumder, R., & Biswas, T. K. (2022). Mental healthcare-seeking behavior during the perinatal period among women in rural Bangladesh. *BMC Health Services Research, 22*(1), 310. https://doi.org/10.1186/s12913-022-07678-z

Edhborg, M., Nasreen, H. E., & Kabir, Z. N. (2011). Impact of postpartum depressive and anxiety symptoms on mothers' emotional tie to their infants 2–3 months postpartum: A population-based study from rural Bangladesh. *Archives of Women's Mental Health, 14*(4), 307–316. https://doi.org/10.1007/s00737-011-0221-7

Ellsberg, M., Jansen, H. A., Heise, L., Watts, C. H., Garcia-Moreno, C., & WHO multi-country study on women's health and domestic violence against women study team. (2008). Intimate partner violence and women's physical and mental health in the WHO multi-country study on women's health and domestic violence: An observational study. *Lancet (London, England), 371*(9619), 1165–1172. https://doi.org/10.1016/S0140-6736(08)60522-X

Esie, P., Osypuk, T. L., Schuler, S. R., & Bates, L. M. (2019). Intimate partner violence and depression in rural Bangladesh: Accounting for violence severity in a high prevalence setting. *SSM – Population Health, 7*, 100368. https://doi.org/10.1016/j.ssmph.2019.100368

Firoz, A. H. M., Karim, M. E., Alam, M. F., Rahman, A. H. M. M., & Zaman, M. M. (2006). Prevalence, medical care, awareness and attitude towards mental illness in Bangladesh. *Bangladesh Journal of Psychiatry, 20*(1), 9–32.

Futterman, I. D., Grace, H., Weingarten, S., Borjian, A., & Clare, C. A. (2023). Maternal anxiety, depression and posttraumatic stress disorder (PTSD) after natural disasters: a systematic review. *The Journal of Maternal-Fetal & Neonatal Medicine, 36*(1). https://doi.org/10.1080/14767058.2023.2199345

Gausia, K., Fisher, C., Algin, S., & Oosthuizen, J. (2007). Validation of the Bangla version of the Edinburgh postnatal depression scale for a Bangladeshi sample. *Journal of Reproductive and Infant Psychology, 25*(4), 308–315. https://doi.org/10.1080/02646830701644896

Gausia, K., Fisher, C., Ali, M., & Oosthuizen, J. (2009). Antenatal depression and suicidal ideation among rural Bangladeshi women: A community-based study. *Archives of Women's Mental Health, 12*(5), 351–358. https://doi.org/10.1007/s00737-009-0080-7

Government of The People's Republic of Bangladesh. (2022). *National Mental Health Strategic Plan, 2020–2030.* https://old.dghs.gov.bd/index.php/bd/home/6171-nmu-2020-2030 (accessed on 21 December, 2024).

Habib, M. A., Begum, F., & Afroz, S. (2011). Psychiatric morbidity after hysterectomy. *TAJ: Journal of Teachers Association, 15*(1), 28–31. https://doi.org/10.3329/taj.v15i1.8378

Hamadani, J. D., Tofail, F., Hilaly, A., Mehrin, F., Shiraji, S., Banu, S., & Huda, S. N. (2012). Association of postpartum maternal morbidities with children's mental, psychomotor and language development in rural Bangladesh. *Journal of Health, Population, and Nutrition, 30*(2), 193–204. https://doi.org/10.3329/jhpn.v30i2.11313

Haque, M. I., Rani, V., Chowdhury, A. A., Akter, T., Hasan, I., Harun, M. G. D., & Zafar Ullah, A. N. (2022). Drug addiction and substance use among the Dalit married adolescent girls in Bangladesh: A cross-sectional survey. *International Journal of Mental Health and Addiction, 20*(5), 3145–3161. https://doi.org/10.1007/s11469-021-00570-7

Hasan, A. B. M. N., Sharif, A. B., Jahan, I., & Begum, M. R. (2023). Mental health status and the quality of life of infertile women receiving fertility treatment in Bangladesh: A cross-sectional study. *PLOS Global Public Health, 3*(12), e0002680. https://doi.org/10.1371/journal.pgph.0002680

Hossain, S. J., Roy, B. R., Hossain, A. T., Mehrin, F., Tipu, S. M. M. U., Tofail, F., Arifeen, S. E., Tran, T., Fisher, J., & Hamadani, J. (2020). Prevalence of maternal postpartum depression, health-seeking behavior and out of pocket payment for physical illness and cost coping mechanism of the poor families in Bangladesh: A rural community-based study. *International Journal of Environmental Research and Public Health, 17*(13), 4727. https://doi.org/10.3390/ijerph17134727

Hossain, M. M., Abdulla, F., Rahman, A., & Khan, H. T. A. (2022). Prevalence and determinants of wife-beating in Bangladesh: Evidence from a nationwide survey. *BMC Psychiatry, 22*(1), 9. https://doi.org/10.1186/s12888-021-03652-x

Insan, N., Weke, A., Forrest, S., & Rankin, J. (2022). Social determinants of antenatal depression and anxiety among women in South Asia: A systematic review & meta-analysis. *PLoS One, 17*(2), e0263760. https://doi.org/10.1371/journal.pone.0263760

Irfan, S. N., Rahman, M. M., Mithun, S., Arafat, S. Y., & Zafreen, F. (2018). Psychological state of selected infertile couples of Bangladesh. *Journal of Armed Forces Medical College, Bangladesh, 14*(1), 41–45. https://doi.org/10.3329/jafmc.v14i1.42720

Irfan, S. D., Khan, M. N. M., & Khan, S. I. (2021). Tales of gender-based oppression and violence: Risks and vulnerabilities of women who inject drugs (WWID) in Dhaka, Bangladesh. *The International Journal on Drug Policy, 92*, 103144. https://doi.org/10.1016/j.drugpo.2021.103144

Islam, M. J., Broidy, L., Baird, K., & Mazerolle, P. (2017). Intimate partner violence around the time of pregnancy and postpartum depression: The experience of women of Bangladesh. *PLoS One, 12*(5), e0176211. https://doi.org/10.1371/journal.pone.0176211

Islam, M. M., Jahan, N., & Hossain, M. D. (2018). Violence against women and mental disorder: A qualitative study in Bangladesh. *Tropical Medicine and Health, 46*, 5. https://doi.org/10.1186/s41182-018-0085-x

Islam, M. J., Broidy, L., Mazerolle, P., Baird, K., Mazumder, N., & Zobair, K. M. (2020). Do maternal depression and self-esteem moderate and mediate the association between intimate partner violence after childbirth and postpartum suicidal ideation? *Archives of Suicide Research, 24*(4), 609–632. https://doi.org/10.1080/13811118.2019.1655507

Kabir, Z. N., Nasreen, H. E., & Edhborg, M. (2014). Intimate partner violence and its association with maternal depressive symptoms 6–8 months after childbirth in rural Bangladesh. *Global Health Action, 7*, 24725. https://doi.org/10.3402/gha.v7.24725

Khan, A. R. (2015). Consequences of domestic violence against women: Some reflections from rural Bangladesh. *Asian Social Work and Policy Review, 9*(3), 210–223. https://doi.org/10.1111/aswp.12059

Khan, A. M., & Flora, M. S. (2017). Maternal common mental disorders and associated factors: A cross-sectional study in an urban slum area of Dhaka, Bangladesh. *International Journal of Mental Health Systems, 11*, 23. https://doi.org/10.1186/s13033-017-0129-3

Khanam, M., Mullick, M. S. I., & Munib, A. A. (1996). Pattern of psychiatric symptoms among the post ligated women. *Bangladesh Journal of Psychiatry, 9*(1), 18–21.

Khanam, M. A. S. U. D. A., Mullick, M. S. I., Naher, J. S., & Salam, M. A. (2000). Psychiatric aspect of hysterectomy. *Bangladesh Journal of Psychiatry, 14*(2), 25–30.

Koly, K. N., Tasnim, Z., Ahmed, S., Saba, J., Mahmood, R., Farin, F. T., Choudhury, S., Ashraf, M. N., Hasan, M. T., Oloniniyi, I., Modasser, R. B., & Reidpath, D. D. (2022). Mental healthcare-seeking behavior of women in Bangladesh: Content analysis of a social media platform. *BMC Psychiatry, 22*(1), 797. https://doi.org/10.1186/s12888-022-04414-z

Koly, K. N., Saba, J., Billah, M. A., McGirr, A., Sarker, T., Haque, M., Mustary, E., Hanifi, S. M. M. A., & Begum, F. (2023). Depressive symptoms and anxiety among women with a history of abortion living in urban slums of Bangladesh. *BMC Psychology, 11*(1), 197. https://doi.org/10.1186/s40359-023-01224-0

Li, J., Imam, S. Z., Jing, Z., Wang, Y., & Zhou, C. (2021). Suicide attempt and its associated factors amongst women who were pregnant as adolescents in Bangladesh: A cross-sectional study. *Reproductive Health, 18*(1), 71. https://doi.org/10.1186/s12978-021-01127-6

Mahbub, F., & Rahman, Z. (2023). The rationale for initiation and continuation of drug abuse among female users: A study of the youth in Dhaka City. *Social Science Review, 40*(1), 21–39. https://doi.org/10.3329/ssr.v40i1.69071

Mahmood, N., Kamruzzaman, M., Rahman, A., Reidpath, D. D., & Akhter, S. (2022). Impact of the COVID-19 lockdown on intimate partner violence: Issues of non-reporting in Bangladesh. *Women's Health (London, England), 18*, 17455057221087888. https://doi.org/10.1177/17455057221087888

Nasreen, H. E., Kabir, Z. N., Forsell, Y., & Edhborg, M. (2011). Prevalence and associated factors of depressive and anxiety symptoms during pregnancy: A population based study in rural Bangladesh. *BMC Women's Health, 11*, 22. https://doi.org/10.1186/1472-6874-11-22

Nishat, J. F., Khan, U. S., Shovo, T., Ahammed, B., Rahman, M. M., & Hossain, M. T. (2023). Patterns, prevalence and risk factors of intimate partner violence and its association with mental health status during COVID-19: A cross-sectional study on early married female adolescents in Khulna district, Bangladesh. *BMJ Open, 13*(11), e072279. https://doi.org/10.1136/bmjopen-2023-072279

Parveen, S., Akteruzzaman, M., Maruf, M. M., Akhter, S., & Tarannum, S. (2015). Factors of psychiatric morbidity during perinatal period. *Bangladesh Journal of Psychiatry, 29*(2), 53–58. https://doi.org/10.3329/bjpsy.v29i2.37850

Rahman, A., Patel, V., Maselko, J., & Kirkwood, B. (2008). The neglected 'm' in MCH programmes – Why mental health of mothers is important for child nutrition. *Tropical Medicine & International Health, 13*(4), 579–583. https://doi.org/10.1111/j.1365-3156.2008.02036.x

Rahman, S., Salehin, F., & Iqbal, A. (2011). Menopausal symptoms assessment among middle age women in Kushtia, Bangladesh. *BMC Research Notes, 4*, 188. https://doi.org/10.1186/1756-0500-4-188

Rahman, M. M., Ahsan, M. A., Monalisa, N. N., & Rahman, K. (2014). Influence of socioeconomic status and BMI on the quality of life after mastectomy in Bangladeshi breast cancer patients in a public hospital. *Japanese Journal of Clinical Oncology, 44*(12), 1150–1157. https://doi.org/10.1093/jjco/hyu144

Rashid Soron, T., Ashiq, M. A. R., Al-Hakeem, M., Chowdhury, Z. F., Uddin Ahmed, H., & Afrooz Chowdhury, C. (2021). Domestic violence and mental health during the COVID-19 pandemic in Bangladesh. *JMIR Formative Research, 5*(9), e24624. https://doi.org/10.2196/24624

Roy, P., Roy, S., Dey, G. S., & Das, M. (2015). Psychiatric disorders following hysterectomy. *Bangladesh Journal of Psychiatry, 29*(2), 44–47.

Saha, A. K., Saifuddin, K., Fatema-Tu-Zohra Binte Zaman, N., & Nisha, J. (2015). Mental health status of infertile women in Bangladesh. *Universal Journal of Psychology, 3*(2), 51–54.

Sharmin, K. N., Sarwar, N., Mumu, S. J., Taleb, D. A., & Flora, M. S. (2019). Postnatal depression and infant growth in an urban area of Bangladesh. *Midwifery, 74*, 57–67. https://doi.org/10.1016/j.midw.2019.03.014

Shaun, M. M. A., Nizum, M. W. R., Shuvo, M. A., Fayeza, F., Faruk, M. O., Alam, M. F., Ahmed, M. S., Zaman, S., Mali, S. K., & Hawlader, M. D. H. (2022). Association between depressive symptoms and poor sleep quality among pregnant women in Northern Rural Bangladesh: A community-based cross-sectional study. *BMC Psychiatry, 22*(1), 201. https://doi.org/10.1186/s12888-022-03839-w

Tasnim, S., Haque, M. A., & Nazmeen, S. (2016). Experience of menopause and menopausal transition among middle aged women attending a Periurban Hospital. *Bangladesh Journal of Obstetrics &; Gynaecology, 31*(1), 10–15. https://doi.org/10.3329/bjog.v31i1.34270

Tasnim, F., Rahman, M., Islam, M. M., & Rahman, M. M. (2021a). Association of pregnancy intention with postpartum depression within six months postpartum among women in Bangladesh. *Asian Journal of Psychiatry, 61*, 102686. https://doi.org/10.1016/j.ajp.2021.102686

Tasnim, F., Rahman, M., Islam, M. M., Hasan, M., Mostofa, M. G., & Rahman, M. M. (2021b). Exposure to domestic violence and the risk of developing depression within 6 months postpartum in Bangladesh. *Social Psychiatry and Psychiatric Epidemiology, 56*(7), 1189–1200. https://doi.org/10.1007/s00127-020-01998-3

Tasnim, F., Abedin, S., & Rahman, M. M. (2023). Mediating role of perceived stress on the association between domestic violence and postpartum depression: Cross-sectional study in Bangladesh. *BJPsych Open, 9*(1), e16. https://doi.org/10.1192/bjo.2022.633

Tran, L. M., Nguyen, P. H., Naved, R. T., & Menon, P. (2020). Intimate partner violence is associated with poorer maternal mental health and breastfeeding practices in Bangladesh. *Health Policy and Planning, 35*(Supplement_1), i19–i29. https://doi.org/10.1093/heapol/czaa106

Valdes, V., Berens, A. E., & Nelson, C. A., 3rd. (2021). Socioeconomic and psychological correlates of postpartum depression at 6 months in Dhaka, Bangladesh. *International Journal of Psychology, 56*(5), 729–738. https://doi.org/10.1002/ijop.12735

Williams, A., Sarker, M., & Ferdous, S. T. (2018). Cultural Attitudes toward Postpartum Depression in Dhaka, Bangladesh. *Medical Anthropology, 37*(3), 194–205. https://doi.org/10.1080/01459740.2017.1318875

World Bank. (2024). *World Bank Country and Lending Groups*. https://datahelpdesk.worldbank.org/knowledgebase/articles/906519-world-bank-country-and-lending-groups (accessed on 02 December, 2024).

Yesmin, S., Muhammad, F., Haque, M. I., & Chowdhury, A. A. (2023). Prevalence of postnatal depression among fathers of newborn babies in Bangladesh. *OIRT Journal of Scientific Research, 3*(1), 7–11.

Ziaei, S., Frith, A. L., Ekström, E. C., & Naved, R. T. (2016). Experiencing lifetime domestic violence: Associations with mental health and stress among pregnant women in rural Bangladesh: The MINIMat randomized trial. *PLoS One, 11*(12), e0168103. https://doi.org/10.1371/journal.pone.0168103

Chapter 4
Women's Reproductive Mental Health in Bhutan

Bushra Zahoor and M. S. Bhatia

1 Introduction

Bhutan, a small, landlocked country in South Asia, is renowned for its unique philosophy of Gross National Happiness (GNH), which prioritizes well-being over material growth. With a population of approximately 800,000, Bhutan's demographic profile reflects a youthful nation, with a significant proportion of individuals in the reproductive age group. Women in the reproductive period (15–49 years) constitute a substantial share of the population, emphasizing the importance of addressing their mental health needs, particularly in the context of reproductive psychiatry. The proportion of Bhutan's population considered to be in the reproductive period (typically defined as women aged 15–49) is relatively high, with recent estimates suggesting a total fertility rate around 1.75 children per woman, indicating a significant portion of the population is within reproductive years; however, this rate has been steadily declining in recent years. The current total fertility rate in Bhutan is around 1.75, which is considered near replacement level. Bhutan has seen a significant drop in fertility rates over the past few decades, with the number of children per woman decreasing considerably (World Fertility, 2024).

B. Zahoor (✉) · M. S. Bhatia
Psychiatry Department, Hamdard Institute of Medical Sciences and Research, Delhi, India

P. Kukreti et al. (eds.), *Women's Reproductive Mental Health in South Asia*, South Asian Perspectives in Mental Health and Psychology,
https://doi.org/10.1007/978-981-96-9219-4_5

2 Epidemiology and Burden of Mental Disorders During the Perinatal Period

Perinatal mental health issues, including depression, anxiety, and postpartum psychosis, are prevalent among women in Bhutan, as they are globally. However, the specific epidemiological data for Bhutan is limited, with much of the understanding drawn from regional and global trends. Factors such as limited access to mental health services, cultural stigmas, and the societal expectations surrounding motherhood contribute to the underreporting and underdiagnosis of these conditions. This highlights the pressing need for targeted interventions and research in this area.

A study was conducted to assess the prevalence of postpartum depression (PPD) among Bhutanese mothers and its associated factors. Conducted in Bhutan's largest hospital, the study found a PPD prevalence of 14.97%, which aligns with regional averages but highlights significant mental health concerns. Risk factors included negative body image perception, with women experiencing this being four times more likely to develop PPD, as well as increased stress levels after delivery, which also nearly quadrupled the risk. Poor relationships with in-laws doubled the risk, aligning with findings in other Asian countries, and negative birth experiences more than doubled the risk. Protective factors against PPD were found to be higher family income, which inversely correlated with risk, and advancing gestational age, as preterm births were linked with higher PPD risk. Other observations revealed that while a history of mental health issues, insufficient antenatal care, and delivery complications showed significance in univariable analyses, they did not after adjustment. The study acknowledged limitations such as the exclusion of biological factors, non-verification of translated tools, and a cross-sectional design (Zangmo et al., 2024).

3 Psychological Effects

3.1 Contraception Use

In Bhutan, a significant 64% of sexually active young women aged 10–24 utilize modern contraceptives, with usage varying by marital status, education level, and region. Injections are the most popular method, followed by oral pills and condoms (National Health Promotion Strategic Plan, 2015–2023). Factors influencing contraceptive use include positive influences such as higher education for women, greater decision-making power in healthcare, and having children, while higher education for husbands and being divorced/widowed act as negative factors. Marital status, women's education, and their healthcare decision-making power are the most significant determinants. Cultural influences, including Hindu and Buddhist beliefs, impact acceptance and specific method preferences, with both generally accepting contraception but emphasizing marital sex and potentially discouraging premarital use of certain methods (Poudel & Dyer, 2013).

3.2 *Medical Termination of Pregnancy (MTP)*

Although medical termination of pregnancy (MTP) is legally permitted in Bhutan under specific circumstances, societal stigma and cultural norms contribute to significant psychological distress for women undergoing the procedure. Many experience feelings of guilt, shame, and isolation, highlighting the need for compassionate and non-judgmental mental health support. In Bhutan, abortion is legal only in cases of rape, incest, to protect the woman's mental health, or to save her life (Penal Code of Bhutan, 2004). However, the exact status of the country's abortion law remains uncertain. According to a United Nations report, "Because the state religion of Bhutan is Buddhism, which disapproves of abortion, it is probable that the procedure is allowed only to save the life of the pregnant woman."

The debate surrounding abortion laws in Bhutan has intensified following reports of several women losing their lives due to unsafe procedures abroad. While the current law allows abortion only in limited circumstances, the reality is that many women—particularly those from economically disadvantaged backgrounds—are resorting to unsafe abortions across the border in India.

The debate over abortion legalization in Bhutan presents strong arguments on both sides. Pro-legalization advocates emphasize women's rights, arguing that women should have the freedom to choose and that illegal abortions lead to unsafe practices and maternal deaths. They also highlight the benefits of addressing unwanted pregnancies through legalization, which would allow for safer procedures, reduce unsafe abortions, and improve data collection for targeted interventions. Conversely, opponents raise ethical and moral concerns, asserting that abortion is morally wrong and that legalizing it would violate the sanctity of life. They also worry about the potential misuse of abortion and the ethical implications of terminating a developing fetus. Instead of legalization, they advocate for prevention-focused solutions such as education, family planning, and addressing the root causes of unwanted pregnancies. Expert opinions remain divided, with some medical professionals supporting legalization to ensure safe procedures and access to medical abortion, while lawmakers hold conflicting views, with some advocating for women's rights and others opposing legalization on ethical and moral grounds. The discussion is further complicated by challenges such as a lack of reliable data on abortion cases, which hinders effective policymaking, and unequal access to quality healthcare, particularly for marginalized women (Oberman & Lehmann, 2023).

Medical termination of pregnancy can have psychological effects, including depression, anxiety, and post-abortion stress. These effects may be more pronounced in women with a history of psychiatric disorders or limited social support. Common psychological symptoms include depression, anxiety, guilt, self-blame, fear of pregnancy, fear of sexual intercourse, nightmares, and, in some cases, suicidal thoughts. Risk factors for experiencing negative psychological outcomes after an abortion include a history of psychiatric disorders, poor social support, and belonging to religious or social groups that do not condone abortion (Reardon, 2018).

3.3 Hysterectomy and Mastectomy

Hysterectomy and mastectomy, often performed for medical reasons, can have profound psychological effects. Women may experience grief, a sense of loss, or diminished self-esteem, particularly in cultures where femininity and motherhood are closely tied to reproductive organs. In Bhutan, the lack of post-surgical psychological support exacerbates these challenges. The study examines the psychological and relational impact of hysterectomy and mastectomy on women, particularly regarding depression, body image, sexual problems, and spouse relationships. Cancer, as a chronic disease, affects not only physical health but also mental well-being, self-perception, and intimate relationships. Women undergoing mastectomy experience higher levels of depression, while hysterectomy patients face greater challenges with sexual function and spouse communication (Keskin & Gumus, 2011). The research, conducted among 94 women receiving cancer treatment, used various standardized scales to assess these impacts. Mastectomy patients reported worse depression scores, while hysterectomy patients showed more issues related to vaginismus, avoidance of sexual intercourse, and communication with their partners. The study underscores the importance of psychological support for cancer patients, as body image disturbances and sexual dysfunction significantly affect emotional well-being and marital relationships (Keskin & Gumus, 2011). Overall, the study highlights the need for holistic care that addresses both the physical and emotional challenges faced by women undergoing these surgeries.

3.4 Domestic Violence

A study on Violence Against Women and Girls (VAW/G) in Bhutan reveals that a quarter of women and girls experience physical or sexual violence, with partner violence affecting 44.6% of women in their lifetime. Controlling behaviors and emotional abuse are most common, and alcohol, jealousy, and affairs are primary triggers. Violence negatively impacts women's health and children, with many children witnessing the violence. A significant portion of victims don't report the abuse. The study recommends a costed national action plan, a stronger legal framework (including raising the marriage age and reviewing punishments for psychological violence), public consultations, and awareness campaigns. It also emphasizes improving services for victims (shelters, counseling, legal aid), building the capacity of service providers, and developing standard procedures. Further research is recommended on risk factors, sexual abuse in the workplace, traditional gender attitudes, and the economic cost of VAW/G. Finally, the study suggests reviewing data collection methods and ensuring regular studies on VAW/G (Choden et al., 2021).

3.5 *Substance Abuse and Suicidal Behaviors During the Reproductive Period*

A study conducted in Bhutan found a relatively low prevalence of drug use among teenagers and young adults compared to other Southeast Asian countries (Wangdi & Jamtsho, 2019). However, the study identified several significant risk factors, including male gender, younger age (18–24 years), single marital status, higher education levels, blue-collar occupations, feelings of loneliness, and prior alcohol and tobacco use. Notably, higher education, which is often associated with reduced drug use in other contexts, was linked to increased drug use in this study, potentially due to increased exposure through media. The study highlights the need for comprehensive drug prevention programs that address these risk factors, particularly among young people, and emphasizes the importance of integrated approaches that combine drug prevention with alcohol and tobacco prevention efforts (Wangdi & Jamtsho, 2019).

A study investigated the prevalence and risk factors of self-reported suicidal behavior among adolescents in Bhutan using data from the 2016 Global School-based Student Health Survey (GSHS). A concerningly high proportion of adolescents reported suicidal ideation (11.6%) and suicide attempts (11.3%). Key risk factors included female gender, bullying, sexual violence, physical attack, loneliness, food insecurity, lack of sleep, substance abuse, and parental smoking. Protective factors included having three or more close friends and high parental engagement. The findings highlight the urgent need for comprehensive suicide prevention strategies in Bhutan, including school-based programs to address bullying and promote mental health, interventions to enhance family support, and efforts to reduce substance abuse and address social determinants of health. These findings underscore the critical need to prioritize the mental well-being of young people in Bhutan (Dema et al., 2019).

Alcohol use disorder (AUD) is a significant problem in Bhutan, despite alcohol being culturally accepted (Wangchuk, 2018). Per capita alcohol consumption is much higher than the global average, and alcohol liver disease is the leading cause of death in the country, though recent numbers show a slight decrease. While drug abuse is less prevalent than in other countries, there's a concerning trend of youth experimenting with volatile substances and then progressing to cannabis and pharmaceutical products. This is particularly alarming given that over 60% of Bhutan's population is under 25 (Ministry of Health, 2023). Bhutan has implemented policies like the National Policy and Strategic Framework to Reduce Harmful Use of Alcohol (2015–2020) and established the Bhutan Narcotic Control Authority (formerly

Agency) to address substance abuse, primarily through the Narcotic Drugs Psychotropic Substances and Substance Abuse Act (revised in 2015 and amended in 2018).

A study that investigated risk factors associated with suicidal ideation and suicide attempts in Bhutan. It used data from the Bhutan STEPS 2014 Survey (Dendup et al., 2020). The key findings were that the prevalence of suicidal ideation and suicide attempt was 3.1% and 0.7%, respectively. The female gender, being unemployed, low and middle household income compared to high household income, and having a family history of suicide were associated with higher odds of having suicidal ideation. Younger age and alcohol consumption were associated with both suicidal ideation and suicide attempts.

4 Current Status of Services

Mental health services in Bhutan are gradually expanding but remain limited in scope and accessibility. The country has a small number of trained psychiatrists and psychologists, with services concentrated in urban centers. Rural areas face significant barriers to accessing mental health care, including geographical isolation and lack of awareness. The establishment of a mental health program in 1997 marked a turning point in psychiatric care in Bhutan (Dorji, 2023). In 2004, an eight-bed psychiatry ward was introduced, transitioning psychiatric care from general medicine wards to a specialized unit. Previously, treating psychiatric clients in general wards posed challenges to patient safety, confidentiality, and privacy, creating discomfort for both patients and healthcare providers. Over time, the psychiatry ward expanded its capacity, increasing to 18 beds in 2012 and 20 beds in 2018 (Dorji, 2023). The Department of Psychiatry at the JDW National Referral Hospital remains Bhutan's only specialized psychiatric unit, spearheading mental health services in the country.

To broaden access to care, mental health services were gradually extended to district hospitals and primary healthcare centers (PHCs) by training general doctors, nurses, and other health professionals. By 2006, the WHO-Assessment Instrument for Mental Health System (WHO-AIMS) reported mental health services were available in 63 outpatient facilities with a total of 100 beds (Tsheten et al., 2023) (WHO and Ministry of Health, 2007). Comprehensive training programs equipped healthcare workers in PHCs to manage psychiatric cases effectively. These centers are now well stocked with psychotropic medications, including antipsychotics, antidepressants, mood stabilizers, antiepileptics, and benzodiazepines, alongside injectable options like chlorpromazine, haloperidol, phenytoin, and diazepam. PHCs and district hospitals also offer pharmacotherapy and counseling services.

Mental health services were further integrated into schools through the deployment of full-time counselors. Civil Society Organizations (CSOs) like RENEW and Nazhoen Lamtoen complement these efforts by providing counseling and psychosocial support. Colleges and CSOs collaborate with the National Mental Health

Table 4.1 Mental health professionals in the Psychiatry Department, Jigme Dorji Wangchuck National Referral Hospital, Bhutan, 2023

Designation	Numbers in total	Regular/Contract
Psychiatrist	4	2/2
Clinical counselor	4	4/0
Clinical nurse	3	1/2
General nursing and midwifery	6	6/0
Occupational therapist	2	2/0
Speech and language pathologist	2	1/1
Health assistant	1	1/0
Peer counselor	4	0/4
Pharmacy technician	1	1/0

Program, managing mental health issues within their institutions (Thimphu, Bhutan: The PEMA, 2023). Additionally, dedicated CSOs focus on rehabilitation, awareness campaigns, and psychosocial support.

A multisectoral approach involving education, health, and CSOs underscores Bhutan's mental health strategy. Recognizing the need for centralized coordination, the PEMA agency was established as the nodal body for mental health. PEMA oversees the planning, implementation, and monitoring of mental health policies and services. A 60-bed hospital, the PEMA Center, is set to become the apex referral, research, and training facility for mental health in the country.

The Department of Psychiatry comprises a multidisciplinary team (Table 4.1) and offers a range of inpatient and outpatient services, including psychiatric consultations, psychotherapy, speech and occupational therapy, and pharmacotherapy (Dorji, 2023). Besides clinical services, it also serves as a consultation and supervising team for the mental health professionals across the country. It also provides training to the resident doctors, medical interns, clinical counselors, and nursing students.

5 Liaison Between Maternal and Mental Health Service Providers

The integration of maternal and mental health services is essential for holistic care. In Bhutan, collaboration between obstetricians, gynecologists, and mental health professionals is nascent. Strengthening this liaison can ensure early identification and management of mental health issues in women (Dorji, 2023).

6 Service Utilization Patterns

Service utilization for reproductive mental health in Bhutan is low, primarily due to stigma, lack of awareness, and limited availability of services. Women often turn to traditional healers or spiritual practices before seeking medical help, reflecting the cultural context of health-seeking behavior (Pradhan & Lhamo, 2023).

7 Country-Specific Challenges

Bhutan's unique challenges include its rugged terrain, which limits access to healthcare, and deeply rooted cultural beliefs that influence perceptions of mental health. Additionally, the shortage of mental health professionals and resources hinders the delivery of comprehensive care.

In Bhutan, mental health is often narrowly associated with clinical depression, limiting public understanding and perpetuating stereotypes. For instance, during the 2021 World Suicide Prevention Day at Sherubtse College, posters depicted victims as primarily female and emphasized seeking counseling, reinforcing stereotypical narratives (Pradhan & Lhamo, 2023). Such representations overlook broader mental health challenges like stress and anxiety.

Cultural stigma further compounds the issue. Mental health is frequently misunderstood as a weakness, deterring individuals from seeking help. Many Bhutanese grow up being told to suppress emotions, contributing to a lack of openness about mental health (Pradhan & Lhamo, 2023).

8 Country-Specific Programs and Policies

Bhutan has made strides in addressing mental health through its National Mental Health Program and integration of mental health into primary healthcare. However, specific programs targeting women's reproductive psychiatry remain underdeveloped. Efforts to align policies with the principles of GNH can create opportunities for innovative interventions.

Bhutan's relatively late entry into modern development has allowed the nation to learn from the experiences and challenges faced by other countries. This is evident in its mental health policies, which prioritize community-based mental health services over large institutional facilities. The approach involves training Primary health care (PHC) workers in basic psychiatric skills and providing essential medications. However, effective implementation remains a challenge due to inadequate monitoring and the preference of health workers to focus on more straightforward health issues.

Although Bhutan lacks a dedicated mental health law, elements of mental health rights and legal provisions are addressed in the Bhutan Penal Code. For instance, individuals with mental disorders who commit crimes can be provided medical treatment instead of incarceration. The absence of specific mental health laws offers flexibility in treatment approaches, especially given the widespread belief in supernatural causes of mental illness. However, this also means patients with severe mental disorders, such as psychosis or bipolar disorder, might not receive necessary care without mandatory legal provisions.

The Bhutan Health Bill, awaiting parliamentary approval, includes several aspects of patient rights and responsibilities. Meanwhile, the Narcotic and Psychotropic Drugs Abuse Act, originally enacted in 2013, has undergone revisions to make it less punitive and more therapeutic. Additionally, a high-level mental health multisectoral steering committee, formed under Her Majesty the Gyaltsuen's secretariat, is working to streamline mental health interventions across relevant agencies (Dorji, 2023).

Bhutan has made significant progress in mental health services since the establishment of the National Mental Health Programme in 1997. This program operates through the district administrative mechanism, delivering services via district hospitals and PHC networks. PHCs are equipped with a variety of psychotropic medications, including antipsychotics, antidepressants, mood stabilizers, anti-epileptics, and other essential drugs.

Despite clear national policy guidelines for integrating mental health services with PHC, service delivery has not met expectations due to resource constraints and limited monitoring. The journey toward specialized mental health care began in 1999 with the first Bhutanese psychiatrist's return after completing training abroad. Subsequent years saw the establishment of a psychiatric ward, the training of more psychiatric professionals, and the introduction of advanced treatments like electroconvulsive therapy in 2012.

By 2019, significant milestones included the consolidation of psychiatry services into a full-fledged department at the Jigme Dorji Wangchuck National Referral Hospital (JDWNRH), the launch of postgraduate psychiatry training, and the graduation of the first batch of clinical counselors (Dorji, 2023). The COVID-19 pandemic further spurred innovation, with online consultations, training, and outreach services becoming critical components of mental health care.

Today, Bhutan's psychiatry department offers comprehensive services, including psychotropic medication, counseling, meditation, yoga, and rehabilitation for both adults and children. The inclusion of traditional medicine practitioners (sowa rigpa) adds a unique dimension to these services.

9 Current Challenges in Reproductive Mental Health and Ways Out

9.1 Geographical Barriers to Access

Bhutan's healthcare system is organized into three tiers: Primary health centers (PHCs) at the grassroots level, district hospitals at the secondary level, and referral hospitals at the tertiary level. The country has 179 PHCs, 49 general and district hospitals, and 3 referral hospitals. The Psychiatry Unit at the JDW National Referral Hospital, located in Thimphu in the western region, provides specialized mental health services (Ministry of Health, 2023). However, the absence of such services at the regional referral hospitals in the eastern and central parts of Bhutan significantly hampers the efficient provision of mental health care that requires specialized expertise. While clinical counselors (psychotherapists) offer psychotherapy services at one referral hospital and seven district hospitals, there are only 16 clinical counselors distributed across various districts and organizations as of 2023. These counselors assess patients with mental health concerns and deliver counseling and psychotherapy. At the primary care level, general doctors and health assistants also provide mental health services.

Clients from remote areas requiring psychiatric consultations and specialized care must travel long distances, often more than 500 km by bus or private car. Some opt for domestic flights, though they are a minority. Due to the high costs associated with such travel, many individuals only seek help in critical situations, limiting access to mental health services for certain populations. Additionally, patients residing far from a clinical counsellor face difficulties in accessing psychotherapy services, making follow-up care a significant challenge.

9.2 Shortage of Human Resources

The Psychiatry Department at JDW National Referral Hospital is understaffed, lacking psychologists, social workers, and professionals with specialized expertise. In addition to one child and adolescent psychiatrist, the hospital does not have psychiatrists, clinical counselors, nurses, or other mental health professionals with subspecialties. Similarly, no mental health professionals are stationed at the central or eastern regional referral hospitals, district hospitals, or PHCs, with the exception of the clinical counselors located in fewer than half of the districts. These counselors are concentrated primarily in the southern and western parts of the country. As of 2023, there are only 160 school counselors serving over 500 schools, which is far below the recommended ratio of one counselor per 400 students. In many schools, a single counselor is responsible for more than 500 students (Katel, 2023).

9.3 Cultural Beliefs and Stigma Surrounding Mental Illness

In Bhutan, traditional beliefs strongly influence public attitudes toward mental illness, creating barriers to accessing mental health care (Nirola et al., 2015). Mental illness is often attributed to karma, spirits, or disruptions to local deities, leading to widespread myths that associate mental illness with personal weakness or a lack of willpower (Nirola et al., 2015). These misconceptions prevent many from seeking help, as they internalize the causes and triggers of mental health conditions (Pradhan & Lhamo, 2023). As a result, a significant portion of the population resorts to religious or traditional forms of treatment. The roles of family dynamics and parenting in mental health are under-researched, further complicating the understanding of psychiatric disorders. Due to low mental health literacy and cultural beliefs, mental illnesses are often stigmatized, with individuals being labeled as "mad" or referred to with derogatory terms like "psycho" or "choelo" (Nirola et al., 2015). This stigma results in marginalization and neglect, creating further barriers to seeking professional assistance.

9.4 Limited Funding for Mental Health

While inadequate funding for mental health is a global issue, it is particularly prevalent in low- and middle-income countries. These countries allocate only 0.5% to 1.9% of their health budgets to the treatment and prevention of mental illness. Bhutan is no exception, with the annual budget for mental health remaining under Nu 3.5 million (approximately US $42,000) over the past five years. This constitutes just 1% of the Ministry of Health's budget, and the allocation has remained unchanged despite growing mental health needs (Tsheten et al., 2023). The World Health Organization recommends that at least 5% of a country's health budget be dedicated to mental health.

10 Way Forward

10.1 Enhancing Human Resources

Expanding the mental health workforce to include psychologists, social workers, and psychiatric nurses is crucial for comprehensive care. Additionally, efforts should focus on increasing the number of mental health professionals beyond the psychiatric unit of the national hospital (Gyeltshen et al., 2024).

Existing policies aim to train primary healthcare providers in mental health, but implementation must be expedited, including clinical supervision and service monitoring (Dorji, 2023). School counselors play a pivotal role in student mental health, yet their numbers fall short of recommended levels (Katel, 2023). Authorities must address this gap by improving both the quality and availability of counselors (Katel, 2023). Regular stakeholder meetings, supervision, and service evaluations are essential for maintaining quality.

10.2 Strengthening Community Mental Health (CMH) Services

Community Mental Health (CMH), as defined by the WHO, involves providing mental health services outside hospital settings. Bhutan initiated CMH services following the formulation of its mental health policy, establishing 63 community-based psychiatric inpatient units nationwide (WHO and Ministry of Health, 2007). Organizations like RENEW, the National Commission for Women and Children, and Nazhoen Lamtoen, alongside the Ministry of Health (MoH), have driven public education and awareness efforts. Links have been established with primary healthcare, child and adolescent health, substance abuse programs, and other sectors.

To strengthen CMH, agencies must supervise and monitor services at primary healthcare centers (PHCs). The PEMA Secretariat should oversee mental health, suicide, and drug prevention programs at the district and PHC levels. Improved coordination among sectors, including health, education, and civil society organizations (CSOs), is necessary. Initiatives like annual mental health screenings through campaigns should be considered to complement ongoing mental health promotion activities.

10.3 Increasing Mental Health Literacy

Improving mental health literacy can reduce stigma and encourage help-seeking behavior. Advocacy programs in schools, institutions, and national media platforms are vital. Educating students about the science of mental health and its connection to physical health—such as the impact of trauma on the brain—can foster emotional resilience and mental well-being. This approach can normalize mental health conversations, reduce stigma, and promote seeking support when needed (Pradhan & Lhamo, 2023).

10.4 Advancing Mental Health Research

There is a significant lack of scientific studies on mental health in Bhutan. Research is essential to understand the national mental health landscape, create context-specific policies, and streamline interventions (Tsheten et al., 2023). Evidence-based approaches will enhance resource allocation, improve health outcomes, and elevate the quality of life for individuals facing mental health challenges. Stakeholders must collaborate to produce data-driven insights that guide targeted interventions and optimize resource utilization (Dorji, 2023).

10.5 Increasing Funding for Mental Health

Globally, mental health funding is insufficient (WHO, 2021), with countries allocating less than 2% of healthcare budgets on average. Bhutan has dedicated only 1% of its health budget to mental health over the past two decades (Tsheten et al., 2023), despite WHO's recommendation of at least 5%. International donors such as UNICEF, WHO, and Health Volunteers Overseas have supported Bhutan's mental health initiatives. To enhance mental health services, partnerships and funding at both domestic and global levels should be fostered (Pradhan & Lhamo, 2023). Increased budget allocation is needed for program implementation, capacity building, infrastructure development, and preventive initiatives.

10.6 Reducing Stigma Associated with Mental Illness

Addressing the stigma surrounding mental illness requires collaborative efforts across sectors (Tsheten et al., 2023). Public education campaigns through social media, national television, arts, and advocacy programs can promote positive perceptions of mental health. Incorporating mental health education into school curricula and integrating mental health services into other medical departments, such as emergency care and oncology, can help normalize mental health treatment and reduce stigma (Pradhan & Lhamo, 2023).

11 Conclusion

To address the problems related to reproductive psychiatry in Bhutan, targeted interventions are needed for high-risk groups, emphasizing multidisciplinary approaches, early screening, and robust protocols. These findings lay the groundwork for future research and maternal health initiatives in Bhutan.

References

Choden, P., Sendall, M. C., & Armstrong, K. (2021). Barriers to help-seeking from intimate partner violence among Bhutanese Women. *Partner Abuse, 12*(4). https://doi.org/10.1891/PA-2020-0034

Dema, T., Tripathy, J. P., Thinley, S., Rani, M., Dhendup, T., Laxmeshwar, C., et al. (2019). Suicidal ideation and attempt among school going adolescents in Bhutan — a secondary analysis of a global school-based student health survey in Bhutan 2016. *BMC Public Health, 19*, 1–12. https://doi.org/10.1186/s12889-019-7791-0

Dendup, T., Zhao, Y., Dorji, T., & Phuntsho, S. (2020). Risk factors associated with suicidal ideation and suicide attempts in Bhutan: An analysis of the 2014 Bhutan STEPS Survey data. *PLoS One, 15*(1), e0225888. https://doi.org/10.1371/journal.pone.0225888

Dorji, C. (2023). Addressing Mental Health in Bhutan. *The Druk Journal, 9*(1), 4–14. https://drukjournal.bt/wp-content/uploads/2023/04/Dr-Chencho-Dorji.pdf.Google Scholar

Gyeltshen, K., Chhetri, B., & Gyeltshen, D. (2024). Delivery of mental health services in Bhutan: Challenges and way forward. *Public Health Challenges, 3*(3), e211. https://doi.org/10.1002/puh2.211

Katel, N. (2023). Addressing Shortage of Counsellors in Schools. *The Bhutanese*. Accessed July 1, 2023, https://thebhutanese.bt/addressing-shortage-of-counsellors-in-schools/

Keskin, G., & Gumus, A. B. (2011). Turkish hysterectomy and mastectomy patients-depression, body image, sexual problems and spouse relationships. *Asian Pacific Journal of Cancer Prevention, 12*(2), 425–432.

Ministry of Health, *Annual Health Bulletin, Thimphu; PPD, MoH.* (Ministry of Health, 2023), https://www.moh.gov.bt/wp-content/uploads/Annual-Health-Bulleti-2023.pdf.Google Scholar

National Health Promotion Strategic Plan. (2015–2023). Ministry of Health. Royal Government of Bhutan. https://www.aidsdatahub.org/sites/default/files/publication/Bhutan_National_Health_Promotion_Strategic_Plan_2015-2023_2016.pdf

Nirola, D. K., Durham, J. C., & Kraus, K. L. (2015). Balancing traditional beliefs and medical science: Mental health care in Bhutan. *Bhutan Health Journal, 1*(1), 66–69. https://doi.org/10.47811/bhj.10

Oberman, M., & Lehmann, L. S. (2023). Doctors' duty to provide abortion infor mation. *Journal of Law and the Biosciences, 10*(2), lsad024. https://doi.org/10.1093/jlb/lsad024

Penal Code of Bhutan. (2004). https://abortion-policies.srhr.org/documents/countries/01-Bhutan-PENAL-CODE-2004.pdf

Poudel, B., & Dyer, J. M. (2013). Contraceptive needs and preferences of Bhutanese women refugees. *Journal of Midwifery & Women's Health, 58*(5), 585–585. https://doi.org/10.1111/jmwh.12120

Pradhan, S., & Lhamo, U. S. (2023). Global crisis, national commitment: Overcoming challenges to inclusive mental health in Bhutan. *The Druk Journal, 9*(1), 71–76. https://drukjournal.bt/wp-content/uploads/2023/07/Global-Crisis-National-Commitment.pdf.Google Scholar

Reardon, D. C. (2018). The abortion and mental health controversy: A comprehensive literature review of common ground agreements, disagreements, actionable recommendations, and research opportunities. *SAGE Open Medicine, 6*, 2050312118807624. https://doi.org/10.1177/2050312118807624

The PEMA Secretariate, *The Institution of "The PEMA" for Mental Health Care for Bhutan* (Thimphu, Bhutan: The PEMA, 2023), http://drukjournal.bt/wp-content/uploads/2023/05/The-Pema-Secretariat.pdf.Google Scholar

Tsheten, T., Chateau, D., Dorji, N., Pokhrel, H. P., Clements, A. C., Gray, D. J., & Wangdi, K. (2023). Impact of COVID-19 on mental health in Bhutan: A way forward for action. *The Lancet Regional Health-Southeast Asia, 11*. https://doi.org/10.1016/j.lansea.2023.100179

Wangchuk, P. (2018). Burden of alcoholic liver disease: Bhutan Scenario. *Euroasian Journal of Hepato-gastroenterology, 8*(1), 81–82. https://doi.org/10.5005/jp-journals-10018-1267

Wangdi, K., & Jamtsho, T. (2019). Drug use among teenagers and young adults in Bhutan. *Indian Journal of Psychological Medicine, 41*(6), 535–540. https://doi.org/10.4103/IJPSYM.IJPSYM_348_19

World Fertility. (2024). United Nations. https://www.un.org/development/desa/pd/sites/www.un.org.development.desa.pd/files/undesa_pd_2025_wfr_2024_final.pdf

World Health Organization. WHO-AIMS report on mental health system in Bhutan. In WHO-AIMS report on mental health system in Bhutan 2007. https://cdn.who.int/media/docs/default-source/mental-health/who-aims-country-reports/bhutan_who_aims_report.pdf?sfvrsn=f082a3c5_3

Zangmo, S., Boonchieng, W., Suvanayos, C., Gyeltshen, K., & Siewchaisakul, P. (2024). Prevalence and factors associated with postpartum depression among Bhutanese mothers: A cross-sectional study. *Women's Health Nursing, 30*(3), 238–249. https://doi.org/10.4069/whn.2024.09.02

Chapter 5
Women's Reproductive Mental Health in India

Rubab Lotiya, Mihika Shidore, and Sundarnag Ganjekar

1 Introduction

India, the seventh largest country in the world, has the highest population of around 1.42 billion individuals. As reported by the World Bank, females constitute approximately 48.4% of India's total population (United Nations Department of Economic and Social Affairs, Population Division (2022)). As per the Sample Registration System (SRS) statistical report 2020, Government of India, the sex ratio at birth was 907 girls for every 1000 boys born (Office of the Registrar General & Census Commissioner, India. 2020). The total fertility rate (TFR) in India is 2.0, with a higher fertility rate in rural women compared to urban. Women during their reproductive period, due to their biological and social roles around menstruation, pregnancy, childrearing practices, and challenges around reproductive activities, are disproportionately vulnerable to developing mental health disorders (Kessler, 2003). Adapting the life cycle approach, this chapter further discusses available literature on women's reproductive psychiatry in India.

2 Epidemiology of Mental Disorders in Reproductive-Age Women in India

Epidemiological studies on mental health among reproductive-age women in India were particularly looked at in certain states such as Goa and Tamil Nadu. The community-based study conducted in Tamil Nadu, Chennai, the Urban Rural

R. Lotiya · M. Shidore · S. Ganjekar (✉)
Department of Psychiatry, National Institute of Mental Health and Neuro Sciences (NIMHANS), Bengaluru, India
e-mail: sundarnag@nimhans.ac.in

P. Kukreti et al. (eds.), *Women's Reproductive Mental Health in South Asia*, South Asian Perspectives in Mental Health and Psychology,
https://doi.org/10.1007/978-981-96-9219-4_5

Epidemiology Study, has shown the prevalence of depression of around 14.8% among women between 20 and 49 years (Poongothai et al., 2009). A community study from Goa, looking at the gender disadvantage, reproductive health, and the risk of common mental disorders (CMD) among reproductive women, found the prevalence of CMDs to be 6.6%. Around 64.8% of these women had mixed anxiety and depression (Patel et al., 2006). Data set from National Family Health Survey-2, examining the married rural women in the age group of 15–39 years, found that the prevalence of CMDs was 10.7% (Shidhaye & Patel, 2010). The National Mental Health Survey (NMHS), India 2016, found that the current and lifetime prevalence of any mental health morbidity among women is 7.5% and 10.8%, respectively. The prevalence of substance use disorder among Indian women is 10.05%, with tobacco being the most common substance of abuse. Among the severe mental illnesses, schizophrenia and other psychotic disorders have a lifetime prevalence of 1.33%, and bipolar disorder 0.42% (Gautham et al., 2020). The prevalence of common mental disorders in women aged between 18 and 49 years was estimated to be around 5.83%, wherein anxiety disorders (4.31%) were most common, followed by depressive disorders (2.67%) (Annajigowda et al., 2023). The prevalence of psychotic disorders among women of reproductive age (18–49 years) in India is not extensively documented in national-level studies. However, the National Mental Health Survey has estimated the prevalence of approximately 4 per 1000 women (0.4%) (National Mental Health Survey, 2016).

3 Menstruation and Mental Health

3.1 Premenstrual Symptoms and Premenstrual Dysphoric Disorder

Menstruation is a complex biological rhythm that begins in adolescence and continues into the fourth or fifth decades of a woman's life. This natural cycle is triggered by a series of hormonal changes that influence various bodily systems, including the brain, emotions, and behavior. One of the well-known entities associated with menstrual cycles is the premenstrual syndrome (PMS), and its severe form, called premenstrual dysphoric disorder (PMDD), has found its separate position in DSM 5 and ICD 11. The pooled prevalence estimates of PMS and PMDD among Indian females were 43% (95% CI: 0.35-0.50) and 8% (95% CI: 0.06-0.10), respectively. There was a variation based on geographical factors, with Delhi showing the highest prevalence for PMS and Kerala the lowest, with PMDD being most prevalent in Puducherry and least in Chandigarh. Heterogeneity could be explained by variable genetic, dietary, familial, socioeconomic, and geographical factors and was as different as customs found in different parts of the country (Dutta & Sharma, 2021). PMDD was shown to significantly impact the quality of life, especially in the domain of social relationships and academic performance in college (Thakrar et al.,

2021). Regarding the symptoms of PMS experienced by Indian women, a study conducted among college-going students in Southern India revealed that physical symptoms such as bloating, breast tenderness, fatigue, and headaches were the most common presentation of PMS, followed by anger and irritability (Bansal et al., 2019). Another study noted pain being the most common physical symptom and feeling depressed as a psychological symptom (Mishra et al., 2015). An epidemiological study done by Chaturvedi et al., in the city of Bangalore in 1994, found that although irritability, sadness, and mood swings were common in women, some also reported a sense of well-being in the premenstrual period (Chandra et al., 1994). Self-report data from an Indian medical college collected from medical students residing in the hostel suggested that PMDD was associated with lifestyle factors like sleep, physical activity, intake of tea/coffee, and food intake under stress (Mishra et al., 2015). A study conducted among college girls analyzed the predictors of PMS and PMDD. It was found to be more common among older girls, probably owing to more academic stress and better understanding of symptoms. Heavy menstrual bleeding and dysmenorrhea showed a positive correlation with PMS and PMDD, as did the presence of a strong family history. It was found that there was poor help-seeking behavior for PMS and PMDD among Indian girls, which could be attributed to poor knowledge among the girls, their parents, and teachers (Durairaj & Ramamurthi, 2019). The menstrual and premenstrual phases are also associated with specific cravings for carbohydrate-containing, tryptophan-rich foods that are associated with a positive impact on the mood. This indicates a possibility that the serotonin deficit hypothesis in this period may hold true (Chandra, 2001).

Treatment of PMDD involves a multifaceted approach targeting both the physical and psychological symptoms that significantly impair functioning. Selective serotonin reuptake inhibitors (SSRIs) are considered the first-line pharmacological treatment, demonstrating rapid efficacy in alleviating mood-related symptoms (Bhatia & Bhatia, 2002). Hormonal interventions, such as oral contraceptives and gonadotropin-releasing hormone (GnRH) agonists, can also be effective in regulating or suppressing the menstrual cycle to reduce symptom severity (Carlini et al., 2022). Non-pharmacological strategies, including cognitive-behavioral therapy (CBT), lifestyle modifications, and stress management techniques, have also shown promise in improving coping mechanisms and quality of life (Modzelewski et al., 2024). An individualized treatment plan that combines pharmacologic and non-pharmacologic methods is often recommended to achieve optimal outcomes in managing PMDD.

3.2 Menstruation and Psychosis

An interesting phenomenon is the occurrence of catamenial (during menstrual bleeding) and premenstrual psychosis. The disorder is characterized by an acute onset of psychotic symptoms, short-lasting, with complete recovery occurring in a previously asymptomatic woman. It is further classified depending on the phase in the cycle when it occurs. It is called premenstrual psychosis if it occurs in the latter half of the cycle and ends with the onset of menstruation; catamenial psychosis if it occurs during menstruation; menstrual (variable in onset with rhythm to the menstrual cycle) and epochal menstrual psychosis in which bipolar illness shows a switch in relation to the menstrual cycle. Indian studies on menstrual psychosis are mostly in the form of case reports and case series, and data in this area is sparse (Ray & Paul, 2020). A strong association was also found between menstrual psychosis and premenstrual migraine. A prospective study done on women with menstrual psychosis revealed that future reproductive events in these women can trigger the onset of psychiatric illnesses like mania, depression, and further episodes of psychosis, indicative of vulnerability to hormonal fluctuations (Chandra, 2001). Most studies have reported estrogen to have a protective effect on the onset of schizophrenia, which may explain the cyclical worsening of psychotic symptoms. An interesting finding from a study conducted in a tertiary care center in India indicated that positive symptoms of schizophrenia showed improvement in the postmenstrual (progestogenic) phase, while negative symptoms and general psychopathology showed improvement during the estrogenic phase of the cycle (Ray et al., 2020).

3.3 Menstruation and Pre-Existing Psychiatric Disorder

Pre-existing psychiatric illnesses have also been found to worsen during the premenstrual phase of the cycle. An inverse relationship has been found between levels of estradiol and severity of psychotic symptoms, with low levels of estradiol indicating increased scores on psychopathology, abnormal ward behavior, and worsening seen in schizophrenia and other psychoses (Kulkarni, 1997). A study conducted on ward admissions among women with regular menstrual cycles, not on contraceptive pills, also showed increased rates of admission in premenstrual, late luteal, and ovulatory phases (Prema et al., 1991). A strong association has been found between the history of depression and PMDD, and it has a bidirectional relationship with stress during menstruation. Studies have implicated trans-diagnostic worsening of psychiatric illnesses in menstrual and premenstrual phases (Handy et al., 2022). A study was conducted in 2007 where 217 autopsies of completed suicides and matched controls were explored for an association between menstruation and suicide. 54.46% of people who died by suicide were menstruating as compared to 6% of controls, indicating a positive association between menstruation and suicide (Dogra et al., 2007). Bipolar disorder (BD) has also shown worsening with certain phases of the reproductive cycle, predominantly postpartum, but also during the premenstrual phase, perimenopausal phase, and menopause. There is mixed evidence on the impact of the menstrual cycle on the course of bipolar disorder, with certain studies reporting frequent premenstrual mood disturbances in these patients.

The challenging part here is the treatment of premenstrual depressive symptoms with antidepressants that can increase the risk of switch in BD patients (Parial, 2015). Pre-existing psychiatric illnesses can also impact the menstrual cycles. Stress-related irregularity of cycles, amenorrhea secondary to anorexia, the effect of physical exercise and negative impact of substance use on reproductive and sexual health are commonplace.

3.4 *Menstruation and Indian Cultural Belief*

In the Indian context, cultural beliefs and social customs significantly contribute to the experience of menstruation. In some Indian societies, women face various restrictions in the form of not entering the kitchen or veneration rooms and not touching or being touched by other members in the family, leading to a sense of discrimination (Singh Malik et al., 2023). Myths around menstruation in India lead to the uniqueness of the experience for Indian women. Beliefs around the origin of menstruation are embedded in concepts of guilt, sin, punishment, and emanation of bad rays, rendering menstruation an "impure" phenomenon. In some parts of India, strict dietary restrictions are followed around menstruation, where it is believed that sour foods like curd, tamarind, and pickles will disrupt or stop the menstrual flow. Exercise is considered to worsen dysmenorrhea, whereas many studies have found that it actually improves it through serotonin release. These norms and values lead most women to associate their bodies with curse and impurity (Garg & Anand, 2015).

An important factor in Indian societies is poor knowledge, attitude, and practices with respect to menstruation. Considered a "taboo," it is rarely ever discussed in homes or schools, and menarche comes as a shock for most girls. Studies done across the country indicate a lack of awareness about menstrual hygiene. Seventy-seven percent of girls and women in India use old cloth, which is often reused, and eighty-eight percent of women resort to using ashes, dried leaves, and husk sand to promote absorption of menstrual blood. Lack of safe, clean sanitary facilities undermines the right to privacy and hygiene during this sensitive phase, leading to illnesses and further stigmatization of this phenomenon. A qualitative study conducted on the experience of menstruation in adolescent girls focused on themes regarding the bizarreness of menarche, the multitude of restrictions, the lack of knowledge and awareness about this, feeling of apprehension, guilt, and shame, and the need for increased awareness as a way of reducing the psychological distress (Jain et al., 2018). Lack of knowledge, illnesses due to poor menstrual hygiene, and overall secrecy and shame around the issue of menstruation are causes of school dropouts and absenteeism among female adolescents, contributing further to the psychological distress (Garg & Anand, 2015).

Overall, a positive relationship has been found to be present between menstrual attitudes and premenstrual changes. The healthiness of attitude depends on the amount of distress experienced during menstruation. It is frequently found that in the aforementioned cultural background, positive and negative experiences may coexist. Menarche is regarded as an auspicious event in India and confers a special position on the young girl. Indian customs of absolving women of their duties during this period and following a host of rituals may occasionally lead to positive attitudes in these women. The presence of positive feelings has been found to protect against premenstrual distress (Chaturvedi & Chandra, 1990, 1991).

As awareness of menstruation and its associated challenges continues to grow, the discussion surrounding menstrual leave has gained prominence. One of the key benefits of such legislation is its ability to address the specific needs of women, reduce the stigma surrounding menstruation, foster a positive work culture, and enhance overall productivity. However, there are potential drawbacks, including the risk of fostering sexism, exacerbating discrimination, and generating resentment among employees, all while imposing financial burdens on small businesses. Currently, India lacks a centralized policy or unified approach regarding paid menstrual leave.

The way forward involves a comprehensive exploration and development of management strategies for psychiatric conditions associated with menstruation. This should be coupled with the implementation of educational and social reforms aimed at enhancing understanding, raising awareness, and reducing the stigma surrounding menstruation. Additionally, creating more inclusive workplaces and fostering a supportive work culture will be essential to addressing the health needs of women during this period.

4 Perinatal Mental Health

4.1 Pre-Conceptional Period

Patients presenting in the pre-conceptional period for mental health support are usually those having difficulty in conception, using artificial reproductive techniques, those who are known cases of a psychiatric illness and on psychotropics, those with traumatic experiences in previous pregnancy, and those facing newly diagnosed illness in current pregnancy. Patients with pre-existing psychiatric illness may need a review for continuation, modification, or discontinuation of treatment during pregnancy. A cross-sectional study in India showed increased levels of overall stress and poor quality of life with poor interpersonal relationships in women undergoing infertility treatment, showing the harmful impact of experiencing infertility in a woman (Prasad et al., 2017). There is also a risk of trivializing women's concerns and reducing their role to "baby-making machines" with the involvement of assisted reproductive technologies (Madge, 2011).

4.2 Mental Health During Pregnancy and Postpartum Period

The perinatal period, which encompasses pregnancy and the first year postpartum, is a time of significant physical, emotional, and psychological change. While many expectant and new mothers experience the joys of welcoming a child, for some, this time is marked by the onset or exacerbation of psychiatric disorders. In the context of psychiatric disorders, the postpartum period is critically important, as it is a time when many women are at increased risk for the onset or exacerbation of mental health conditions. Although typically the first 6 weeks define the postpartum period for most disorders, with respect to psychiatric disorders, it may extend up to a year. This allows a larger window for identification of these disorders as well as addressing the multi-fold impact on diverse areas of life, including bonding with the baby.

Postpartum experiences can vary from temporary mood swings, irritability, and crying episodes to more severe symptoms such as intense agitation, delusions, confusion, and delirium.

4.3 Severe Mental Illnesses During Pregnancy and Postpartum

Postpartum psychosis is observed in 1–2/1000 childbearing women within the first 2–4 weeks following delivery. It can be seen as early as 2–3 days following delivery and is characterized by elation, labile mood, disorganized behavior, rambling speech, hallucinations, and delusions. It has an acute onset of florid symptoms with a variable and fluctuating course. Most studies recognize postpartum psychosis as a form of bipolar disorder with distinct clinical characteristics. The psychopathology is poorly understood, but factors like primiparity, hormonal changes, difficult labor, and genetic predisposition have been suggested as etiological factors. The final pathway appears to be sleep disruption, highlighting the importance of adequate sleep as a preventive measure (Sharma & Mazmanian, 2003).

A study done among 200 women with postpartum psychosis found that 20% of them have symptoms of catatonia, with the most common feature being mutism. Most women showed a good response to the lorazepam trial. It was also observed that a longer duration of untreated catatonia was associated with poor response. Those who did not respond to lorazepam showed response to ECT. Catatonia was more commonly seen in the early postpartum period (initial 4 weeks) (Nahar et al., 2017). Another study found thyroid volumetric and free T4 level changes to be associated with postpartum psychosis (Sethy et al., 2021). Other conditions, like cerebral venous thrombosis (Brockington, 2007; Louis et al., 2024) and various autoimmune conditions, may clinically present with psychotic symptoms in the early postpartum period. Hence, there is a need to rule out organic conditions that may mimic postpartum psychosis.

Regarding the onset of symptoms, another study involving 76 women admitted for postpartum and pregnancy-related mental illness found that 10% had prepartum onset (Chandra, 2001).

Women with bipolar disorder are at a much higher risk of relapse during and after pregnancy, about three times more likely than nonpregnant women who are not on mood stabilizers and are stable at the time of conception. Postpartum depression also bears a higher risk of bipolarity (Harsha & Acharya, 2019).

As against a study by McNeil (1998), which stated a higher prevalence of affective psychosis among the early postpartum group (onset within 3 weeks), Indian studies have found a higher prevalence of affective symptoms in the late-onset group (beyond 3 weeks) (Kulkarni, 1997).

Around 40% of the women suffering from postpartum psychosis had a family history of psychiatric illness, with 75% of the affected members having affective disorders and 30% of cases having mothers or sisters with a history of postpartum psychiatric illness (Chandra, 2001).

An interesting study done in an inpatient setting comparing clinical features, severity, and short-term outcomes of postpartum and non-postpartum onset mania showed that symptoms of anxiety and depression are more common and severe in postpartum onset mania as compared to more typical features in non-postpartum onset mania, although there is no significant difference between the two groups with respect to duration of hospital stay or short term outcomes (Ganjekar et al., 2013).

Postpartum depression (PPD) is an important reason for postpartum distress. Genetic liability, hormonal fluctuations, birth trauma, and psychosocial factors may be associated with postpartum depression. The prevalence in India is found to be 22%, with higher prevalence in the South Indian regions (Panolan & Benson Thomas, 2024). Another recent scoping review done in India, evaluating the prevalence of postpartum depression (PPD), showed prevalence rates variable across studies, ranging from 4% to 48.5% and around 18% on average across all research. A community study found that PPD was prevalent among new moms at a rate of 21.5%. The awareness rate among the family members and moms struggling with PPD was found to be 54%. Studies in this review pointed to a lack of social support post-delivery being an important risk factor for mental illnesses in these women. Women undergoing cesarean section were found to have a greater risk as compared to those undergoing vaginal delivery. Traumatic childbirth, complications at childbirth, low socioeconomic status, adverse life events, partner abuse, and history of anxiety and depression were found among the other important risk factors (Rajeev et al., 2024).

4.4 Consequences of Severe Mental Illnesses During the Perinatal Period

Among 82 women with postpartum psychosis interviewed in a tertiary care mental health facility, 38% reported suicidal ideation and 18% had attempted suicide in the current episode. It was more frequent in women with severe depression, those with insidious onset, and higher scores on the depressive dimension. Suicidal ideation was also associated with ideas of harm to the infant (Babu et al., 2008). A study was done in 2016 to assess the prevalence and predictors of suicidality among 462 healthy pregnant women in South India. The prevalence was found to be 7.6%, with 2.4% of the women having suicidal plans and 1.7% having attempted suicide in the current pregnancy. Younger age, poor perceived support, middle socioeconomic status, domestic violence, depressive symptoms, and past history of suicidality were found to predict suicidal ideation during the current episode. Lifetime history of suicidality and severity of depression were found to be the strongest predictors. This urges the health systems to be more active in screening women in this vulnerable period (Supraja et al., 2016).

In a study done in 2002, among 50 women admitted with a severe psychiatric illness in the postpartum period, 36% reported infanticidal behavior and 34% reported both infanticidal ideas and behavior. It was associated with depression in the mother, psychotic ideas toward the infant, and an adverse reaction to separation from the infant. Infanticidal behavior was also associated with having a female infant. The presence of depression and psychotic ideas predicted infanticidal ideas, whereas the presence of psychotic ideas toward the infant predicted infanticidal behavior (Chandra et al., 2002).

4.5 Common Mental Illnesses During the Perinatal Period

Despite the significant morbidity and, in some cases, mortality caused by severe mental illnesses, women are most commonly afflicted by conditions like anxiety and depression, with prevalence rates of 15–20% in low- and middle-income countries. The prevalence in India was found to be 21.87% (Kalra et al., 2021). The common risk factors seen were young age, being unmarried, unintended pregnancy, socioeconomic disadvantage, poor family support and emotional support, birth of a female child, and a history of psychiatric illness in the past. Belonging to the ethnic majority, having a supportive partner, good education, and a permanent job were found to protect against developing a mental illness (Fisher et al., 2012).

Anxiety disorders are highly prevalent in pregnancy and postpartum. Despite this, they haven't received as much of a focus as perinatal depression. Anxiety during pregnancy and postpartum can be in the form of tokophobia (fear of giving birth), concerns about the wellbeing of the fetus, sudden panic about new responsibilities as a mother, fear of cot death, fear of adverse health conditions in the newborn, and anxiety about being inadequate as a mother. This can be worsened by poor social support and financial worries. Pressure to have a male child, alcohol use, and physical violence can be other factors causing anxiety (Jyothi Kantipudi et al., 2020).

In a study done on 380 women in their early pregnancy (under 24 weeks) availing antenatal care at a facility in Bangalore, 55.7% of women had pregnancy-related anxiety. Low social support, poor socioeconomic conditions, and depression emerged as major determinants of anxiety (Nath et al., 2019). Perinatal anxiety, stress, and depression have worsened following COVID-19 and have been found to be 50.3% in HIV-positive pregnant women. Lack of partner support and known HIV status during pregnancy are significantly associated with anxiety (Easwaran et al., 2025).

Anxiety and depression can have negative outcomes during pregnancy and childbirth. This is supported by a community study done in urban Bengaluru, wherein birth outcomes were recorded in 583 pregnant women along with anxiety and depression symptoms. Twenty-three infants were born preterm and 15.6% had low birth weight (LBW). Female infants had an increased chance of LBW with an increase in maternal anxiety in each trimester, while male infants had a higher chance of LBW with higher baseline depression scores and an increase in scores from the first to second trimester (Chandra et al., 2021). It can also lead to negative neurodevelopmental, cognitive, and emotional outcomes in the child (Jagtap et al., 2023).

Perinatal OCD appears to be more common than in the general population during pregnancy and the postpartum period. It is manifested as the obsession with contamination and fear of harm to the baby. Untreated, it can cause significant distress, impair care toward infants, and affect mother-baby bonding. A systematic review done in 2024 examined the negative feto-maternal outcomes with OCD and found OCD to be associated with pre-eclampsia, antepartum and postpartum hemorrhage, emergency C-section, preterm birth, LBW, low APGAR score, neonatal hypoglycemia, respiratory distress, and congenital malformations (Aujla et al., 2024).

Although childbirth is considered to be a happy experience for most women, some of them may have traumatic experiences. A study was conducted in South India that showed an association between negative childbirth experience and post-traumatic stress disorder (PTSD) and a prevalence of 9% (Shiva et al., 2021). Further research on the prevalence and consequence of perinatal PTSD and other outcomes of perinatal stress, like functional neurological disorders, is still in a nascent stage in India (Desai & Chandra, 2023).

Loss of a child can be a very difficult event for a mother and may in many cases go, unaddressed, as the presentation may be different from grief caused by other losses (Davoudian et al., 2021). In a study done in the city of Chhattisgarh, India, it was found that perinatal grief was significantly higher in women who experienced stillbirth. Younger age, lack of support, and maternal agreement with norms were associated with higher grief (Roberts et al., 2012). Another study showed that women's position in the house, social support, rural background, and norms also affected the experience of perinatal grief (Roberts et al., 2021). Mothers, in most cases, openly express grief reaction but a qualitative interview depicted that most fathers coped with avoidance of discussion and engagement in work (Das et al., 2021). This emphasizes the need for bereavement support for both mothers and fathers with measures like mindfulness-based interventions that have shown merit (Roberts & Montgomery, 2015).

One very important outcome of maternal, perinatal psychopathology is the disruption of maternal-fetal attachment and mother-infant bonding. Development of bonding disorder can occur even in the absence of psychiatric illness, as these are two different entities. A study found the prevalence of bonding disorders to be 24% in healthy mother-baby dyads as compared to 45.2% in mothers with psychiatric disorders. Twenty percent of the mothers with psychiatric disorders had infant-related anxiety, with Indian mothers having a clinging/over-involvement subtype of anxiety (Vengadavaradan et al., 2019). Another cross-sectional study done in Kerala in 2024 stated the prevalence of mother-infant bonding disorders to be 12.3%. It was associated with postpartum complications, maternal depression, and temperamental difficulties in the infant (Thamby et al., 2024). Early identification of bonding disorders is necessary, as it adversely affects the development of the quality of physical life of the infant (Narayan et al., 2023).

Underlying these bonding difficulties may be the understanding deficits in recognition of infant emotions in mothers with mental illness. The infant facial emotion recognition (InFER) tool has shown to be a promising tool in Indian settings for understanding maternal recognition of infant emotions (Pantoji et al., 2024).

Assessment of bonding disorders may become complex owing to the formal training required to use most available assessment tools, especially in low-resource, low- and middle-income countries. The NIMHANS maternal behavioral scale (NIMBUS) has proven to be useful in assessing bonding in mothers with postpartum severe mental illnesses in these settings where observations are made by family members and health assistants rather than perinatal nurses (Ganjekar et al., 2020). An intervention in bonding disorders is video-based feedback of mother-infant interaction and has proven to be efficacious for mothers with schizophrenia in a low-resource setting (Reddy et al., 2014).

4.6 Cultural Aspects of Perinatal Mental Illnesses

In the Indian context, cultural undercurrents affect the experience of pregnancy and childbirth. Different explanatory models (EM) given by patients and families suffering from perinatal illnesses were explored in an Indian study. Patients attributed their illness to being subjected to interpersonal issues and violence, poor social support, gender preference, and various supernatural causes like black magic, possession by evil spirits, karma, unfulfilled vows, and more. Understanding these EMs helps to develop a more holistic understanding of the illness, helps in establishing better rapport, and helps in providing well-rounded solutions (Thippeswamy et al., 2015).

4.7 Interventions for Perinatal Mental Illnesses

Interventions for perinatal mental illness can be pharmacological or non-pharmacological (including psychotherapy and neuromodulation techniques).

Depending on the conditions, the use of certain antipsychotics, antidepressants, mood stabilizers, and sedatives is advised in pregnancy after a detailed discussion with the patient on the advantages and disadvantages of continuing these medications and the effect of medications and maternal illness on the fetus during pregnancy and the infant during breastfeeding. Certain medications like valproate and carbamazepine are contraindicated during pregnancy due to their teratogenic potential, and lithium and clozapine are best avoided during breastfeeding due to difficulty in infant monitoring and risk of agranulocytosis, respectively (Bharadwaj et al., 2022).

A study was conducted in the mother-baby unit of a tertiary care hospital in India to evaluate the short-term outcomes of atypical antipsychotic exposure in breastfed infants. The occurrence of side effects was quite low (17.8%), more commonly in the form of constipation and sedation. Some of these infants showed developmental delay at the first follow-up, but this finding was confounded by other factors like advanced maternal age and low birth weight (Sinha et al., 2021).

The use of neuromodulation techniques like ECT during pregnancy and postpartum may be lifesaving in certain cases if given under adequate monitoring (Bharadwaj et al., 2022). Common indications include catatonia, augmentation of medication suicidality, and it has not been shown to have any adverse outcomes in breastfed infants (Grover et al., 2018). Hence, ECT has been shown to be an effective and safe option in the postpartum period with good response and minimal side effects (Grover et al., 2018).

Few studies have been done on the use of repetitive transcranial magnetic stimulation (rTMS) in pregnancy and have not reported any adverse maternal or infant outcomes (Hebel et al., 2020). An interesting yet complex case was reported in an Indian setting where a woman suffering from tokophobia with depression was treated safely and successfully with rTMS (Nanjundaswamy et al., 2019).

4.8 Decision Making in the Perinatal Period

A study in India reviewed factors that influence decision-making regarding planning pregnancy for women with psychiatric illness. Around 88% of the women who underwent in-depth interviews reported autonomy over pregnancy-related decision-making. Stigma was one of the major contributory factors. Nearly 80% reported not using contraception despite medical advice because of a lack of control over contraception use. About 50% of the women believed that taking psychotropics would harm the fetus or that illness would not recur if medicines were stopped in pregnancy. This study revealed that many socio-cultural factors affect decision-making in women coming from low-resource settings like India (Bagadia et al., 2020).

To address the sensitive treatment needs in this population, various Western countries have established inpatient mother-baby units. This ensures that the mother-baby bonding is not disrupted during the period when the mother is being treated. In India, this dedicated service first started in 2009 at the National Institute of Mental

Health and Neurosciences and is the only one of its kind in the entire country (Chandra et al., 2015). It caters to a variety of psychiatric illnesses, focuses on reinstituting lactation, uses a multidisciplinary approach to cover the psychosocial needs of the patients, focuses on bonding intervention, and overall encompasses a holistic approach that improves patient experience and chances of recovery.

4.9 *Female Dhat Syndrome*

Female Dhat Syndrome represents a psychosomatic condition rooted in cultural misconceptions and sexual health anxieties in Indian women. The common symptoms with which women in their reproductive period present, include excessive concern about vaginal discharge, fatigue, weakness, anxiety, and low mood. Women may complain of frequent headache, backache, and loss of appetite. There could be feelings of sexual inadequacy and associated guilt feelings. Though not formally recognized in diagnostic manuals like the DSM-5, female Dhat syndrome has been proposed by Indian psychiatrists to describe psychosomatic distress related to vaginal discharge, perceived as pathologic and debilitating (Chaturvedi et al., 1993). Subsequently, isolated case (Singh et al., 2001) and case series (Grover et al., 2014) were published on female Dhat syndrome. Systematic evaluation of 26 women using a self-rated questionnaire modified from the Comprehensive Questionnaire for Assessment of Dhat Syndrome for complaints of non-pathological vaginal discharge along with depressive and somatic complaints found that phenomenologically, females can have similar symptoms as male patients with dhat syndrome (Grover et al., 2016). In another study, 70 females with non-pathological vaginal discharge visiting gynecological outpatient services were assessed using the Scale for Assessment of Female Dhat Syndrome. It was found that phenomenologically non-pathological vaginal discharge in women was similar to that of Dhat syndrome in males (Joshi et al., 2022).

5 Women and Addiction

Substance use among women is a complex and often overlooked issue that spans across social, psychological, and biological dimensions. From the pressures of modern life to the silent struggles behind closed doors, women's relationship with substances is shaped by unique challenges. Yet, despite its growing prevalence, the narrative surrounding women and addiction remains largely untold.

5.1 Prevalence

The traditional use of various varieties of drugs among women is not unheard of. Alcohol use is common in women in many tribal populations, as is chewing betel leaf with lime paste, keeping a wad of tobacco in the mouth, and consuming a drink made from cannabis leaves (bhang) during festivals like Holi and Shivaratri. However, the trends of problematic substance use beyond these cultural contexts have now become a rising predicament.

Until the early 90s, studies done in India indicated that drug abuse was predominantly a male phenomenon. This, when compared to the current drug prevalence reports, has shown a considerable change from old studies that said the drug use prevalence in women is negligible (Ministry of Social Justice and Empowerment, Government of India, 2002).

Although most studies measure substance use in women across a wide age range, an extensive study conducted in 2008 found that most women using substances were in their 20s or 30s with 6.2% of women being under 20 years of age. This study showed high rates of use of tobacco (79.1%), alcohol (77.4%), heroin (33.5%), dextropropoxyphene (25.9%), sleeping pills (22.4%), and cannabis (22.7%). Other than solvents, tobacco was the main drug of initiation in the late teens. Tobacco and sleeping pills were taken alone, alcohol and opiates with a partner or alone, and solvents mainly in groups (United Nations Office on Drugs and Crime, 2008).

According to the GENACIS study done in 2005, the prevalence of alcohol use in women was found to be 5.9% (World Health Organization, 2012).

Half of the respondents in the Bangalore mall study that investigated the non-medical use of sedatives among people in the age group of 18–40 years were females (Nattala et al., 2014).

According to the National Mental Health Survey (NMHS), the prevalence of substance use disorders is 10.05% in women, out of which the maximum prevalence is for tobacco use (9.78%), followed by alcohol use (0.48%) and other substances (0.09%) (Gururaj & Varghese, 2016). The findings from these surveys tell us that substance use does exist among Indian women, but the magnitude of the problem is much smaller than in men.

5.2 Clinical Profile of Women with Substance Use

It has been found that almost 80% of women seeking help for substance use had alcohol use disorder (AUD) (Malik et al., 2015). Detailed clinical evaluation indicated that in these women, initiation of alcohol use was started in their 20s and they developed AUD by 30 (Malik et al., 2017a, 2017b). As against this, a chart review conducted in North India found that only 10% of women reported alcohol being their primary substance and opioids being the main substance (Ambekar et al., 2017). This reveals regional differences in substance use across India. Another study conducted to identify patterns of substance use in adolescent girls in the northern part of the country found that almost 60% of these girls engaged in illicit opioid use, mainly in injectable form, and belonged predominantly to urban background (Mandal et al., 2019). In the NMHS, participants from UP seemed to have a high prevalence of alprazolam use. (National Mental Health Survey, 2016). A study that was conducted at NIMHANS, Bangalore, in 1995 showed that male-to-female ratio of alcohol use was 57:1. These women had higher rates of family and spousal alcohol dependence. Psychiatric comorbidity was present in almost 34% of women, with depression being the most common and the rates of physical comorbidity were high (Murthy et al., 1995). Yet another study conducted at a university hospital in Manipal almost 15 years later (2010) showed that the male-to-female ratio of alcohol use now was 39.5:1, showing a changing trend. Most of these women had a later age of onset, presenting to the hospital in their forties. Most women were single, belonging to a nuclear family with identifiable stressors in the background of alcohol use. Help-seeking from local urban dwellers was less, suggesting the possibility of stigma. The late onset secondary alcohol dependence suggests the role of exogenous non-genetic factors, which seemed to play a greater role in alcohol dependence in women (Ashutosh et al., 2010). Tobacco dependence was found to be the most common psychiatric comorbidity in women with alcohol use. Women with alcohol use disorders have a higher prevalence of affective disorders, self-harm behaviors, and borderline personality disorder (Malik et al., 2017a, 2017b; Sutradhar et al., 2023; Yadav et al., 2021a, 2021b).

A rapid assessment survey was conducted in 2000–2001 for difficult-to-reach populations. Alcohol was found to be the most common drug of initiation, followed by cannabis (especially in Goa). There was a variation with geographical locations, with heroin being the drug of initiation in some parts of Mumbai and Imphal, and tranquilizers and sedatives being more prominent in Amritsar (Ministry of Social Justice and Empowerment, Government of India, 2002). Abuse of heroin is reported more commonly in cities like Delhi, Imphal, and Dimapur, with polydrug use in states like Kerala. The women in this study were mostly well-educated, employed single women with early onset of drug use, high levels of drug use in families, many friends using drugs, and early initiation into sex (Ministry of Social Justice and Empowerment, Government of India, 2002). Studies show that women have also been involved in the production and marketing of opiates. There have been cases where the drug mafia in Mumbai has used women whose husbands are in jail as drug couriers, taking advantage of their vulnerability (Ministry of Social Justice and Empowerment, Government of India, 2002). In the RAS study, it was found that most women had been introduced to drug use at an early age, and opiates, alcohol, and tranquilizers were the common substances of use. Forty percent of these women were intravenous drug users (United Nations International Drug Control Programme, Regional Office for South Asia, 2002).

There is a variation in the prevalence of women using alcohol according to geographical location in the country. The rate was to be higher in areas where women were subjected to poverty, marginalization, and a high ST/SC population. The prevalence was found to be more clustered in the eastern, southeastern, and northeastern parts of India (Roy et al., 2024). The use of opium was found to be significantly high in tribal communities of Arunachal Pradesh and was introduced to women, most commonly by their spouses (Chaturvedi et al., 2013).

5.3 Risk Factors of Substance Use in Women

Biologically, women are at a higher risk of alcohol intoxication and adverse effects due to low levels of alcohol dehydrogenase, less body water, and low levels of antidiuretic hormone, with increased consumption seen in those with premenstrual syndrome. Women also report different responses to opiates, with higher rates of nausea and analgesia (Frezza et al., 1992; Seitz et al., 1993; Van Thiel et al., 1988). Another important phenomenon is the development of medical and psychological impairment earlier in women, known as the phenomenon of "telescoping." This is more commonly seen in alcohol use, but a similar phenomenon is found with tobacco, opioids, and cocaine (Patton et al., 1998; Powis et al., 1996; Randall et al., 1999). In women, initiation of substance use is shaped by environmental factors, but progression to abuse/dependence is determined by genetic influences (Kendler & Prescott, 1998a, 1998b). Marital discord and interpersonal conflicts were identified to be one of the significant causes of initiation and maintenance of substance use in women (Malik et al., 2015), as was the influence of spouse or partner and elder males. Initiation was also influenced by factors like curiosity, positive expectancies regarding the benefits of alcohol, and working in an alcohol joint (Chaturvedi et al., 2013).

A study done in 2017 explored adverse experiences among women using substances. Most women had experienced physical, emotional, and sexual abuse early in life. The earlier the age of experience, the worse the psychopathology and severity of addiction (Malik et al., 2017a).

In most adult women, alcohol was used as a 'self-medication' to deal with the stress from intimate partner violence, financial concerns, and difficult living circumstances. A bidirectional relationship was found between alcohol use and adverse life experiences, making women with substance use further prone to multiple adversities (Malik et al., 2017a). Other risk factors included poor education status, unemployment, young age at work, early marriage, and poor social support (Rajat, R. 2004); women from marginalized societies, sex workers, and partners of males using substances (Ministry of Social Justice and Empowerment, Government of India, 2002). A study found increased levels of alcohol and other substance use in sex workers before sexual activity (Gupta et al., 2009).

5.4 Substance Use During the Perinatal Period

A systematic review done in 2025 on the prevalence of tobacco and alcohol use among pregnant women in India also found a high prevalence of tobacco use in pregnant women, especially those above 25 years of age, limited awareness about the adverse effects of tobacco use, and the presence of a close contact using tobacco (Dhir et al., 2025). Use of solvents and inhalants is more often found in young girls living off the street (Ministry of Social Justice and Empowerment, Government of India, 2002).

A systematic review was published in 2024 on alcohol use in pregnancy utilizing the data from the National Family Health Survey (NFHS). It showed that the national prevalence of alcohol use in pregnancy was 1.26%, with regional variations. Arunachal Pradesh, Chhattisgarh, and Assam were the states with the maximum prevalence. The alcohol use correlated with tobacco use, lack of education, and being a part of a scheduled tribes (Ghosh et al., 2025). Alcohol use has been shown to be deeply embedded in the daily rituals of tribal women. Low alcohol literacy, easy access to alcohol, and lack of social monitoring appeared to play a role in alcohol use among pregnant women in certain tribal populations of Odisha (Pati et al., 2018). The impact of alcohol use in pregnancy is immense, with one of the worst consequences being the occurrence of fetal alcohol spectrum disorders in the baby, characterized by minor physical anomalies, behavioral problems, and poor intellectual functioning (Nayak et al., 2012).

A study examined the outcomes of the consumption of recreational drugs in pregnant women. Pregnant women using cocaine and/or opioids during pregnancy had 3.88 times higher odds of developing adverse neonatal outcomes (Kandhasamy et al., 2025).

5.5 *Outcomes of Substance Use*

Women using substances are also more vulnerable to sexual exploitation and intimate partner violence (United Nations Office on Drugs and Crime, 2008). Women have been found to develop more severe pneumonia, TB, lung complications, hepatitis, HIV and AIDS, other STDs, irregular menstrual cycles, and termination of pregnancies (Kumar & Sharma, 2008). The presence of IPV, domestic conflicts, and the neglect of children leads them to engage in deviant behavior (Ministry of Social Justice and Empowerment, Government of India, 2002). These women have high levels of depression, anxiety, low confidence, and self-esteem (United Nations Office on Drugs and Crime, 2008). They also have a higher incidence of suicidal attempts (United Nations Office on Drugs and Crime, 2008). A high proportion of these women are found to be involved in peddling, sex work, pickpocketing, and theft and face legal consequences, including incarceration in prisons (Rajat, 2004).

5.6 *Help Seeking for Substance Use Among Women*

Studies have found fewer women from affluent societies accessing care at established drug treatment centers. Drug centers have shown to lack the gender sensitivity required to address women's needs. This could be secondary to the significant stigma associated with drug abuse, especially in women, low social support, and prioritization of concerns for their children and family over the concerns for their treatment (Ministry of Social Justice and Empowerment, Government of India, 2002). There are also negative attitudes toward women seeking help and poor decision-making in women that make it difficult for women to access care. Data from treatment centers in Delhi, Jodhpur, and Lucknow, collected between 1989 and 1991, showed that 1–3% of those seeking treatment were women. Similarly, the Drug Abuse Monitoring System indicates that women make up about 2.3–3% of new treatment seekers (Ray & Chopra, 2012).

Studies that have used relapse as an outcome measure have found that women tend to have better outcomes than men. Findings from Project MATCH revealed that women not only have a lower likelihood of relapse but also are more likely to seek help after a relapse. It was suggested that the differences in outcomes based on gender and treatment modality may influence the results (Cutler & Fishbain, 2005; Greenfield et al., 2007). A study conducted at a tertiary care center in India among women with opioid use indicated that women with onset of opioids beyond 25 years of age, with medical comorbidities, and using opioids for pain relief had a greater chance of treatment completion (Dayal et al., 2017). Another study found that better education status in women positively influenced abstinence at follow-up (Dayal et al., 2017; Nebhinani et al., 2013).

6 Medical Disorders and Mental Health

6.1 Polycystic Ovarian Syndrome

Polycystic Ovarian Syndrome (PCOS) is a complex endocrine disorder that affects millions of women of reproductive age worldwide. While its clinical manifestations are primarily associated with reproductive, metabolic, and dermatological issues, the psychological burden of PCOS is often overlooked. Emerging research highlights a strong link between PCOS and mental health concerns, including depression, anxiety, mood disorders, and reduced quality of life, making PCOS a multi-system disorder. The interplay between hormonal imbalances, insulin resistance, chronic inflammation, and the psychosocial impact of symptoms such as weight gain, hirsutism, and infertility contributes to the increased mental health risks in women with PCOS. This section examines the bidirectional link between PCOS and mental health, highlighting key mechanisms, contributing factors, and the need for a holistic management approach.

In PCOS, other than the obvious psychological impacts secondary to the physical and gynecological symptoms, there is direct biological vulnerability noted due to dysregulation in the hypothalamic-pituitary-ovarian (HPO) and hypothalamic-pituitary-adrenal (HPA) axes. The neuroendocrine imbalance and downregulation of hormone signaling are noted to have an impact on mood. Evidence shows that there is an imbalance in levels of FSH, LH, and free testosterone in women with PCOS, which is linked with higher rates of anxiety and depression. Additionally, they are also found to have altered serotonin, dopamine, and adrenergic signaling linked with multiple disorders of mood, impulse control, and cognition. The role of the gut-brain axis, pro-inflammatory mechanisms, obesity, and insulin resistance needs further investigation in the pathogenesis of mental health disorders in PCOS (Maliszewska et al., 2024).

6.2 Mood Disorders and PCOS

The prevalence of depression and anxiety in females with PCOS is variable, with a wide range of prevalence of depression varying from 11 to 93.5%. The prevalence of depression varied across studies depending on the assessment tool used. Using the Patient Health Questionnaire-9 (PHQ-9), Bhattacharya et al. reported a prevalence of 64.1%, while Habib et al. found 20% with the application of the Hamilton Depression Rating (HAM-D) scale, Chaudhari et al. reported 25.7%, whereas Prathap et al. found 93.5%. The prevalence was 11% with HADS and 49.19% with Depression Anxiety and Stress Scale (DASS)-21. Using the Mini International Neuropsychiatric Interview (MINI) 5.0.0, major depressive disorder was reported in 23% of cases, while dysthymia was observed in 1.8% (Bhattacharya & Jha, 2010; Chaudhari et al., 2018; Habib et al., 2021).

The prevalence of anxiety among Indian women with PCOS ranged from 15.45% to 100%, depending on the assessment tool used. A study using the Hospital Anxiety and Depression Scale (HADS) reported a 28% prevalence. Among studies using the Hamilton Anxiety (HAM-A) scale, Chaudhari et al. found a prevalence of 38.6%, while Prathap et al. reported 100%. With DASS-21, anxiety was observed in 70.7% of participants. The MINI 5.0.0 assessment indicated a 15.45% prevalence for both generalized anxiety disorder and panic disorder, whereas the Generalized Anxiety Disorder (GAD)-7 scale showed a 25% prevalence of major anxiety. Additionally, one study found higher baseline state and trait anxiety scores in adolescent girls with PCOS compared to healthy controls but did not calculate prevalence rates. An assessment of anxiety severity in another study reported that 62.9% had mild anxiety, 29.6% had moderate anxiety, and 7.4% had severe anxiety (Chaudhari et al., 2018; Prathap et al., 2018).

Higher prevalence was noted in patients visiting tertiary care centers with more gynecological complications. Acne, hirsutism, infertility, menstrual abnormalities, and alopecia were associated with depression and anxiety with poor quality of life (Chaudhari et al., 2018; Kanagarajan et al., 2023; Prathap et al., 2018).

A study done in Kolkata, on women visiting the clinic for gynecological concerns, showed no correlation between depression and any socio-demographic, clinical, and biochemical parameters, contrary to global literature (Bhattacharya & Jha, 2010).

6.2.1 Other Mental Health Disorders

Another study done in North India showed the prevalence of bipolar disorder, panic disorder, OCD, dysthymia, and suicidality was reported to be 2.72%, 15.45%, 6.36%, 1.87%, and 8.1%, respectively, using MINI 5.0.0. Yet another study revealed a 3% prevalence of anorexia or bulimia with a higher risk of eating disorders in depressive females (Balaji et al., 2015; Habib et al., 2021; Hussain et al., 2015).

6.3 Mastectomy

Breast cancer is the most common malignancy among women, accounting for nearly one-fourth of total cancer cases in women (Zhang et al., 2025). The tiresome and long journey of cancer treatment includes radiotherapy, chemotherapy, surgery, and hormonal treatment. The physical and psychological burden of the illness and treatment significantly impacts the quality of life of the women. The various alterations in the bodily appearance of women have shown detrimental effects on self-esteem, poor self-concept, and poor self-concept and self-image, which lead to anxiety, depression, and poor quality of life. There are very limited studies in India assessing the mental health impacts on women with breast cancer.

A cross-sectional study in North India showed the prevalence of depression in 47.5% of women diagnosed with cancer; the majority of the patients (56.7%) had mild depression, followed by moderate (33.3%) and severe depression (10%) (Thakur et al., 2019). A cross-sectional study in Kerala on 270 women revealed a 21.5% prevalence of depression assessed using PHQ-9 and ICD guidelines. In this study, 7% had moderate depression, 8% had moderately severe to severe depression, and 6% had mild depression (Purkayastha et al., 2017). A prospective follow-up study in Varanasi on 200 patients showed the prevalence of anxiety in 37% and depression in 28%, the prevalence of anxiety in 37%, and depression in 28% of women. The wide gap in the prevalence rates can be attributed to the heterogeneity in the sample based on socio-demographic differences, clinical status, and phase of assessment, with higher rates of mood symptoms noted in single, lower socio-economic status, rural background, and earlier in the course of the disease and poor social support (Srivastava et al., 2015). A cross-sectional study at a tertiary care center in North India on 165 women who underwent mastectomy for breast cancer showed the rates of depression, anxiety, and stress were 27·8%, 31·5%, and 24·8%, respectively, with higher rates of depression in newly diagnosed women. The study also identified higher scores on the body image scale, pointing toward higher body image issues in women who underwent mastectomy, with improving scores with the passage of time (Thakur et al., 2022). A qualitative study done in Gujarat revealed that often during the post-surgical period, the stressors and mental health concerns were overlooked and untreated. Contacting previous survivors who underwent surgery and family support were identified as positive coping mechanisms (Trivedi et al., 2016). A 5-year follow-up study in Mumbai found no statistically significant difference in quality-of-life scores in women who underwent radical mastectomy versus women with breast-conservative surgery at 5-year follow-up.

A study done in Mumbai evaluating mastectomized vs. lumpectomized women shared some insight into the difference in mood symptoms and coping skills among the two groups and found no significant difference in the anxiety and depression scores among the two groups; however, the study revealed that women's perception of their femininity, sexual attractiveness, and desire was linked to their breasts, resulting in disturbances in sexual functions and body image issues. The coping, fear of relapse, and adaptive process were found to be poorer in the mastectomized group, implying the trauma and distress associated with the mutilating process (Mahapatro & Parkar, 2005).

Overall, the majority of studies showed that risk of relapse and recurrence, treatment-related concerns, and fear of the future were some of the common concerns in women irrespective of the mode of treatment. However, dysfunction related to body image issues, sexuality, and reproductive concerns was seen more frequently in women undergoing mastectomy. Hence, psychological impact of mastectomy extends beyond physical recovery, deeply affecting body image, self-esteem, and emotional well-being. Cultural perceptions of femininity, societal expectations, and limited mental health support further contribute to distress among patients, highlighting the need for collaborative care.

6.4 Hysterectomy

Hysterectomy, one of the most common gynecological surgeries, has significant physical and psychological implications for women. In India, where cultural beliefs and societal norms deeply influence perceptions of womanhood and reproductive health, the mental health impact of hysterectomy is particularly profound. Women undergoing this procedure may experience a range of emotional responses, including relief from medical symptoms, but also grief, anxiety, depression, and concerns about femininity, aging, and marital relationships. This chapter explores the mental health consequences of hysterectomy in India, examining the interplay between biological, psychological, and socio-cultural factors.

Hysterectomy is the surgical removal of the uterus for the treatment of multiple benign conditions, including fibroids, cysts, endometriosis, and pelvic organ prolapse. The psychiatric manifestations associated with hysterectomy are considered to emerge secondary to hormonal dysfunction that arises due to decline in ovarian function. Higher rates of physical and psychological morbidity were seen in women where hysterectomy is accompanied by oophorectomy (Subramaniam et al., 1982). A systematic review in 2022 showed that there was a negative impact on mental health and cognitive functions in women with premature menopause and premature ovarian failure (Sathiyaseelan et al., 2022).

There is limited evidence for the association between mental health disorders and hysterectomy. The studies have shown a link between psychosis, anxiety, depression, psychosexual dysfunction, and insomnia with hysterectomy. However, there is contradictory evidence linking the two.

Two Indian studies done in the 1990s reported completely contrasting findings. Vyas et al. identified a statistically significant rise in neurotic disorders after hysterectomy, whereas Bhatia et al. concluded that the procedure rarely resulted in psychiatric disorders (Bhatia et al., 1990; Was et al., 1989). Secondary analysis of data from the Longitudinal Ageing Survey of India (LASI) conducted during the year 2017–2018 reported around 28.1% prevalence of depression in post-hysterectomy women. The analysis showed higher prevalence in the older age group of >70 years of age and increased likelihood of depression in rural populations with lower education and socio-economic background, in divorced and unmarried women (Ambika, 2025). A comparative study done in 2018 in women who underwent hysterectomy and other gynecological surgery revealed no significant difference in the prevalence of anxiety or depression in women at 6 months post-surgery. There was no significant difference in quality of life, marital adjustment and sexual functioning (Mathur, 2018).

A prospective study done in Bangalore showed a decrease in depression and anxiety assessed by structured clinical interview post hysterectomy. There was a decrease in depression from 90% to 41.7%, and anxiety reduced from 63.3% to 5% (Malyam et al., 2020). The results also correlated with another Indian survey done in rural North India, which showed that women stopped bothering about their menses and also that women started visiting religious places, and women started to show interest in day-to-day activities like mopping and washing utensils, indicating that they were much better after hysterectomy. However, around 39.5% of women reported a sense of emptiness and losing their sense of being women. Interestingly, laywomen also complained of clothes not fitting properly due to the removal of abdominal organs (Singh & Arora, 2008).

Current evidence is inconclusive and lacking in explanation of the causality of psychiatric disorders in women undergoing hysterectomies.

The connection between these medical conditions and mental well-being requires further investigation to facilitate timely identification and early intervention. Addressing the psychological impact of these conditions is crucial for enhancing the overall quality of life of affected women and minimizing morbidity and functional impairment. A comprehensive, multidisciplinary approach that integrates medical, psychological, and social support can help mitigate the emotional distress associated with these conditions. Future research and awareness initiatives are essential to bridge gaps in mental health care, ensuring that women receive holistic treatment that prioritizes both their physical and emotional well-being.

6.5 Contraception

Contraception is a crucial aspect of reproductive health, offering individuals the ability to make informed choices about family planning. It empowers people to control the timing and size of their families, promoting physical and emotional well-being. With various methods available, contraception ensures a safer, healthier future for individuals and communities.

The concept of contraception in India was introduced in 1952, marking the beginning of the country's family planning efforts. However, due to deeply rooted cultural and religious beliefs, contraception remains a taboo in certain parts of India. Access and usage often vary, influenced by economic factors, social status, and the level of education and affordability. At the London Summit on Family Planning in 2012, the Government of India made a significant global commitment to expand access to family planning services. They pledged to reach an additional 48 million new users by 2020 (Muttreja & Singh, 2018).

Multiple methods of contraception are available to women. A mixed-method study to evaluate the type of contraception used by women in the country found that around 76% of women used female sterilization, followed by barrier method, contraceptive pills, and IUD in that order. The methods changed from short-acting to permanent as women aged. The women with more accepting attitudes toward domestic violence and low levels of social independence had a higher reliance on permanent methods of contraception (Ewerling et al., 2021). Female sterilization dominates contraceptive use in the country, with a considerable number of women being in the age group of 25–28. The rates of male sterilization methods were significantly low as compared to female sterilization rates (Samal & Dehury, 2015; Vinoda Thulaseedharan, 2018). A recent study found that half of sterilizations occur before women complete their reproductive years, influenced by their education, access to information, and media influence. Female sterilization is the most common method in both urban and rural areas. There is a high rate of intrauterine device (IUD) use in urban areas, but rural women have high parity scores at sterilization, showing a later preference for family planning. Women with higher education levels and wealthier couples showed a preference for male condoms and reversible methods like IUDs and periodic abstinence, while uneducated women belonging to low socioeconomic status predominantly relied on sterilization (Sharma & Gupta, 2024).

Contraceptive use in India varies significantly by religion and social group. Christians tend to favor IUDs (7.93%) and withdrawal (7.58%), while Sikhs have the highest male condom usage (17.68%). Female sterilization is most common among Hindus (50%) and Buddhists/Neo-Buddhists (33.87%). Muslims and Sikhs have lower adoption rates of sterilization, influenced by religious beliefs. General caste couples prefer male condoms (12.11%), while sterilization is more prevalent among Scheduled Castes (47.86%) and OBCs (48.09%). Scheduled Tribes show higher use of IUDs (4.56%) and withdrawal (5.71%). Awareness and healthcare access contribute to earlier sterilization among General caste women with lower median age, marital duration, and parity. Married couples typically use more effective methods like pills (5.56%) and male condoms (7.73%), while sterilization rates are highest among widowed women (45.69%) as they complete their family size. Timing, marital duration, and parity at sterilization are also influenced by marital status and life circumstances (Sharma & Gupta, 2024).

Many states in India still rely on the traditional methods of contraception like coitus interruptus, the rhythm method, abstinence, and having intercourse during periods of lactational amenorrhea. These methods are prevalent both in high-fertility states like Uttar Pradesh and Assam, as well as low-fertility states like West Bengal and Kerala (Ram et al., 2014).

A study (part of a district-level household survey) examining contraceptive knowledge and use in over six lakh women identified that modern, even traditional, methods are practiced quite frequently in the country. The education levels in the couple and socio-economic class emerged as factors determining contraceptive use (Sharma, 2012).

A study showed that condoms were the most prominent method of contraception between April and June 2020. Diaphragms were not used very commonly by women unless they were trained to use them, and many women found it to be messy (Jain & Muralidhar, 2020).

An oral contraceptive was developed indigenously by the name "centchorman." It is a nonsteroidal, weakly estrogenic but potently antiestrogenic and was found to be safe and effective and is now being marketed in India since 1991 as a "once-a-week pill." Twenty-five percent of women of reproductive age use "progesterone pills" only, and they are usually effective in 99% of cases (Sharma et al., 2001).

The intrauterine contraceptive device is commonly used in India, but the discontinuation rate is 62.8%, with most removals due to associated side effects (Kumar et al., 2019). Implant rates are highly effective, with a failure rate of less than 1% (Samal & Dehury, 2015). Injectable contraceptives like DMPA and NET-EN, with DMPA being more widely used, are 97–99% effective in preventing pregnancies. Despite demand from women and healthcare workers, many discontinue due to side effects such as menstrual irregularities, vaginal discharge, and weight changes. Other reasons for discontinuation include method preference and the inconvenience of regular clinic visits. Improved counseling is needed, as many women are not fully informed about potential side effects and proper use. Hormonal patches are also largely used in India (Jain & Muralidhar, 2020).

The vaginal ring was introduced in India in 2009, with 94.2% of women (195/207) expressing satisfaction with its use. 76.2% of women reported regular menstrual bleeding, and it is particularly popular among women over 18 due to fewer contraindications compared to other methods. However, discontinuation rates were noted, with 36% of women experiencing menstrual irregularities and 6% reporting vaginal irritation (Sharma et al., 2001).

7 Menopause and Mental Health

Menopause signifies the shift from the reproductive to the non-reproductive phase in a woman's life. It acts as a natural safeguard against reproductive health risks in aging women while also contributing to the aging process and elevating the risk of noncommunicable diseases. Menopause marks a significant transition in a woman's life, bringing about complex physical, hormonal, and psychological changes. In India, where cultural attitudes toward aging and womanhood play a crucial role in shaping health experiences, menopause is often accompanied by misconceptions, stigma, and limited healthcare access. While some women view it as a natural phase of life, others experience distress due to symptoms such as hot flashes, sleep disturbances, mood swings, and cognitive change. This chapter explores the relationship between menopause and mental health, examining how menopause influences emotional regulation, cognitive function, and overall well-being, while also addressing their impact on diagnosis and treatment.

Around the age of 40, there is accelerated loss of primordial follicles from the ovary, which coincides with a selective rise in follicle stimulating hormone (FSH). The FSH levels gradually increase even in women who menstruate regularly. During menopause, there is a change in cycle frequency or menstrual flow, after which gonadotrophins, oestradiol, and inhibin show a marked degree of variability with abrupt changes from typical postmenopausal patterns to those characteristic of the reproductive age group. During menopause, FSH levels are markedly elevated, luteinizing hormone (LH) levels moderately so, while estradiol and inhibin levels are low or undetectable. The usual age of menopause is 45 to 55 years. The average age of Indian women at menopause is 46 years (Burger, 1996).

A study done in 1981 on 105 women in the perimenopausal period identified 21 (20%) women to have "possible cases." The most commonly reported symptoms were depression, somatic symptoms, anxiety, and fatigue (Jai Prakash et al., 1981). A meta-analysis done in 2021 showed 42.47% (95% CI: 28.73–57.49) of perimenopausal and postmenopausal women have some form of depression (V. Yadav et al., 2021a, 2021b). Based on a case-control study published in 2022, around 47.1% of women in the study group were found to have some mental health diagnosis, with 18% suffering from depression and 10% having a diagnosis of anxiety disorder. A cross-sectional study conducted in a tertiary care hospital on perimenopausal women published in 2024 revealed some interesting findings: The risk factors for psychological disturbances were identified as single, widowed, or separated women; housewives, low education status, domestic violence, and substance abuse in partners. The surprising finding was higher severity of menopausal and somatic symptoms in married women (Aziz et al., 2024). A cross-sectional study in 2023 assessing cognition and mood symptoms in postmenopausal women showed 13.33% of women having mild cognitive impairment (Nagda et al., 2023). A study done in the Gynaecology department in 2011 reported vasomotor symptoms in 75.3% of women, psychological symptoms in 62.01%, physical ailments in 32%, and genitourinary symptoms in 15.53%. Multiple studies done in India on quality of life using a standardized menopause-specific QOL (MENQOL) questionnaire consisting of physical, vasomotor, psychosocial, and sexual domains have shown higher scores in physical and vasomotor symptoms and relatively lower scores in the sexual domain, which could be attributable to social, cultural, economic, and educational factors.

A study in rural South India found that 59% of postmenopausal and 38% of premenopausal women experienced reduced sexual desire. Additionally, 54% and 32%, respectively, were not sexually active, while 34% and 24% did not enjoy sex, with some finding it intolerable. Many attributed this to a lack of privacy and the presence of adolescent children, leading to a decline in sexual activity (Aaron et al., 2002). A cross-sectional study in a hospital-based perimenopausal population on McCoy's scoring index confirmed a significant decline in sexual function after menopause in Indian women. The survey also revealed discomfort in discussing sexual issues, highlighting the influence of sociocultural factors (Mundhra et al., 2024). Previous studies have reported reluctance to acknowledge vaginal atrophy and sexual dysfunction, often delaying medical care. However, women often reported feeling relieved when doctors initiated the conversation and offered help. This underscores the need for greater awareness of menopause and sexual and emotional well-being in perimenopausal women (Meeta et al., 2021).

In the Indian context, the experience of menopause is affected by sociocultural factors, where menopause is considered a loss of sense of self associated with grief of losing the reproductive capacity, including childbearing and decreased sexual drive. The Indian multicenter study revealed that there was an association between the symptom profile and socio-demographics of the women. With predominant physical and somatic complaints like multiple-site body aches and cognitive impairment in rural women and more psychological impact like a loss of sense of self in urban women. The coping mechanisms adapted by these women vary as well based on the above details, with urban women found to have better coping due to better access to information, with more concern about the cognition and emotional as well as social changes like "how husband would see her" as reason of worry (Durairaj & Venkateshvaran, 2022; Krishnamoorthy et al., 2018; Sharma & Mahajan, 2015; Singla et al., 2016).

However, today, women are more vocal and aware of menopause, resulting in improved service-seeking behavior. Currently, menopausal care is understudied, with limited studies in India about menopause and mental health implications. However, due to increasing evidence about the role of mood symptoms, stress, and psychological well-being on the physical, vasomotor symptoms and gynecological symptoms and treatment-seeking more research needs to be encouraged focusing on the multidisciplinary approach to promote good quality care and empowering women for navigating this transition with resilience and grace.

8 Violence Against Women

Gender-based Violence against women is one of the common evils in the community, affecting women across the globe. Violence is defined as "any action causing physical, sexual, or mental harm to women, including threats, coercion, or unjust deprivation of liberty, whether in public or private settings" (Declaration on the Elimination of Violence against Women, United Nations General Assembly, 1993). Additional behaviors included in DV in India are honor killings, unwarranted dowry demands, and related harassment by husband and/or in-laws (Sabri & Young, 2022). As per WHO, around 1 in 3 women experience some form of violence (Declaration on the Elimination of Violence against Women, United Nations General Assembly,

1993). Violence during critical reproductive periods can have long-lasting effects, contributing to complications like unwanted pregnancies, unsafe abortions, sexually transmitted infections (STIs), and postpartum depression. This chapter explores the intricate relationship between violence against women and reproductive mental health in India, highlighting the socio-cultural determinants, psychological consequences, and the need for a multidisciplinary approach to intervention. It aims to shed light on the systemic challenges and propose strategies for prevention, support, and policy reform to protect and empower women.

As per the fifth National Family Health Survey round 2019–2021, the weighted prevalence of domestic violence in India is estimated to be 31.2% (International Institute for Population Sciences (IIPS) & ICF, 2021). With the proportion of 28.5%, 13.1%, and 5.7% of women reporting experiences of physical, emotional, and sexual violence, respectively. The findings from the survey were interesting, showing socio-cultural influence on the incidence of DV across the country. Decrease in rates of DV with an increase in educational levels, higher chances of DV in working women, rural regions, lower socio-economic states, and those with a history of substance use in spouse (Sabri et al., 2014).

A survey done in urban slums revealed that earlier age of marriage, working status, violence being justified by the wife, and the husband's use of alcohol were significantly associated with domestic violence. In India, cultural aspects like dowry, witnessing violence as a child, higher population, forced sex, gender roles, normalization of violence, and media portrayal play a role in the perpetuation of violence (Campbell & Sabri, 2015). Despite such high prevalence, due to the perception of DV and cultural aspects, DV has been minimized to "social crime" and labeled as a private matter by law enforcers and policymakers. Based on a systematic review, protective factors were identified; at the sociocultural and community levels were better gender equality and social support. At the interpersonal/relationship level, empowerment, financial control, access to an account, and involvement in decision-making. At the individual level, higher education, >18 years of age at marriage, sexual and financial autonomy, and freedom of movement and employment (Donta et al., 2015; Jeyaseelan et al., 2007; Martin et al., 1999; Vindhya, 2000).

Reproduction is an important event associated with the status of women in Indian society; adverse reproductive experiences, like child death or unwanted pregnancy, were associated with an increased risk of intimate partner violence, while positive reproductive experiences like having a first child were associated with a lower risk of initiation and continuation of violence. There have been conflicting results on the risk of violence and gender preference for male children. Studies show a higher risk of physical and sexual violence and loss of autonomy with higher birth orders. There is a higher proportion of sterilization in women experiencing DV (Abraham, 2000; Dalal & Lindqvist, 2012; Niaz, 2003; Nigam, 2016; Pandey et al., 2009; Sabri et al., 2014).

Based on a community study, nearly 95% of women facing physical violence exhibited symptoms of depression on the DASS-21 scale. Additionally, 80% reported anxiety, and nearly 94% suffered from some form of psychological distress. Post-traumatic stress disorder (PTSD) was observed in 68.8% of women.

Another study revealed that a history of sexual violence in the past 1 year was significantly related to unhealthy mental status (OR 3.11, 95% CI 2.04–4.74) and suicidal thoughts (OR 14.89, 95% CI 6.91–32.05). A hospital survey in Bangalore reported that sexual coercion correlated positively ($r = 0.39$) with PTSD severity (Chandra et al., 2009; Das Gupta & Mari Bhat, 1997; Jejeebhoy, 1998; Nigam, 2016; Sabarwal et al., 2012; Sathe et al., 2024; Sharma et al., 2019; Weitzman, 2020).

Due to its high prevalence, domestic and intimate partner violence demands early identification and timely interventions. A pilot study in Pune evaluated "Ghya Bharari Ekatra (GBE)," a couples-based primary prevention intervention among newly married couples, and showed a decrease in rates of psychological abuse in the study group (Kalokhe et al., 2021). Other promising interventions that showed significant positive outcomes for future violence were *Counselling Men to Achieve Reproductive Health and Marital Equality* (*CHARM*), *Raising HIV Awareness in Non-HIV-Infected Indian Wives (RHANI)* wives' intervention, a sexual risk reduction intervention for couples, an individual and couples-based intervention for IPV, contraceptive use, and a community mobilization intervention (Saggurti et al., 2014).

A systematic review showed the effective components of integrated domestic violence (DV) and reproductive health interventions include:

(a) **Psychoeducation/Education**: Raising awareness to challenge gender-inequitable norms, promoting understanding of the health impacts of DV, and providing strategies for safety and prevention. (b) **Skill-Building**: Developing various competencies to enhance coping and resilience. (c) **Engaging Male Spouses**: Involving partners in the intervention to foster supportive relationships. (d) **Counseling**: Offering information, emotional support, and crisis intervention. (e) **Engaging Stakeholders**: Collaborating with healthcare providers, law enforcement, and other key figures. (f) **Using Trained Lay Peer Facilitators**: Utilizing community-based facilitators for outreach and support.

Additionally, integrated health components—such as education on sexual negotiation, communication, decision-making, and addressing alcohol misuse—may have contributed to addressing intimate partner violence (IPV) due to the interconnected nature of these issues in relationships (Donta et al., 2015; Jones et al., 2013; Sabri et al., 2024).

STREE MANORAKSHA is a recently launched initiative aimed at integrating training and supervision in psychosocial and mental health care for One Stop Centre (OSC) staff to support women facing violence. Implemented by the National Institute of Mental Health and Neurosciences (NIMHANS), Bangalore, with funding from the Ministry of Women and Child Development, Government of India, the project seeks to train around 1400 counselors and over 2000 OSC staff in trauma-informed care. By equipping OSC functionaries with the necessary tools and techniques to handle cases sensitively, the initiative aims to enhance the mental health and well-being of women experiencing violence and distress, ensuring they receive compassionate and practical support (Project Stree Manoraksha - NIMHANS STREEMANORAKSHA, 2022).

Despite limited evidence on the efficacy of community-based interventions for reducing intimate partner violence (IPV) in India, existing evaluations show promise. To build on this progress, future initiatives should strengthen the evidence base by leveraging established community health worker (CHW) networks and women's groups, addressing key predictors of IPV victimization and perpetration, and incorporating culturally sensitive assessment tools. Additionally, adopting a community-based participatory framework in the design and evaluation of interventions can enhance their effectiveness and sustainability. By integrating these strategies, efforts to combat IPV and support survivors can become more impactful and contextually relevant.

9 Conclusion

The reproductive health landscape in India is intricately linked with mental health outcomes across various life stages—from menarche and pregnancy to the postpartum period and menopause. Each phase presents unique psychological challenges, often exacerbated by limited awareness, inadequate healthcare infrastructure, and social stigma. Reproductive health issues such as infertility, menstrual disorders, and complications during pregnancy not only impact physical health but also contribute significantly to emotional distress, anxiety, and depression. Moreover, substance use among women—often rooted in trauma, social neglect, or coping with untreated mental health conditions—requires urgent, gender-sensitive interventions. The chapter also emphasizes the pervasive influence of gender-based violence, entrenched socio-cultural norms, and widespread myths and misconceptions, all of which contribute to the marginalization and psychological vulnerability of women. These complex and intersecting factors highlight the critical need for an integrated approach that prioritizes both mental and reproductive health. A comprehensive public health response must include community education, accessible mental health services, and policies that empower women with knowledge and support throughout their reproductive journey. Ultimately, addressing these issues with sensitivity and equity is essential for improving the overall well-being of women and fostering a healthier, more inclusive society.

References

Aaron, R., Muliyil, J., & Abraham, S. (2002). Medico-social dimensions of menopause: A cross-sectional study from rural South India. *The National Medical Journal of India, 15*(1), 14–17.

Abraham, Margaret. (2000). Speaking the unspeakable : marital violence among South Asian immigrants in the United States. 234.

Ambekar, A., Parmar, A., Therthani, S., & Mandal, P. (2017). Profile of women substance users seeking treatment at tertiary care treatment center in India: A retrospective chart review study. *Journal of Substance Use, 22*(5), 507–510. https://doi.org/10.1080/14659891.2016.1255792

Ambika, A. (2025). Prevalence of depressive symptoms among women who had hysterectomy in India: Evidence from Lasi. *International Journal of Indian Psychology*. https://doi.org/10.25215/1301.133

Annajigowda, H. H., Nirisha, L. P., Ganjekar, S., Rao, G. N., Gururaj, G., Varghese, M., & Benegal, V. (2023). Common mental disorders among women in reproductive age group: An analysis of national mental health survey, India 2016. *Indian Journal of Psychiatry, 65*(12), 1238. https://doi.org/10.4103/INDIANJPSYCHIATRY.INDIANJPSYCHIATRY_832_23

Ashutosh, C., Radhika, B., Hema, T., Mrigaya, S., Sudhindra, C., & Narsimha, S. P. S. V. (2010). Alcohol dependence syndrome in women: An Indian perspective. *International Psychiatry, 7*(1), 15. https://doi.org/10.1192/s1749367600000953

Aujla, S., Sandeep, M., Aparnavi, P., Padhi, B. K., Shamim, M. A., Sahoo, S., Gangane, N., & Gandhi, A. P. (2024). Effect of maternal obsessive-c disorder (OCD) on feto-maternal outcomes: A systematic review and meta-analysis. *International Journal of Gynecology & Obstetrics, 167*(3), 949–956. https://doi.org/10.1002/IJGO.15792

Aziz, S., Kelkar, P., Chaudhury, S., & Saldanha, D. (2024). Prevalence of psychiatric morbidity and somatic symptoms in perimenopausal women. *Medical Journal of Dr. D.Y. Patil Vidyapeeth, 17*(3), 580–586. https://doi.org/10.4103/mjdrdypu.mjdrdypu_1090_22

Babu, G., Subbakrishna, D., & Chandra, P. (2008). Prevalence and correlates of suicidality among Indian women with post-partum psychosis in an inpatient setting. *The Australian and New Zealand Journal of Psychiatry, 42*(11), 976–980. https://doi.org/10.1080/00048670802415384

Bagadia, A., Nanjundaswamy, M. H., Ganjekar, S., Thippeswamy, H., Desai, G., & Chandra, P. S. (2020). Factors influencing decision-making around pregnancy among women with severe mental illness (SMI): A qualitative study. *International Journal of Social Psychiatry, 66*(8), 792–798. https://doi.org/10.1177/0020764020925104

Balaji, S., Amadi, C., Prasad, S., Bala Kasav, J., Upadhyay, V., Singh, A. K., Surapaneni, K. M., & Joshi, A. (2015). Urban rural comparisons of polycystic ovary syndrome burden among adolescent girls in a hospital setting in India. *BioMed Research International, 2015*. https://doi.org/10.1155/2015/158951

Bansal, D., Raman, R., & Rao, T. S. S. (2019). Premenstrual dysphoric disorder: Ranking the symptoms and severity in Indian college students. *Journal of Psychosexual Health, 1*(2):159–163. https://doi.org/10.1177/2631831819827183

Bharadwaj, B., Endumathi, R., Parial, S., & Chandra, P. (2022). Management of psychiatric disorders during the perinatal period. *Indian Journal of Psychiatry, 64*(8), S414–S428. https://doi.org/10.4103/INDIANJPSYCHIATRY.INDIANJPSYCHIATRY_12_22

Bhatia, M. S., Kaur, N., Bohra, N., & Goyai, U. (1990). Psychiatric reactions in hysterectomy. *Indian Journal of Psychiatry, 32*(1), 52. https://pmc.ncbi.nlm.nih.gov/articles/PMC2989570/

Bhatia, S. C., & Bhatia, S. K. (2002). Diagnosis and treatment of premenstrual dysphoric disorder. *American Family Physician, 66*(7), 1239–1249. https://www.aafp.org/pubs/afp/issues/2002/1001/p1239.html

Bhattacharya, S. M., & Jha, A. (2010). Prevalence and risk of depressive disorders in women with polycystic ovary syndrome (PCOS). *Fertility and Sterility, 94*(1), 357–359. https://doi.org/10.1016/J.FERTNSTERT.2009.09.025

Brockington, I. F. (2007). Cerebral vascular disease as a cause of postpartum psychosis. *Archives of Women's Mental Health, 10*(4), 177–178. https://doi.org/10.1007/S00737-007-0187-7

Burger, H. G. (1996). The endocrinology of the menopause. *Maturitas, 23*(2), 129–136. https://doi.org/10.1016/0378-5122(95)00969-8

Campbell, J., & Sabri, B. (2015). Intimate partner violence against women in slums in India. *Indian Journal of Medical Research, 141*(6), 757. https://doi.org/10.4103/0971-5916.160693

Carlini, S. V., Di Scalea, T. L., McNally, S. T., Lester, J., & Deligiannidis, K. M. (2022). Management of premenstrual dysphoric disorder: A scoping review. *International Journal of Women's Health, 14*, 1783–1801. https://doi.org/10.2147/IJWH.S297062

Chandra, P. S. (2001). The interface between psychiatry and women's reproductive and sexual health. *Indian Journal of Psychiatry, 43*(4), 295–305.

Chandra, P. S., Bajaj, A., Desai, G., Satyanarayana, V. A., Sharp, H. M., Ganjekar, S., Supraja, T. A., Jangam, K. V., Venkatram, L., & Kandavel, T. (2021). Anxiety and depressive symptoms in pregnancy predict low birth weight differentially in male and female infants-findings from an urban pregnancy cohort in India. *Social Psychiatry and Psychiatric Epidemiology, 56*(12), 2263–2274. https://doi.org/10.1007/S00127-021-02106-9

Chandra, P. S., Chaturvedi, S. K., & Gururaj, G. (1994). Identification and assessment of premenstrual symptoms and syndromes in women: An epidemiological approach to investigation. *NIMHANS Journal, 12*(1), 1–8. https://psycnet.apa.org/record/1995-29808-001

Chandra, P. S., Desai, G., Reddy, D., Thippeswamy, H., & Saraf, G. (2015). The establishment of a mother-baby inpatient psychiatry unit in India: Adaptation of a Western model to meet local cultural and resource needs. *Indian Journal of Psychiatry, 57*(3), 290–294. https://doi.org/10.4103/0019-5545.166621

Chandra, P. S., Satyanarayana, V. A., & Carey, M. P. (2009). Women reporting intimate partner violence in India: Associations with PTSD and depressive symptoms. *Archives of Women's Mental Health, 12*(4), 203–209. https://doi.org/10.1007/S00737-009-0065-6

Chandra, P. S., Venkatasubramanian, G., & Thomas, T. (2002). Infanticidal ideas and infanticidal behavior in Indian women with severe postpartum psychiatric disorders. *The Journal of Nervous and Mental Disease, 190*(7), 457–461. https://doi.org/10.1097/00005053-200207000-00006

Chaturvedi, H. K., Mahanta, J., Bajpai, R. C., & Pandey, A. (2013). Correlates of opium use: Retrospective analysis of a survey of tribal communities in Arunachal Pradesh, India. *BMC Public Health, 13*(1). https://doi.org/10.1186/1471-2458-13-325

Chaturvedi, S. K., & Chandra, P. S. (1990). Stress-protective functions of positive experiences during the premenstrual period. *Stress Medicine, 6*, 53–55. https://doi.org/10.1002/smi.2460060111

Chaturvedi, S. K., & Chandra, P. S. (1991). Sociocultural aspects of menstrual attitudes and premenstrual experiences in India. *Social Science and Medicine, 32*(3), 349–351. https://doi.org/10.1016/0277-9536(91)90114-r

Chaturvedi, S. K., Chandra, P. S., Issac, M. K., & Sudarshan, C. Y. (1993). Somatization misattributed to non-pathological vaginal discharge. *Journal of Psychosomatic Research, 37*(6), 575–579. https://doi.org/10.1016/0022-3999(93)90051-G

Chaudhari, A. P., Mazumdar, K., & Mehta, P. D. (2018). Anxiety, depression, and quality of life in women with polycystic ovarian syndrome. *Indian Journal of Psychological Medicine, 40*(3), 239. https://doi.org/10.4103/IJPSYM.IJPSYM_561_17

Cutler, R. B., & Fishbain, D. A. (2005). Are alcoholism treatments effective? The project MATCH data. *BMC Public Health, 5*. https://doi.org/10.1186/1471-2458-5-75

Dalal, K., & Lindqvist, K. (2012). A national study of the prevalence and correlates of domestic violence among women in India. *Asia-Pacific Journal of Public Health, 24*(2), 265–277. https://doi.org/10.1177/1010539510384499

Das Gupta, M., & Mari Bhat, P. N. (1997). Fertility decline and increased manifestation of sex bias in India. *Population Studies, 51*(3), 307–315. https://doi.org/10.1080/0032472031000150076

Das, M. K., Arora, N. K., Gaikwad, H., Chellani, H., Debata, P., Rasaily, R., Meena, K. R., Kaur, G., Malik, P., Joshi, S., & Kumari, M. (2021). Grief reaction and psychosocial impacts of child death and stillbirth on bereaved north Indian parents: A qualitative study. *PLoS One, 16*(1). https://doi.org/10.1371/JOURNAL.PONE.0240270

Davoudian, T., Gibbins, K., & Cirino, N. H. (2021). Perinatal loss: The impact on maternal mental health. *Obstetrical & Gynecological Survey, 76*(4), 223–233. https://doi.org/10.1097/OGX.0000000000000874

Dayal, P., Sarkar, S., Pal, Y., & Balhara, S. (2017). Predictors of inpatient treatment completion among females with opioid use disorder: Findings from a tertiary care drug dependence treatment centre of India. *Indian Journal of Psychological Medicine, 39*(4), 464–468. https://doi.org/10.4103/0253-7176.211769

Desai, G., & Chandra, P. (2023). Perinatal mental health in India: Time to deliver! *Journal of Psychiatry Spectrum, 2*(1), 1. https://doi.org/10.4103/JOPSYS.JOPSYS_3_23

Dhir, D., Kumari, S., Devi, V., Chaudhary, V., Murti, K., Dhingra, S., Yanadaiah, P., & Pal, B. (2025). Prevalence of tobacco and alcohol use among pregnant women in India: A systematic review and meta-analysis. *Journal of Substance Use*. https://doi.org/10.1080/14659891.2024.2448806

Dogra, T. D., Leenaars, A. A., Raintji, R., Lalwani, S., Girdhar, S., Wenckstern, S., & Lester, D. (2007). Menstruation and suicide: An exploratory study. *Psychological Reports, 101*(2), 430–434. https://doi.org/10.2466/PR0.101.2.430-434

Donta, B., Nair, S., Prakasam, C., & Begum, S. (2015). Socio-demographic factors associated with domestic violence in urban slums, Mumbai, Maharashtra, India. *Indian Journal of Medical Research, 141*(6), 783. https://doi.org/10.4103/0971-5916.160701

Durairaj, A., & Ramamurthi, R. (2019). Prevalence, pattern and predictors of premenstrual syndrome (PMS) and premenstrual dysphoric disorder (PMDD) among college girls. *New Indian Journal of OBGYN, 5*(2), 93–98. https://doi.org/10.21276/obgyn.2019.5.2.6

Durairaj, A., & Venkateshvaran, S. (2022). Determinants of menopausal symptoms and attitude towards menopause among midlife women: A cross-sectional study in South India. *Cureus*. https://doi.org/10.7759/cureus.28718

Dutta, A., & Sharma, A. (2021). Prevalence of premenstrual syndrome and premenstrual dysphoric disorder in India: A systematic review and meta-analysis. *Health Promotion Perspectives, 11*(2), 161–170. https://doi.org/10.34172/HPP.2021.20

Easwaran, V., Orayj, K., Goruntla, N., Mekala, J. S., Bommireddy, B. R., Mopuri, B., Mantargi, M. J. S., Bhupalam, P., Thammisetty, D. P., & Bandaru, V. (2025). Depression, anxiety, and stress among HIV-positive pregnant women during the COVID-19 pandemic: A hospital-based cross-sectional study in India. *BMC Pregnancy and Childbirth, 25*(1), 1–17. https://doi.org/10.1186/S12884-025-07261-4/TABLES/4

Ewerling, F., McDougal, L., Raj, A., Ferreira, L. Z., Blumenberg, C., Parmar, D., & Barros, A. J. D. (2021). Modern contraceptive use among women in need of family planning in India: An analysis of the inequalities related to the mix of methods used. *Reproductive Health, 18*(1), 1–12. https://doi.org/10.1186/S12978-021-01220-W/TABLES/2

Fisher, J., de Mello, M. C., Patel, V., Rahman, A., Tran, T., Holton, S., & Holmesf, W. (2012). Prevalence and determinants of common perinatal mental disorders in women in low- and lower-middle-income countries: A systematic review. *Bulletin of the World Health Organization, 90*(2), 139–149. https://doi.org/10.2471/BLT.11.091850

Frezza, M., di Padova, C., Pozzato, G., Terpin, M., Baraona, E., & Lieber, C. S. (1990). High blood alcohol levels in women. The role of decreased gastric alcohol dehydrogenase activity and first-pass metabolism. *The New England Journal of Medicine*, 322(2), 95–99. https://doi.org/10.1056/NEJM199001113220205

Gururaj, G, & Varghese, M. (2016). *National mental health survey*. https://indianmhs.nimhans.ac.in/phase1/nmhs-results.php.

Ganjekar, S., Desai, G., & Chandra, P. S. (2013). A comparative study of psychopathology, symptom severity, and short-term outcome of postpartum and nonpostpartum mania. *Bipolar Disorders, 15*(6), 713–718. https://doi.org/10.1111/bdi.12076

Ganjekar, S., Prakash, A., Thippeswamy, H., Desai, G., & Chandra, P. S. (2020). The NIMHANS (National Institute of Mental Health and Neuro Sciences) Maternal Behaviour Scale (NIMBUS): Development and validation of a scale for assessment of maternal behaviour among mothers with postpartum severe mental illness in low resource settings. *Asian Journal of Psychiatry, 47*. https://doi.org/10.1016/J.AJP.2019.101872

Garg, S., & Anand, T. (2015). Menstruation related myths in India: Strategies for combating it. *Journal of Family Medicine and Primary Care, 4*(2), 184. https://doi.org/10.4103/2249-4863.154627

Gautham, M. S., Gururaj, G., Varghese, M., Benegal, V., Rao, G. N., Kokane, A., Chavan, B. S., Dalal, P. K., Ram, D., Pathak, K., Lenin Singh, R. K., Singh, L. K., Sharma, P., Saha, P. K., Ramasubramanian, C., Mehta, R. Y., Shibukumar, T. M., Deuri, S. P., Krishnatreya, M., et al. (2020). The National Mental Health Survey of India (2016): Prevalence, socio-demographic correlates and treatment gap of mental morbidity. *The International Journal of Social Psychiatry, 66*(4), 361–372. https://doi.org/10.1177/0020764020907941

Ghosh, A., Verma, A., Choudhury, S., & Dhawan, P. (2025). Regional disparities and correlates of alcohol use during pregnancy in India: Insights from the National Family Health Survey-5. *Drug and Alcohol Review, 44*(2), 576–587. https://doi.org/10.1111/DAR.13995

Greenfield, S. F., Brooks, A. J., Gordon, S. M., Green, C. A., Kropp, F., McHugh, R. K., Lincoln, M., Hien, D., & Miele, G. M. (2007). Substance abuse treatment entry, retention, and outcome in women: A review of the literature. *Drug and Alcohol Dependence, 86*(1), 1–21. https://doi.org/10.1016/J.DRUGALCDEP.2006.05.012

Grover, S., Avasthi, A., Gupta, S., Hazari, N., & Malhotra, N. (2016). Do female patients with nonpathological vaginal discharge need the same evaluation as for Dhat syndrome in males? *Indian Journal of Psychiatry, 58*(1), 61. https://doi.org/10.4103/0019-5545.174376

Grover, S., Kate, N., Avasthi, A., Rajpal, N., & Umamaheswari, V. (2014). Females too suffer from Dhat syndrome: A case series and revisit of the concept. *Indian Journal of Psychiatry, 56*(4), 388–392. https://doi.org/10.4103/0019-5545.146537

Grover, S., Sahoo, S., Chakrabarti, S., Basu, D., Singh, S. M., & Avasthi, A. (2018). ECT in the postpartum period: A retrospective case series from a tertiary health care center in India. *Indian Journal of Psychological Medicine, 40*(6), 562. https://doi.org/10.4103/IJPSYM.IJPSYM_105_18

Gupta, J., Raj, A., Decker, M. R., Reed, E., & Silverman, J. G. (2009). HIV vulnerabilities of sex-trafficked Indian women and girls. *International Journal of Gynaecology and Obstetrics: The Official Organ of the International Federation of Gynaecology and Obstetrics, 107*(1), 30–34. https://doi.org/10.1016/J.IJGO.2009.06.009

Habib, S., Anwar, A., Hoda, F., Verma, R., Akhtar, M., & Najmi, A. K. (2021). Prevalence of depression, anxiety and quality of life among north Indian polycystic ovary syndrome women: Evidence from a prospective observational study. *International Journal of Basic & Clinical Pharmacology, 10*(12), 1360–1367. https://doi.org/10.18203/2319-2003.IJBCP20214500

Handy, A. B., Greenfield, S. F., Yonkers, K. A., & Payne, L. A. (2022). Psychiatric symptoms across the menstrual cycle in adult women: A comprehensive review. *Harvard Review of Psychiatry, 30*(2), 100. https://doi.org/10.1097/HRP.0000000000000329

Harsha, G. T., & Acharya, M. S. (2019). Trajectory of perinatal mental health in India. In *Indian Journal of Social Psychiatry* (Vol. 35, pp. 47–54). Wolters Kluwer Medknow Publications. https://doi.org/10.4103/ijsp.ijsp_30_18

Hebel, T., Schecklmann, M., & Langguth, B. (2020). Transcranial magnetic stimulation in the treatment of depression during pregnancy: A review. *Archives of Women's Mental Health, 23*(4), 469–478. https://doi.org/10.1007/S00737-019-01004-Z

Hussain, A., Chandel, R., Ganie, M. A., Dar, M., Rather, Y., Wani, Z., Shiekh, J., & Shah, M. (2015). Prevalence of psychiatric disorders in patients with a diagnosis of polycystic ovary syndrome in kashmir. *Indian Journal of Psychological Medicine, 37*(1), 66–70. https://doi.org/10.4103/0253-7176.150822

International Institute for Population Sciences (IIPS) & ICF (2021). National Family Health Survey (NFHS-5), 2019-21: India: Volume 1. Mumbai: IIPS.. https://mohfw.gov.in/sites/default/files/NFHS-5_Phase-II_0.pdf.

Jagtap, A., Jagtap, B., Jagtap, R., Lamture, Y., & Gomase, K. (2023). Effects of prenatal stress on behavior, cognition, and psychopathology: A comprehensive review. *Cureus, 15*(10), e47044. https://doi.org/10.7759/CUREUS.47044

Jai Prakash, I., Vinoda, N., & Murthy, P. D. (1981). Psychiatric morbidity and the menopause. *Indian Journal of Psychiatry, 23*(3), 242.

Jain, P., Kumar Tiwari, G., Awasthi, I., & Chaubey, A. (2018). Menstrual experiences of adolescent girls: A qualitative study. *International Journal of Indian Psychology, 6*(1). https://doi.org/10.25215/0601.087

Jain, R., & Muralidhar, S. (2020). A detail study on contraceptives and its status in India. *IOSR Journal of Pharmacy And Biological Sciences (IOSR-JPBS), 15*(5), 1–16. https://doi.org/10.9790/3008-1505010116

Jejeebhoy, S. J. (1998). Wife-beating in rural India: A husband's right? Evidence from survey data. *Economic and Political Weekly, 33*(15) http://www.jstor.org/stable/4406642

Jeyaseelan, L., Kumar, S., Neelakantan, N., Peedicayil, A., Pillai, R., & Duvvury, N. (2007). Physical spousal violence against women in India: Some risk factors. *Journal of Biosocial Science, 39*(5), 657–670. https://doi.org/10.1017/S0021932007001836

Jones, D., Bagga, R., Nehra, R., Deepika, S. S., Walia, K., Kumar, M., Villar-Loubet, O., Lopez, M., & Weiss, S. M. (2013). Reducing sexual risk behavior among high-risk couples in northern India. *International Journal of Behavioral Medicine, 20*(3), 344–354. https://doi.org/10.1007/S12529-012-9235-4

Joshi, S., Tripathi, A., Agarwal, S., Singh, N., Gupta, B., Nischal, A., & Kar, S. K. (2022). Phenomenology, disability and sexual functioning in female Dhat syndrome: A study of tertiary care gynaecology outpatients. *General Psychiatry, 35*(5), e100863. https://doi.org/10.1136/gpsych-2022-100863

Jyothi Kantipudi, S., Kannan, G. K., Viswanathan, S., Ranganathan, S., Menon, J., & Ramanathan, S. (2020). Antenatal depression and generalized anxiety disorder in a tertiary Hospital in South India. *Indian Journal of Psychological Medicine, 42*(6), 513–518. https://doi.org/10.1177/0253717620928440

Kalokhe, A. S., Iyer, S., Gadhe, K., Katendra, T., Kolhe, A., Rahane, G., Stephenson, R., & Sahay, S. (2021). A couples-based intervention (Ghya Bharari Ekatra) for the primary prevention of intimate partner violence in India: Pilot feasibility and acceptability study. *JMIR Formative Research, 5*(2). https://doi.org/10.2196/26130

Kalra, H., Tran, T. D., Romero, L., Chandra, P., & Fisher, J. (2021). Prevalence and determinants of antenatal common mental disorders among women in India: A systematic review and meta-analysis. *Archives of Women's Mental Health, 24*(1), 29–53. https://doi.org/10.1007/S00737-020-01024-0

Kanagarajan, S., Varshney, P., Ganjekar, S., Muralidhar, A., & Desai, G. (2023). Psychiatric comorbidities among Indian women with polycystic ovary syndrome: A scoping review. *Journal of Psychiatry Spectrum, 2*(1), 7. https://doi.org/10.4103/JOPSYS.JOPSYS_30_22

Kandhasamy, S., Lepigeon, K., Baggio, S., Céline, R., Ceulemans, M., Winterfeld, U., Jenkinson, S. P., Francini, K., Maisonneuve, E., & Panchaud, A. (2025). Risk of adverse obstetrical and neonatal outcomes in women consuming recreational drugs during pregnancy. *BMC Pregnancy and Childbirth, 25*(1), 1–15. https://doi.org/10.1186/S12884-024-07062-1

Kendler, K. S., & Prescott, C. A. (1998a). Cannabis use, abuse, and dependence in a population-based sample of female twins. *The American Journal of Psychiatry, 155*(8), 1016–1022. https://doi.org/10.1176/AJP.155.8.1016

Kendler, K. S., & Prescott, C. A. (1998b). Cocaine use, abuse and dependence in a population-based sample of female twins. *The British Journal of Psychiatry: The Journal of Mental Science, 173*(OCT.), 345–350. https://doi.org/10.1192/BJP.173.4.345

Kessler, R. C. (2003). Epidemiology of women and depression. *Journal of Affective Disorders, 74*(1), 5–13. https://doi.org/10.1016/S0165-0327(02)00426-3

Krishnamoorthy, Y., Sarveswaran, G., Jayaseelan, V., Sakthivel, M., Arivarasan, Y., & Bharathnag, N. (2018). Assessment of quality of life based on psychological, somatovegetative, and urogenital health problems among postmenopausal women in urban Puducherry, South India: A cross-sectional observational study. *Journal of Mid-Life Health, 9*(4), 173. https://doi.org/10.4103/jmh.JMH_61_18

Kulkarni, J. (1997). Women and schizophrenia: A review. *Australian & New Zealand Journal of Psychiatry, 31*(1), 46–56. https://doi.org/10.3109/00048679709073798

Kumar, M. S., & Sharma, M. (2008). Women and substance use in India and Bangladesh. *Substance Use & Misuse, 43*(8–9), 1062–1077. https://doi.org/10.1080/10826080801918189

Kumar, S., Srivastava, A., Sharma, S., Yadav, V., Mittal, A., Kim, Y. M., Nash-Mercado, A., Reijneveld, S. A., & Sood, B. (2019). One year continuation of post-partum intrauterine contraceptive device: Findings from a retrospective cohort study in India. *Contraception, 99*(4), 212–216. https://doi.org/10.1016/J.CONTRACEPTION.2018.12.003

Louis, F., Yelwatkar, S., Sathe, H., & Karia, S. (2024). Psychosis as initial clinical presentation for cerebral venous thrombosis: A case report. *Indian Journal of Private Psychiatry, 18*(1), 39–41. https://doi.org/10.5005/jp-journals-10067-0144

Madge, V. (2011). Infertility, women and assisted reproductive technologies. *Indian Journal of Gender Studies, 18*(1), 1–26. https://doi.org/10.1177/097152151001800101

Mahapatro, F., & Parkar, S. (2005). A comparative study of coping skills and body image: Mastectomized vs. lumpectomized patients with breast carcinoma. *Indian Journal of Psychiatry, 47*(4), 198. https://doi.org/10.4103/0019-5545.43051

Malik, K., Benegal, V., Murthy, P., Chand, P., & Suman, L. N. (2015). Clinical audit of women with substance use disorders: Findings and implications. *Indian Journal of Psychological Medicine, 37*(2). https://doi.org/10.4103/0253-7176.155620

Malik, K., Chand, K., Marimuthu, P., & Suman, L. N. (2017a). Stressful and traumatic experiences among women with alcohol use disorders in India. *Indian Journal of Psychological Medicine, 39*(5), 611–618. https://doi.org/10.4103/IJPSYM.IJPSYM_411_16

Malik, K., Chand, P. K., Marimuthu, P., & Suman, L. N. (2017b). Addiction severity and comorbidity among women with alcohol use disorders: A hospital-based study from India. *Asian Journal of Psychiatry, 28*, 67–72. https://doi.org/10.1016/J.AJP.2017.03.028

Maliszewska, B., Tokarzewska, A., Łasica, M., Małyszek, M., Łaba, Ł., Dziurda, S., Łomża-Łaba, A. W., & Łuczyński, D. (2024). Psychiatric disorders in women with polycystic ovary syndrome. *Journal of Pre-Clinical and Clinical Research*. https://doi.org/10.26444/JPCCR/192128

Malyam, V., Gopalkrishna, V., Parameshwaraiah, S. T., Sannappa, A. C., & Bhaskara, A. (2020). Anxiety and psychological aspects of hysterectomy-A prospective study. *International Journal of Indian Psychology, 8*(2), 340–349. https://doi.org/10.25215/0802.041

Mandal, P., Parmar, A., Ambekar, A., & Dhawan, A. (2019). Substance use among treatment seeking Indian adolescent girls: Are they unique? *Asian Journal of Psychiatry, 41*, 17–19. https://doi.org/10.1016/J.AJP.2019.03.007

Martin, S. L., Tsui, A. O., Maitra, K., & Marinshaw, R. (1999). Domestic violence in northern India. *American Journal of Epidemiology, 150*(4), 417–426. https://doi.org/10.1093/OXFORDJOURNALS.AJE.A010021

Mathur, G. (2018). Psychological well-being, marital adjustment and quality of life after hysterectomy: A comparative study. *International Journal of Reprod Contracept Obstetrics and Gynecology, 7*(12), 4960–4965. https://doi.org/10.18203/2320-1770.ijrcog20184948

Meeta, M., Majumdar, S., Tanvir, T., Sharma, S., Shah, J., Aggarwal, N., Olayi, R., Ahuja, M., & Joshi, S. A. (2021). Effects of menopause on sexual function in Indian women. *Journal of Mid-Life Health, 12*(2), 144–154. https://doi.org/10.4103/jmh.jmh_95_21

Mishra, A., Banwari, G., & Yadav, P. (2015). Premenstrual dysphoric disorder in medical students residing in hostel and its association with lifestyle factors. *Industrial Psychiatry Journal, 24*(2), 150. https://doi.org/10.4103/0972-6748.181718

Ministry of Social Justice and Empowerment, Government of India & United Nations Office on Drugs and Crime, Regional Office for South Asia. Rapid assessment survey of drug abuse in India (2002). Retrieved from https://www.unodc.org/pdf/india/RAS.pdf

Modzelewski, S., Oracz, A., Żukow, X., Iłendo, K., Śledzikowka, Z., & Waszkiewicz, N. (2024). Premenstrual syndrome: New insights into etiology and review of treatment methods. *Frontiers in Psychiatry, 15*, 1363875. https://doi.org/10.3389/FPSYT.2024.1363875

Mundhra, R., Bahadur, A., Khoiwal, K., Kumar, M., Chhetri, S. S., & Chaturvedi, J. (2024). Female sexuality across the menopausal age group: A cross sectional study. *European Journal of Obstetrics & Gynecology and Reproductive Biology: X, 21*, 100287. https://doi.org/10.1016/j.eurox.2024.100287

Murthy, N. V., Benegal, V., & Murthy, P. (1995). Murthy, N. V., Benegal, V., & Murthy, P. (1995). Alcohol dependent females: A clinical profile. In scientific papers presented at the 47th annual national conference of the Indian Psychiatric Society. Indian J Psychiatry (Vol. 37, No. 2).

Muttreja, P., & Singh, S. (2018). Family planning in India: The way forward. *The Indian Journal of Medical Research, 148*(Suppl), 1–9. https://doi.org/10.4103/IJMR.IJMR_2067_17

Nagda, A. L., Datar, M. C., Naphade, N. M., & Shetty, J. V. (2023). A cross-sectional assessment of depression, anxiety, and cognition in perimenopausal and menopausal women. *Journal of Mid-Life Health, 14*(2), 117–122. https://doi.org/10.4103/JMH.JMH_34_23

Nahar, A., Kondapuram, N., Desai, G., & Chandra, P. S. (2017). Catatonia among women with postpartum psychosis in a mother-baby inpatient psychiatry unit. *General Hospital Psychiatry, 45*, 40–43. https://doi.org/10.1016/J.GENHOSPPSYCH.2016.12.010

Nanjundaswamy, M. H., Varshney, P., Thanki, M. V., Arunya, B., Rai, V., Mehta, U. M., Arumugham, S. S., Sudhir, P. M., & Chandra, P. S. (2019). Theta burst stimulation for tokophobia during pregnancy. *Brain Stimulation, 12*(5), 1322–1324. https://doi.org/10.1016/j.brs.2019.06.018

Narayan, S., Kishore, M. T., Satyanarayana, V., Bhaskarapillai, B., Desai, G., & Chandra, P. (2023). Bonding and infants' development and quality of life: A study among mothers with severe mental illnesses in remission. *Indian Journal of Psychological Medicine, 45*(3), 250–256. https://doi.org/10.1177/02537176231164732

Nath, A., Venkatesh, S., Balan, S., Metgud, C. S., Krishna, M., Venkata, G., & Murthy, S. (2019). The prevalence and determinants of pregnancy-related anxiety amongst pregnant women at less than 24 weeks of pregnancy in Bangalore, southern India. *International Journal of Women's Health, 11*, 241. https://doi.org/10.2147/IJWH.S193306

Nattala, P., Murthy, P., Thennarasu, K., & Cottler, L. (2014). Nonmedical use of sedatives in urban Bengaluru. *Indian Journal of Psychiatry, 56*(3), 246. https://doi.org/10.4103/0019-5545.140619

Nayak, R., Murthy, P., Girimaji, S., & Navaneetham, J. (2012). Fetal alcohol spectrum disorders—a case-control study from India. *Journal of Tropical Pediatrics, 58*(1), 19–24. https://doi.org/10.1093/TROPEJ/FMR015

Nebhinani, N., Sarkar, S., Gupta, S., Mattoo, S. K., & Basu, D. (2013). Demographic and clinical profile of substance abusing women seeking treatment at a de-addiction center in North India. *Industrial Psychiatry Journal, 22*(1), 12. https://doi.org/10.4103/0972-6748.123587

Niaz, U. (2003). Violence against women in south Asian countries. *Archives of Women's Mental Health, 6*(3), 173–184. https://doi.org/10.1007/S00737-003-0171-9

Nigam, S. (2016). Is domestic violence a lesser crime? Countering the backlash against section 498A, IPC. *SSRN Electronic Journal*. https://doi.org/10.2139/SSRN.2876041

NIMHANS Stree Manoraksha. (2025). Project Stree Manoraksha. Retrieved August 7, 2025, from https://nimhansstreemanoraksha.in/project-stree-manoraksha/.

Office of the Registrar General & Census Commissioner, India. (2020). Sample registration system statistical report 2020 [SRS_STAT_2020]. Ministry of Home Affairs, Government of India. https://censusindia.gov.in/nada/index.php/catalog/44376

Pandey, G. K., Dutt, D., & Banerjee, B. (2009). Partner and relationship factors in domestic violence: Perspectives of women from a slum in Calcutta, India. *Journal of Interpersonal Violence, 24*(7), 1175–1191. https://doi.org/10.1177/0886260508322186

Panolan, S., & Benson Thomas, M. (2024). Prevalence and associated risk factors of postpartum depression in India: A comprehensive review. *Practice, 15*(1), 1. https://doi.org/10.25259/JNRP_584_2023

Pantoji, M. V., Ganjekar, S., Mehta, U. M., Chandra, P. S., & Thippeswamy, H. (2024). Development of a tool for infant facial emotion recognition (InFER) for postpartum mothers with mental illnesses. *Infant Mental Health Journal, 45*(3), 318–327. https://doi.org/10.1002/IMHJ.22111

Parial, S. (2015). Bipolar disorder in women. *Indian Journal of Psychiatry, 57*, 252–263. https://doi.org/10.4103/0019-5545.161488

Patel, V., Kirkwood, B. R., Pednekar, S., Pereira, B., Barros, P., Fernandes, J., Datta, J., Pai, R., Weiss, H., & Mabey, D. (2006). Gender disadvantage and reproductive health risk factors for common mental disorders in women: A community survey in India. *Archives of General Psychiatry, 63*(4), 404–413. https://doi.org/10.1001/ARCHPSYC.63.4.404

Pati, S., Chauhan, A. S., Mahapatra, P., Hansdah, D., Sahoo, K. C., & Pati, S. (2018). Weaved into the cultural fabric: A qualitative exploration of alcohol consumption during pregnancy among tribal women in Odisha, India. *Substance Abuse Treatment, Prevention, and Policy, 13*(1), 9. https://doi.org/10.1186/S13011-018-0146-5

Patton, G. C., Carlin, J. B., Coffey, C., Wolfe, R., Hibbert, M., & Bowes, G. (1998). Depression, anxiety, and smoking initiation: A prospective study over 3 years. *American Journal of Public Health, 88*(10), 1518–1522. https://doi.org/10.2105/AJPH.88.10.1518

Poongothai, S., Pradeepa, R., Ganesan, A., & Mohan, V. (2009). Prevalence of depression in a Large urban south Indian population—the Chennai urban rural epidemiology study (cures – 70). *PLoS One, 4*(9), e7185. https://doi.org/10.1371/JOURNAL.PONE.0007185

Powis, B., Griffiths, P., Gossop, M., & Strang, J. (1996). The differences between male and female drug users: Community samples of heroin and cocaine users compared. *Substance Use & Misuse, 31*(5), 529–543. https://doi.org/10.3109/10826089609045825

Prasad, S., Kumar, Y., Nayar, P., Prasad, S., & Sharma, G. (2017). A prospective study to assess the mental health and quality of life in women undergoing assisted reproduction. *Fertility Science and Research, 4*(2), 117. https://doi.org/10.4103/FSR.FSR_7_18

Prathap, A., Subhalakshmi, T. P., & Joseph Varghese, P. (2018). A cross-sectional study on the proportion of anxiety and depression and determinants of quality of life in polycystic ovarian disease. *Indian Journal of Psychological Medicine, 40*(3), 257. https://doi.org/10.4103/IJPSYM.IJPSYM_221_17

Prema, S. V., Chandra, P. S., & Chaturvedi, S. K. (1991). Psychiatric admissions and the menstrual cycle: Is there a relationship? *NIMHANS Journal, 9*(2), 91–96. https://psycnet.apa.org/record/1992-32707-001

Purkayastha, D., Venkateswaran, C., Nayar, K., & Unnikrishnan, U. G. (2017). Prevalence of depression in breast cancer patients and its association with their quality of life: A cross-sectional observational study. *Indian Journal of Palliative Care, 23*(3), 268–273. https://doi.org/10.4103/IJPC.IJPC_6_17

Rajat, R. (2004). The extent, pattern and trends of drug abuse in India: National Survey. Ministry of Social Justice and Empowerment, Government of India & United Nations Office on Drugs and Crime, Regional Office for South Asia. https://books.google.co.in/books/about/The_Extent_Pattern_and_Trends_of_Drug_Ab.html?id=pB5iGwAACAAJ&redir_esc=y.

Rajeev, S. P., Nair, G. M., Krishna, K. K., & Maria, C. (2024). India's silent struggle: A scoping review on postpartum depression in the land of a billion mothers. *Indian Journal of Psychological Medicine.* https://doi.org/10.1177/02537176241245773

Ram, F., Shekhar, C., & Chowdhury, B. (2014). Use of traditional contraceptive methods in India & its socio-demographic determinants. *The Indian Journal of Medical Research, 140*(Suppl 1), S17. https://pmc.ncbi.nlm.nih.gov/articles/PMC4345748/

Randall, C. L., Roberts, J. S., Del Boca, F. K., Carroll, K. M., Connors, G. J., & Mattson, M. E. (1999). Telescoping of landmark events associated with drinking: A gender comparison. *Journal of Studies on Alcohol, 60*(2), 252–260. https://doi.org/10.15288/JSA.1999.60.252

Ray, P., Mandal, N., & Sinha, V. K. (2020). Change of symptoms of schizophrenia across phases of menstrual cycle. *Archives of Women's Mental Health, 23*(1), 113–122. https://doi.org/10.1007/S00737-019-0952-4

Ray, R., & Chopra, A. (2012). Monitoring of substance abuse in India—initiatives & experiences. *The Indian Journal of Medical Research, 135*(6), 806.

Ray, R., & Paul, I. (2020). Menstrual psychosis: A not so forgotten reality. *Indian Journal of Psychiatry, 62*(5), 585–587. https://doi.org/10.4103/PSYCHIATRY.INDIANJPSYCHIATRY_883_20

Reddy, P. D., Desai, G., Hamza, A., Karthik, S., Ananthanpillai, S. T., & Chandra, P. S. (2014). Enhancing mother infant interactions through video feedback enabled interventions in women with schizophrenia: A single subject research design study. *Indian Journal of Psychological Medicine, 36*(4), 373–377. https://doi.org/10.4103/0253-7176.140702

Roberts, L. R., & Montgomery, S. B. (2015). Mindfulness-based intervention for perinatal grief after stillbirth in rural India. *Issues in Mental Health Nursing, 36*(3), 222. https://doi.org/10.3109/01612840.2014.962676

Roberts, L. R., Montgomery, S., Lee, J. W., & Anderson, B. A. (2012). Social and cultural factors associated with perinatal grief in Chhattisgarh, India. *Journal of Community Health, 37*(3), 572. https://doi.org/10.1007/S10900-011-9485-0

Roberts, L. R., Renati, S. J., Solomon, S., & Montgomery, S. (2021). Perinatal grief among poor rural and urban women in central India. *International Journal of Women's Health, 13*, 305. https://doi.org/10.2147/IJWH.S297292

Roy, S., Majumder, S., Bose, A., & Chowdhury, I. R. (2024). Understanding geographical variability of women's alcohol prevalence in India using spatial regression models: Evidence from national representative survey. *Regional Science Policy & Practice, 16*(6), 100040. https://doi.org/10.1016/J.RSPP.2024.100040

Sabarwal, S., McCormick, M. C., Subramanian, S. V., & Silverman, J. G. (2012). Son preference and intimate partner violence victimization in India: Examining the role of actual and desired family composition. *Journal of Biosocial Science, 44*(1), 43–56. https://doi.org/10.1017/S002193201100037X

Sabri, B., Mani, S. S., & Kaduluri, V. P. S. (2024). Integrated domestic violence and reproductive health interventions in India: A systematic review. *Reproductive Health, 21*(1), 1–28. https://doi.org/10.1186/S12978-024-01830-0

Sabri, B., Renner, L. M., Stockman, J. K., Mittal, M., & Decker, M. R. (2014). Risk factors for severe intimate partner violence and violence-related injuries among women in India. *Women & Health, 54*(4), 281–300. https://doi.org/10.1080/03630242.2014.896445

Sabri, B., & Young, A. M. (2022). Contextual factors associated with gender-based violence and related homicides perpetrated by partners and in-laws: A study of women survivors in India. *Health Care for Women International, 43*(7–8), 784–805. https://doi.org/10.1080/07399332.2021.1881963

Saggurti, N., Nair, S., Silverman, J. G., Naik, D. D., Battala, M., Dasgupta, A., Balaiah, D., & Raj, A. (2014). Impact of the RHANI wives intervention on marital conflict and sexual coercion. *International Journal of Gynaecology and Obstetrics, 126*(1), 18. https://doi.org/10.1016/J.IJGO.2014.01.015

Samal, J., & Dehury, R. K. (2015). Family planning practices, programmes and policies in India including implants and injectables with a special focus on Jharkhand, India: A brief review. *Journal of Clinical and Diagnostic Research, 9*(11), LE01–LE04. https://doi.org/10.7860/JCDR/2015/16152.6714

Sathe, H. S., Maliye, C. H., Varma, P. S., Garg, B. S., Shahare, K., & Rathod, R. (2024). Intimate partner violence and mental health problems in married women in rural central India: A community-based cross-sectional study. *Indian Journal of Community Medicine : Official Publication of Indian Association of Preventive & Social Medicine, 49*(6), 866–872. https://doi.org/10.4103/IJCM.IJCM_677_22

Sathiyaseelan, A., Chaudhury, S., & Patangia, B. (2022). Cognitive and biological challenges of menopausal women in India. *Life Res, 5*(3), 23. https://doi.org/10.53388/2022-0622-401

Seitz, H. K., Egerer, G., Simanowski, U. A., Waldherr, R., Eckey, R., Agarwal, D. P., Goedde, H. W., & Von Wartburg, J. P. (1993). Human gastric alcohol dehydrogenase activity: Effect of age, sex, and alcoholism. *Gut, 34*(10), 1433–1437. https://doi.org/10.1136/GUT.34.10.1433

Sethy, R. R., Garg, S., Ram, D., & Tikka, S. K. (2021). Thyroid function in postpartum psychosis: An exploratory study. *Asia-Pacific Psychiatry, 13*(2). https://doi.org/10.1111/APPY.12465

Sharma, H. L., & Gupta, A. (2024). Discover social science and health effective contraceptive methods and sterilization in India: Some results on socio-demographic differentials. *Discover Social Science and Health, 4*, 78. https://doi.org/10.1007/s44155-024-00139-4

Sharma, K., Vatsa, M., Kalaivani, M., & Bhardwaj, D. (2019). Mental health effects of domestic violence against women in Delhi: A community-based study. *Journal of Family Medicine and Primary Care, 8*(7), 2522. https://doi.org/10.4103/JFMPC.JFMPC_427_19

Sharma, R. S., Rajalakshmi, M., & Jeyaraj, D. A. (2001). Current status of fertility control methods in India. *Journal of Biosciences, 26*(4 Suppl), 391–405. https://doi.org/10.1007/BF02704741

Sharma, S., & Mahajan, N. (2015). Menopausal symptoms and its effect on quality of life in urban versus rural women: A cross-sectional study. *Journal of Mid-Life Health, 6*(1), 16. https://doi.org/10.4103/0976-7800.153606

Sharma, V., & Mazmanian, D. (2003). Sleep loss and postpartum psychosis. *Bipolar Disorders, 5*(2), 98–105. https://doi.org/10.1034/J.1399-5618.2003.00015.X

Shidhaye, R., & Patel, V. (2010). Association of socio-economic, gender and health factors with common mental disorders in women: A population-based study of 5703 married rural women in India. *International Journal of Epidemiology, 39*(6), 1510–1521. https://doi.org/10.1093/IJE/DYQ179

Shiva, L., Desai, G., Satyanarayana, V. A., Venkataram, P., & Chandra, P. S. (2021). Negative childbirth experience and post-traumatic stress disorder—a study among postpartum women in South India. *Frontiers in Psychiatry, 12*. https://doi.org/10.3389/FPSYT.2021.640014

Singh, A., & Arora, A. K. (2008). Why hysterectomy rate are lower in India. *Indian Journal of Community Medicine, 33*(3), 196. https://doi.org/10.4103/0970-0218.42065

Singh, G., Avasthi, A., & Pravin, & D. (2001). DHAT syndrome in a female-a CASE report. *Indian Journal of Psychiatry, 43*(4), 345–348.

Singh Malik, V., Singh, V., Kumar, H., Kumar, S., Yadav, H., Kumar, K., Kumar Behmani, R., & Malik, S. (2023). Menstruation, menstrual distress and mental health: A literature review menstruation, menstrual distress and mental health: A literature review a literature review-Vandana. *Indian Journal of Social Sciences and Literature Studies, 9*. https://www.researchgate.net/publication/372646945

Singla, M., Sharma, A., Samuel, C., & George, J. M. (2016). To compare sociodemographic profile, attitude, coping strategies and psychiatric morbidity among rural and urban menopausal women. *International Journal of Medical and Dental Sciences, 5*(1), 1016. https://doi.org/10.19056/IJMDSJSSMES/2016/V5I1/83545

Sinha, S. K., Thomas Kishore, M., Thippeswamy, H., Kommu, J. V. S., & Chandra, P. S. (2021). Adverse effects and short-term developmental outcomes of infants exposed to atypical antipsychotics during breastfeeding. *Indian Journal of Psychiatry, 63*(1), 52–57. https://doi.org/10.4103/PSYCHIATRY.INDIANJPSYCHIATRY_45_20

Srivastava, V., Ahmad Ansari, M., Kumar, A., Gautam Shah, A., Kumar Meena, R., Sevach, P., Prakash Singh, O., & Author, C. (2015). Study of anxiety and depression among breast cancer patients from North India. *Clinical Psychiatry, 2*(1). https://doi.org/10.21767/2471-9854.100017

Subramaniam, D., Subramaniam, K., Charles, S. X., Abraham Verghese, F., Psych, F., & Cp, F. Z. (1982). Psychiatric aspects of hysterectomy. *Journal of Psychiatry, 24*(1), 75–79.

Supraja, T. A., Thennarasu, K., Satyanarayana, V. A., Seena, T. K., Desai, G., Jangam, K. V., & Chandra, P. S. (2016). Suicidality in early pregnancy among antepartum mothers in urban India. *Archives of Women's Mental Health, 19*(6), 1101–1108. https://doi.org/10.1007/S00737-016-0660-2

Sharma, S. (2012). Contraceptive choices among Indian women: Is the role of women's education overemhasized? *International Journal of Current Research, 4*(12), 180–186. https://www.journalcra.com/sites/default/files/issue-pdf/Download%202725.pdf

Sutradhar, B., Mukherjee, D., & Pathak, K. (2023). An observational study on deliberate self-harm in individuals with alcohol dependence syndrome. *Industrial Psychiatry Journal, 32*(2), 369–374. https://doi.org/10.4103/IPJ.IPJ_50_23

Thakrar, P., Bhukar, K., & Oswal, R. (2021). Premenstrual dysphoric disorder: Prevalence, quality of life and disability due to illness among medical and paramedical students. *Journal of Affective Disorders Reports, 4*, 100112. https://doi.org/10.1016/J.JADR.2021.100112

Thakur, M., Gupta, B., Kumar, R., Mishra, A., Gupta, S., & Kar, S. (2019). Depression among women diagnosed with breast cancer: A study from North India. *Indian Journal of Medical and Paediatric Oncology, 40*(3), 347–352. https://doi.org/10.4103/IJMPO.IJMPO_43_18

Thakur, M., Sharma, R., Mishra, A. K., Singh, K., & Kar, S. K. (2022). Psychological distress and body image disturbances after modified radical mastectomy among breast cancer survivors: A cross-sectional study from a tertiary care Centre in North India. *The Lancet Regional Health - Southeast Asia, 7*, 100077. https://doi.org/10.1016/J.LANSEA.2022.100077

Thamby, A., Bajaj, A., Manoj, L., Sunil Kumar, G., Gokul, G. R., Thennarasu, K., & Jaisoorya, T. S. (2024). Impaired mother-infant bonding: A community study from India. *Journal of Reproductive and Infant Psychology, 42*(3), 528–539. https://doi.org/10.1080/02646838.2022.2125938

Thippeswamy, H., Dahale, A., Desai, G., & Chandra, P. S. (2015). What is in a name? Causative explanatory models of postpartum psychosis among patients and caregivers in India. *International Journal of Social Psychiatry, 61*(8), 818–823. https://doi.org/10.1177/0020764015597016

Trivedi, P., Soni, M., & Saxena, D. (2016). Mental health of females after mastectomy: A qualitative case study, Gujarat, India. *International Journal of Medical Science and Public Health, 5*(11), 2244. https://doi.org/10.5455/IJMSPH.2016.02042016448

UN General Assembly, Declaration on the Elimination of Violence against Women, A/RES/48/104, UN General Assembly, 20 December 1993. https://www.refworld.org/legal/resolution/unga/1993/en/10685

United Nations Office on Drugs and Crime. (2008). Women and drug use in India: Substance, Women and High – Risk Assessment Study. United Nations Office on Drugs and Crime, Regional Office for South Asia and Ministry of Social Justice and Empowerment. Retrieved from https://www.unodc.org/documents/southasia/reports/UNODC_Book_Women_and_Drug_Use_in_India_2008.pdf

United Nations Department of Economic and Social Affairs, Population Division (2022). World Population Prospects 2022: Summary of Results. UN DESA/POP/2022/TR/NO. 3.

UNODC_Book_Women_and_Drug_Use_in_India_2008 (1). (2008). https://www.unodc.org/documents/southasia/reports/UNODC_Book_Women_and_Drug_Use_in_India_2008.pdf

Van Thiel, D. H., Tarter, R. E., Rosenblum, E., & Gavaler, J. S. (1988). Ethanol, its metabolism and gonadal effects: Does sex make a difference? *Advances in Alcohol & Substance Abuse, 7*(3–4), 131–169. https://doi.org/10.1300/J251V07N03_21

Vengadavaradan, A., Bharadwaj, B., Sathyanarayanan, G., & Durairaj, J. (2019). Frequency and correlates of mother-infant bonding disorders among postpartum women in India. *Asian Journal of Psychiatry, 44*, 72–79. https://doi.org/10.1016/J.AJP.2019.07.004

Vindhya, U. (2000). "Dowry Deaths" in Andhra Pradesh, India. *Violence Against Women, 6*(10), 1085–1108. https://doi.org/10.1177/10778010022183532

Vinoda Thulaseedharan, J. (2018). Contraceptive use and preferences of young married women in Kerala, India. *Open Access Journal of Contraception, 9*, 1–10. https://doi.org/10.2147/OAJC.S152178

Vyas, J. N., Rathore, R. S., Sharma, P., & Singhal, A. K. (1989). A study of psychiatric aspects of hysterectomy. *Indian Journal of Psychiatry, 31*(1), 83–89.

Weitzman, A. (2020). The sex of firstborn children and intimate partner violence in India. *Violence Against Women, 26*(6–7), 590–613. https://doi.org/10.1177/1077801219833823

Yadav, P., Saini, R., Chauhan, V. S., & Sood, S. (2021a). Personality traits associated with alcohol dependence syndrome and its relapse. *Medical Journal, Armed Forces India, 79*(1), 80. https://doi.org/10.1016/J.MJAFI.2021.01.025

Yadav, V., Jain, A., Dabar, D., Goel, A. D., Sood, A., Joshi, A., Agarwal, S. S., & Nandeshwar, S. (2021b). A meta-analysis on the prevalence of depression in perimenopausal and postmenopausal women in India. *Asian Journal of Psychiatry, 57*, 102581. https://doi.org/10.1016/J.AJP.2021.102581

Zhang, Y., Ji, Y., Liu, S., Li, J., Wu, J., Jin, Q., Liu, X., Duan, H., Feng, Z., Liu, Y., Zhang, Y., Lyu, Z., Song, F., Song, F., Yang, L., Liu, H., & Huang, Y. (2025). Global burden of female breast cancer: New estimates in 2022, temporal trend and future projections up to 2050 based on the latest release from GLOBOCAN. *Journal of the National Cancer Center.* https://doi.org/10.1016/J.JNCC.2025.02.002

Chapter 6
Women's Reproductive Mental Health in Nepal

Pawan Sharma and Sulochana Joshi

1 Introduction

Nepal, a landlocked country in South Asia and home to over 29 million people, has a little over half of its population consisting of women; most of them marry young, and a small percentage face diverse disabilities. The 2021 National Population and Housing Census Nepal identifies that 51.1% of its 29,164,578 population are females, among whom 64.3% are married, with 35.9% getting married at the age of 18–20 years. Overall, 2% of females are reported to be disabled (National Population and Housing Census, 2021). Nepalese society is patriarchal. The prevalent socio-cultural norms discriminate against women, favor male children, contribute to high female school dropout rates, and encourage early marriages among females (Nepal, UNFPA, 2017). This male-dominated structure often leads to gender-based violence and inequality, granting men disproportionate privilege and power. Thus, gender appears to be a strong factor influencing different aspects of women's health, behavior, and the sociocultural and financial lives in Nepal.

In this chapter, we plan to explore the epidemiology of mental disorders among females in Nepal within the scope of reproductive mental health. We also aim to explore the impact of pregnancy, postpartum, and menopause; assess available services, highlight socio-cultural challenges, and provide evidence-based recommendations to improve women's mental health care in the context of Nepal.

P. Sharma (✉) · S. Joshi
Department of Psychiatry, Patan Academy of Health Sciences, Lalitpur, Nepal

P. Kukreti et al. (eds.), *Women's Reproductive Mental Health in South Asia*, South Asian Perspectives in Mental Health and Psychology,
https://doi.org/10.1007/978-981-96-9219-4_6

2 Epidemiology

According to the National Mental Health Survey of 2020 in Nepal, the lifetime prevalence of any mental disorder among females was 8%, while the current prevalence was 5.1% (Dhimal et al., 2021). Mental health challenges, particularly anxiety and depression, are prevalent among women in Nepal, with various factors contributing to gender disparities. According to the Nepal Demographic and Health Survey (NDHS) 2022, 22% of women aged 15–49 had symptoms of anxiety, and 5% had symptoms of depression (Ministry of Health and Population, Nepal & ICF, 2023). The gender disparities in the prevalence of anxiety and depression were influenced by age, geographical areas, level of education, and household wealth. Women, especially of reproductive age, were more likely to experience anxiety and depression. However, no difference was observed in the rates of seeking care for anxiety or depression (Shawon et al., 2024). Substance use among women remains a significant public health concern, with various surveys revealing notable trends in alcohol and tobacco consumption. The mental health survey 2020 reported 0.8% of females with substance use disorder (Dhimal et al., 2021). The STEPwise approach to NCD risk factor surveillance (STEPS) survey 2019 showed 10.8% of women were current drinkers, and 11.6% of women had at least one form and pattern of tobacco use (Dhimal et al., 2020). As per a nationally representative household survey among 9000 married women of reproductive age, the prevalence of alcohol consumption was 24.7% in the last 12 months (Thapa et al., 2016).

2.1 Depression Among Maternal Population in Nepal

Antenatal depression and psychological distress are common among perinatal women in Nepal. Among 239 perinatal women in a study, 12 (5%) were teenagers, and 3% of them had depressive symptoms (Pokharel et al., 2023). The prevalence of antenatal depression was found to be 24.8% in a study done among 250 randomly selected pregnant women in the community. Multigravida, unintended pregnancy, male sex preference of child by the family, and intimate partner violence were found to predict antenatal depression (Chalise et al., 2022). In a study done on 115 pregnant women attending the obstetric unit of a tertiary hospital, psychological distress was found in 2.6% and was significantly associated with occupation, fear of ANC visit, fear of visits to the hospital for other health problems, and fear of being alone or without help around delivery. Emotion-focused coping was the most used coping strategy. Psychological distress and overall coping strategies were found to correlate positively (Rimal et al., 2022).

Different studies in Nepal have shown the prevalence of postpartum depression ranging from 14.7% to 20.2% (Pradhananga et al., 2020; Bhusal et al., 2016; Chalise et al., 2020; Bhusal et al., 2023). The incidence of postpartum depression varied in the postpartum period, i.e., 19.4% (6 weeks postpartum) and 22.22% (10th week postpartum), respectively (Budhathoki et al., 2012). Other studies showed depressive symptoms ranging from 17.1% to 33.7% among the maternal population (Bhusal & Bhandari, 2018; Singh et al., 2021; Kumwar et al., 2015).

Various risk factors were identified in different studies for postpartum depressive symptoms. They were women without adequate rest during pregnancy, abortion history, poor relationship with husband, marital dissatisfaction, stressful life events, lower income, migration of husband for employment, location of the nearest health facility, delivery of the last child by cesarean section, fewer ANC care, age, smoking, pressure to conceive a child, intent of pregnancy, delivery related problems, sex of newborn, and pregnancy-induced health problems (Chalise et al., 2020; Bhusal & Bhandari, 2018; Singh et al., 2021; Kumwar et al., 2015). A prospective cohort study among 1222 institutional deliveries showed a prevalence of depressive symptoms to be 4.4%, and women who had been exposed to mistreatment during childbirth were almost 50% more likely to have postpartum depressive symptoms, and women giving birth to female infants were 30% more likely to have postpartum depressive symptoms (Gurung & Bask, 2024).

2.2 Anxiety Among the Maternal Population in Nepal

As per the nationally representative Nepal Demographic and Health Survey (NDHS) 2022, the prevalence of anxiety was 22.2% among women of reproductive age. The predictors of anxiety were self-reported health status, experience of emotional violence and pregnancy termination, husband's alcohol consumption, genital discharge, and household wealth status (Tohan et al., 2025). Available estimates from Nepal reveal a significant prevalence of anxiety among pregnant women, with nearly half (46.4%) at risk of anxiety and a prevalence rate of 32.6% (Paudel et al., 2020). Factors such as age, type of family, gravida, history of abortion, and maternal desires regarding the pregnancy were associated with anxiety (Shrestha & Pun, 2018). In addition, concerns about the sex of the fetus were found to be strongly associated with higher anxiety levels (Paudel et al., 2020). It is interesting to note that there was not much change in anxiety levels during the COVID-19 pandemic. A study among 273 pregnant women from a tertiary hospital showed a mild level of anxiety (Shrestha et al., 2021a, 2021b). However, the anxiety symptoms increased with the time nearing delivery, as per another study, where it was 44.6% in the third trimester, followed by 31.4% in the second trimester, and 29.4% in the first trimester during the pandemic (Shrestha et al., 2021a, 2021b).

2.3 Suicide Among the Maternal Population in Nepal

As per the National Mental Health Survey of Nepal, suicidality in females was two times more than in males (9.2% for females and 4.8% for males). In females, suicidal thoughts were 8.5% and suicidal attempts were 1.2%. Suicidal behavior in females (1%) was higher compared to males (0.8%) (Dhimal et al., 2021). Suicide (16%) was the leading cause of death among women of reproductive age, with 21% of suicideS occurring below the age of 18 years, as per the 2008–2009 government survey done among more than 86,000 women of reproductive age in eight districts and of different ethnicities and levels of development. Rather than maternal-related issues (12%), suicide was the single leading cause of death (Suvedi et al., 2009).

Poisoning has been the most common means of suicide. The contributing factors for suicide and deliberate self-harm among women in Nepal are abuse, interpersonal conflicts, marital disputes, relationship problems, adjustment problems, unpaid loans and financial losses, mood disorder, adjustment disorder, and substance abuse disorder (Kasaju et al., 2021).

2.4 Substance use Among the Maternal Population in Nepal

Substance use, particularly alcohol use, by women during pregnancy is well-documented in Nepal. A significant proportion of women consume home-brewed alcohol during pregnancy, with one-third drinking it daily. Factors such as low education levels, lack of awareness about the harmful effects of alcohol on both mother and child, being from marginalized groups like Dalits, disadvantaged communities, and Janajatis, as well as the husband's drinking habits and home brewing of alcohol, are strongly associated with increased alcohol consumption during pregnancy (Aryal et al., 2016). During postpartum, 43% of women consumed home-brewed alcohol. Factors similar to antepartum were associated with drinking during postpartum, like ethnicity, education, and husband's drinking (Aryal et al., 2016). A community-based cross-sectional study in 52 clusters of Dhanusha District of Nepal among 426 pregnant women in the second trimester showed that 21.3% and 13.3% had tobacco use and harmful alcohol drinking, respectively (Paudel et al., 2018). A study among 436 women in the mountain district of Nepal showed the prevalence of tobacco use during pregnancy to be 17.2% and illiteracy, alcohol use during the last pregnancy, and having tobacco users within the family, were the associated factors (Barakoti et al., 2017).

3 Domestic Violence During Pregnancy in Nepal

Violence against women has been seen since old times in Nepal. Several factors, such as ethnicity, age, rural residence, exposure to paternal violence against mothers, and characteristics of husbands or partners, including unemployment, controlling behavior, and alcohol use, influence the violence (Dhital et al., 2024). A significant proportion of women in the reproductive age group have experienced various forms of violence, with 23% reporting physical violence, 8% experiencing sexual violence, and 6% enduring violence during pregnancy, as per the National

Demographic and Health Survey 2022. The survey also showed that the rate increased from 14% in 2016 to 17% in 2022. The violence increased sharply with increasing age, from 13% among 15–19-year-olds to 30% among 40–49-year-olds. The emotional violence of married women was not being cared for when ill during pregnancy, delivery, or the postpartum period (Ministry of Health and Population Nepal & ICF, 2023). The prevalence of domestic violence during and around the time of pregnancy ranges from 6% to 29% in Nepal (Ministry of Health and Population Nepal & ICF, 2023; Rishal et al., 2018; Singh et al., 2018). The prevalence of violence during pregnancy is twice as high among women with three or four children than women with one or two children. A study done among 140 pregnant women attending a tertiary hospital showed that the lifetime prevalence of domestic and family violence was found to be 27.7%, followed by 17.1% of women fearing someone in their family. Domestic violence was significantly associated with anxiety, depression, quality of life, and perceived social support. However, there was significantly low use of safety measures by the women (Sapkota et al., 2021). Several factors put women at a higher risk of violence during pregnancy. They include refusing to have sex, fetal gender identification during pregnancy, giving birth to a female child, and partners with alcohol use disorder (Deuba et al., 2016).

4 Psychiatric Aspects of Menarche and Menopause in Nepal

Menstrual restriction and sometimes seclusion have persisted in Nepalese society for centuries. One of the most severe forms of menstrual restriction, known as Chaupadi, is a practice in which females are secluded and forced to stay separately in makeshift huts or animal sheds during menstruation, which has led to many psychological effects (Dahal et al., 2023). However, this has been prohibited by the Muluki Criminal Code, 2017 (Nepal Law Commission, 2017). Apart from that, there are provisions of restrictions on touching food, cooking food, touching plants with holy belief, livestock or animals, eating together with family, participating in cultural rituals, sleeping in any bed, using common toilet, or common taps during menstruation. These practices lead to higher perceived stress in women (Dahal et al., 2023; Joshi & Acharya, 2022). A study conducted among 270 adolescent girls in a community showed that low perceived family and friend support during menstruation and experiencing moderate/severe dysmenorrhea were associated with higher scores of anxiety, depression, and perceived stress (Niroula et al., 2025).

A hospital-based descriptive study among 243 women aged between 45 and 55 years showed that the psychological symptoms were present in 69.5% (Dongol et al., 2021). A community-based study among 355 menopausal women showed the prevalence of depression to be 31.5%, whereas another study among 203 women showed the prevalence of depressive mood to be 35% (Sharma et al., 2021). As compared to 15–29-year-old women, the 45–69-year-old age group was five times more likely to be tobacco users in Nepal (Bista et al., 2013). A community study done among 390 menopausal women showed that the prevalence of alcohol consumption in the past month is 18.2% (Khatri et al., 2024).

5 Current Status of Services in Maternal Mental Health in Nepal

Antenatal and postnatal care are provided by doctors (medical officers), health officers, nurses, or midwives in primary health centers. There are no psychiatrists or psychologist available at this level. Most of the health care providers have received Mental Health Gap Action Program (mhGAP) training in different modules as a part of the integration of mental health services in primary care settings (Sharma et al., 2024). The psychiatrists are only available in the tertiary care hospitals and some district hospitals. Only those mothers who come with their symptoms of psychiatric illnesses are referred, and screening is not done on a regular basis.

The Paropakar Maternity and Women's Hospital (PMWH), Nepal's only government-run tertiary care maternity hospital, launched its first-ever Mental Health Outpatient Unit in 2024 and has been considered a landmark initiative (WHO, 2024). In all the teaching institutes of Nepal, the department of psychiatry manages the cases of women's reproductive psychiatry who come to outpatient or inpatient care; however, there are no specialized clinics as such and no provision of mandatory screening for mental disorders.

There are some other trainings that are provided to health care workers like auxiliary nurses, who are key maternity care providers in rural areas (Mahato et al., 2018; Ireland et al., 2021). These programs are short-term NGO initiatives which are not sustainable.

6 Service Utilization Patterns for Maternal Mental Health Services in Nepal

The utilization of maternal health services in the context of Nepal has improved over the decades; however, it is well below than that of the neighboring countries like India, Sri Lanka, Bhutan, and the Maldives, and only marginally better than Pakistan, Afghanistan, and Bangladesh (Ali et al., 2023). Hence, the utilization of maternal mental health is also poor, as these are interconnected. The health professionals who provide antenatal services care are not trained to deliver mental health services under the routine government healthcare service. The data on service utilization patterns for mental health services among the maternal population is not available for Nepal. A study among randomly selected women in a community showed that the barriers to antenatal care were being from a disadvantaged ethnicity, lower women's autonomy, poor knowledge of health, less media exposure related to health services, and lower wealth rank (Deo et al., 2015). Similar factors might be true for the mental health service utilization for pregnant women. Regarding the service utilization for gender-based violence, it was seen that only 28% of women have sought help to stop the violence. These women sought support from their close family members, including in-laws, and mostly tolerated and accepted the husbands' abuse because of economic dependence (Ministry of Health and Population Nepal & ICF, 2023).

7 Programs and Policies for Maternal Mental Health in Nepal

The constitution of Nepal states that "Every woman shall have the right to safe motherhood and reproductive health." There are acts like the Labour Act 2017 that have the provision of maternity leave and engaging pregnant females in easier work, and the Public health Service Act 2018 that has the provision of access to and certainty of health services for maternal health (Nepal Law Commission, 2017; Family Welfare Division, 2018). The Domestic Violence Act 2009 identifies mental harm as one of the forms of violence and has provision of punishment for the perpetrator (Ankita, 2013).

Currently, the mental health policy of Nepal is governed by the National Health Policy and mental health is mentioned in Sect. 6.17.5. The National Mental Health Strategy and Action Plan (2020) of Nepal have mentioned maternal mental health as a priority via integration of maternal mental health with ongoing maternal health programs like *Ama Surakshya Yojana*. The action plan also emphasizes on the screening and management of depression and suicide during pregnancy along with awareness programs (WHO, 2024; Sharma et al., 2024).

Nepal introduced the "One Stop Crisis Management Centre" (OCMC) in 2010, which provides integrated health, security, legal, rehabilitation, and psychological services through a one-door system as a part of comprehensive support to the people who are facing gender-based violence. The major service utilizers are women of reproductive age. It is available in 94 different hospitals throughout the nation (Joshi et al., 2023; Atreya et al., 2020).

8 Available Research and Gaps in Maternal Mental Health in Nepal

One of the landmark studies conducted to assess maternal deaths and complications related to pregnancy and childbirth in Nepal was the Nepal Maternal Mortality and Morbidity Study (MMM) 2008/2009 among 86,000 women of reproductive age in eight districts. According to this study, the leading individual cause of death in the reproductive age group was suicide, i.e., 16%. The factors associated with suicide were family/marriage, mental health issues, and other illness. The two main methods used by women to commit suicide were consuming poison, mainly pesticides (57%), and hanging (39%). This study played a crucial role in raising awareness about the mental health aspects of maternal mortality in Nepal and highlighted the need for mental health interventions in maternal healthcare policies.

Most of the research done among the maternal population in Nepal is cross-sectional. The bulk of the literature is on the prevalence of depression, especially in the clinical setting. The studies have reported a wide variation which could be due to due to methodological variation like types of screening tools used, gestational time point when screened for symptoms, sample size, and sample characteristics. There is a lack of studies on the longitudinal observation and outcome of the interventions. Some of the qualitative studies done in the community have also provided baseline evidences in maternal mental health. The widely used Edinburgh Postnatal Depression Scale, which is a screening tool for postpartum depression, has been validated in the Nepalese population (Bhusal et al., 2016). Though many cases of postpartum psychosis are seen in a clinical setting, there are minimal studies, and this needs to be addressed.

9 Current Challenges in Reproductive Mental Health and Ways Out

9.1 Stigma and Low Mental Health Literacy

The stigma and its manifestations regarding mental disorders are more prevalent among women (Gurung et al., 2022). The self-stigma regarding mental illness was also found to be more among the female patients (Maharjan & Panthee, 2019). Similarly, the mental health literacy among the people of Nepal is low, and this is a challenge that causes a huge treatment gap. Hence, it is necessary to develop policies and campaigns to reduce stigma and promote mental health awareness in Nepal. It is seen that the interventions like outreach worker's visits, radio programs on maternal health, health information disseminated through various mass media sources, and raising women's status through education have improved the awareness and maternal health care utilization, similar programs on mental health could help to deal with the challenges faced (Sharma et al., 2007).

9.2 Service Availability

The services for mental illness are limited and are mainly concentrated in the big cities. This has been a major challenge not only for maternal mental health but also for all groups of people. A paper on stakeholder perspective emphasized the limited availability and accessibility of maternal health services, which potentially caused immense distress among pregnant women (Sah et al., 2024). The mental health services are not available at the community level, making it hard for both the service users and service providers. Hence, it is important to scale up mental health services for the maternal population by building the clinical capacity of the primary health care workers with supervision and quality assurance. One of the tested interventions has been the use of the Community Informant Detection Tool (CIDT) by the female community health volunteers for raising awareness and promoting the identification of mental health problems (Subba et al., 2024). Similar interventions are needed that are culturally contextualized and acceptable. One of the ways out would be the use of digital mental health and tele-psychiatry, considering the dearth of experts in rural area.

9.3 Specialized Training and Specialized Services

There is no psychiatrist who is specifically trained in women's reproductive psychiatry in Nepal. The burden of assessing and handling this special population lies on the general psychiatrists working in government and private setups. One of the ways out would be to include this area in the curriculum of the postgraduate psychiatry and clinical psychology courses. Further, funding is needed for capacity building and research activities in this field.

9.4 Integration of Maternal and Mental Health

There has been tremendous improvement in mental health and maternal health services in Nepal, but both have been going independently. In a review of nursing curriculum, it was seen that basic material was included on both mental health and maternity care but little or nothing on the combination of the two topics, suggesting the lack of integration (van Teijlingen et al., 2015). The government policy and programs also need integration, and it is imperative that all maternal health programs include mental health. There is also a need for the integration of maternal mental health in all the maternal health programs at the primary care level as well as the tertiary care level.

9.5 Social Dynamics

One of the major challenges that pregnant women in Nepal face is inadequate social support from family/relatives, neighbors, and the community (Sah et al., 2024). A study among 271 pregnant females from a tertiary care center showed that the others lacked support from family and spouses, impeding daily life and newborn care. There would be traditional superstitions above medical advice leading to risks (Neupane et al., 2024). One of the ways to deal with this social challenge would be a bottom-up communication system, community sensitization, communication skills for midwives, and community-based health education for pregnant women (Gurung, 2024).

10 Conclusion

There is a high burden of mental health disorders, especially depression, anxiety, and suicide, among reproductive-aged women in Nepal. The socio-cultural norms, gender-based violence, and limited healthcare access make this area complex. Current mental health services in Nepal remain primarily urban-centric, with inadequate outreach to rural and marginalized communities. The scarcity of trained professionals in women's reproductive psychiatry poses a significant barrier to effective care delivery. Although there are some government initiatives, implementation gaps remain. Future strategies should focus on scaling up primary healthcare capacity, integrating mental health education into antenatal and postnatal services, and using digital health solutions to improve accessibility. By integrating mental health into mainstream reproductive healthcare, Nepal can make significant strides in ensuring the mental well-being of the maternal population.

References

Ali, S., Thind, A., Stranges, S., Campbell, M. K., & Sharma, I. (2023). Investigating health inequality using trend, decomposition and spatial analyses: A study of maternal health service use in Nepal. *International Journal of Public Health, 68*, 1605457. https://doi.org/10.3389/ijph.2023.1605457

Ankita, K. C. (2013). An analysis on domestic violence (offence and punishment) act of Nepal, 2009. *Kathmandu School of Law Review*, 159–170.

Aryal, K. K., Thapa, N., Mehata, S., Thapa, P., Alvik, A., & Stray-Pedersen, B. (2016). Alcohol consumption during pregnancy and postpartum period and its predictors in Sindhupalchowk District, Nepal. *Journal of Nepal Health Research Council, 14*(34), 143–153.

Atreya, A., Shrestha, R., Nepal, B., Nepal, S., Shrestha, D., & Mahato, S. (2020). When sexual offence is an unexpected diagnosis—exploration of medical, legal and social aspects in Nepalese scenario. *Medico-Legal Journal, 88*(4), 192–195. https://doi.org/10.1177/0025817220935878

Barakoti, R., Ghimire, A., Pandey, A. R., Baral, D. D., & Pokharel, P. K. (2017). Tobacco use during pregnancy and its associated factors in a Mountain District of eastern Nepal: A cross-sectional questionnaire survey. *Frontiers in Public Health, 5*. https://doi.org/10.3389/fpubh.2017.00129

Bhusal, B. R., & Bhandari, N. (2018). Identifying the factors associated with depressive symptoms among postpartum mothers in Kathmandu, Nepal. *International Journal of Nursing Sciences, 5*(3), 268–274. https://doi.org/10.1016/j.ijnss.2018.04.011

Bhusal, B. R., Bhandari, N., Chapagai, M., & Gavidia, T. (2016). Validating the Edinburgh postnatal depression scale as a screening tool for postpartum depression in Kathmandu,

Nepal. *International Journal of Mental Health Systems, 10*, 71. https://doi.org/10.1186/s13033-016-0102-6

Bhusal, C. K., Bhattarai, S., Shrestha, A., & Sharma, H. R. (2023). Depression and its determinants among postpartum mothers attending at Universal College of Medical Sciences and Teaching Hospital, Bhairahawa, Rupandehi, Nepal. *International Journal of Pediatrics, 2023*, 1331641. https://doi.org/10.1155/2023/1331641

Bista, B., Mehata, S., Aryal, K. K., Thapa, P., Pandey, A. R., Pandit, A., Dhakal, P., Dhimal, M., & Karki, K. B. (2015). Socio-demographic Predictors of Tobacco Use among Women of Nepal: Evidence from Non Communicable Disease Risk Factors STEPS Survey Nepal 2013. *Journal of Nepal Health Research Council, 13*(29), 14–19.

Budhathoki, N., Dahal, M., Bhusal, S., Ojha, H., Pandey, S., & Basnet, S. (2012). Violence against women by their husband and postpartum depression. *Journal of Nepal Health Research Council, 10*(22), 176–180.

Chalise, A., Shrestha, G., Paudel, S., & Poudyal, A. K. (2022). Antenatal depression and its associated factors among women of Godawari Municipality, Lalitpur, Nepal: A cross-sectional study. *BMJ Open, 12*, e063513. https://doi.org/10.1136/bmjopen-2022-063513

Chalise, M., Karmacharya, I., Kaphle, M., Wagle, A., Chand, N., & Adhikari, L. (2020). Factors associated with postnatal depression among mothers attending at Bharatpur Hospital, Chitwan. *Depression Research and Treatment, 2020*, 9127672. https://doi.org/10.1155/2020/9127672

Dahal, A., Sapkota, K. P., Bhatta, D. K., & Acharya, A. (2023). Breaking barriers: A cross-sectional study on menstrual restrictions and perceived stress among adolescent girls in Kailali, Nepal. *Medrxiv*. https://doi.org/10.1101/2023.03.31.23287836

Deo, K. K., Paudel, Y. R., Khatri, R. B., Bhaskar, R. K., Paudel, R., Mehata, S., & Wagle, R. R. (2015). Barriers to utilization of antenatal care services in Eastern Nepal. *Frontiers in Public Health, 3*. https://doi.org/10.3389/fpubh.2015.00197

Deuba, K., Mainali, A., Alvesson, H. M., & Karki, D. K. (2016). Experience of intimate partner violence among young pregnant women in urban slums of Kathmandu Valley, Nepal: A qualitative study. *BMC Women's Health, 16*, 11. https://doi.org/10.1186/s12905-016-0293-7

Dhimal, M., Bista, B., Bhattarai, S., Dixit, L., Hyder, M., Agrawal, N., Rani, M., & Jha, A. (2020). Report of non communicable disease risk factors: Steps survey Nepal 2019. Nepal Health Research Council.

Dhimal, M., Dahal, S., Adhikari, K., Koirala, P., Bista, B., Luitel, N., Pant, S., Marahatta, K., Shakya, S., Sharma, P., Ghimire, S., Gyanwali, P., Ojha, S. P., & Jha, A. K. (2021). A nationwide prevalence of common mental disorders and suicidality in Nepal: Evidence from National Mental Health Survey, 2019-2020. *Journal of Nepal Health Research Council, 19*(04), 740–747. https://doi.org/10.33314/jnhrc.v19i04.4017

Dhital, R., Khatri, R., (Dahal) Paudel, S., Yangchen Sherpa, L., & Edmeades, J. (2024). *Determinants of violence against women perpetrated by intimate partners and nonpartners, 2022 Nepal DHS*. https://dhsprogram.com/publications/publication-FA154-Further-Analysis.cfm.

Dongol, A., Deoju, S., Shikharakar, S., Rayamajhi, S. J., Pradhan, N., & Tripathi, P. (2021). Menopausal symptoms in premenopausal women among the cohort of gynecological patients attending outpatient Department of Dhulikhel Hospital. *Journal of Lumbini Medical College, 9*(2) Article 2. https://doi.org/10.22502/jlmc.v9i2.467

Family Welfare Division. (2018). The-Public-Health-Service-Act-2075-2018 |. Retrieved April 1, 2025, from https://fwd.gov.np/cms/the-public-health-service-act-2075-2018/.

Gurung, D., Poudyal, A., Wang, Y. L., Neupane, M., Bhattarai, K., Wahid, S. S., Aryal, S., Heim, E., Gronholm, P., Thornicroft, G., & Kohrt, B. (2022). Stigma against mental health disorders in Nepal conceptualised with a 'what matters most' framework: A scoping review. *Epidemiology and Psychiatric Sciences, 31*, e11. https://doi.org/10.1017/S2045796021000809

Gurung, R. (2024). Co-creating respectful maternity care intervention to improve perinatal mental health in Nepal. https://urn.kb.se/resolve?urn=urn:nbn:se:uu:diva-540880.

Gurung, R., & Bask, M. (2024). Does mistreatment during institutional childbirth increase the likelihood of experiencing postpartum depressive symptoms? A prospective cohort study in Nepal. *Global Health Action, 17*(1), 2381312. https://doi.org/10.1080/16549716.2024.2381312

Ireland, J., Havelock, D., Lawrie, A., & Ghimire, S. (2021). Facilitating learning for auxiliary nurse midwives around maternal mental health in southern Nepal. *Journal of Midwifery Association of Nepal, 2*(1) .

Joshi, S., & Acharya, Y. (2022). Women's extreme seclusion during menstruation and children's health in Nepal. *PLOS Global Public Health, 2*(7), e0000355. https://doi.org/10.1371/journal.pgph.0000355

Joshi, S., Baniya, S., Bhandari, A. R., & Shakya, R. (2023). Hospital based one-stop crisis management centre at patan academy of health sciences: New avenues for the mental health professionals. *Journal of Psychiatrists' Association of Nepal, 12*(2) Article 2. https://doi.org/10.3126/jpan.v12i2.63409

Kasaju, S. P., Krumeich, A., & Van der Putten, M. (2021). Suicide and deliberate self-harm among women in Nepal: A scoping review. *BMC Women's Health, 21*(1), 407. https://doi.org/10.1186/s12905-021-01547-3

Khatri, S., Yadav, D. K., Ghimire, A., Baral, D., Yadav, B. K., & Pokharel, P. K. (2024). Behavioural and metabolic risk factors of cardiovascular diseases among post-menopausal women: A cross-sectional study in Itahari sub-metropolitan city of Nepal. *PLoS One, 19*(11), e0310725. https://doi.org/10.1371/journal.pone.0310725

Kumwar, D., Corey, E. K., Sharma, P., & Risal, A. (2015). Screening for postpartum depression and associated factors among women who deliver at a university hospital, Nepal. *Kathmandu University Medical Journal (KUMJ), 13*(49), 44–48. https://doi.org/10.3126/kumj.v13i1.13752

Maharjan, S., & Panthee, B. (2019). Prevalence of self-stigma and its association with self-esteem among psychiatric patients in a Nepalese teaching hospital: A cross-sectional study. *BMC Psychiatry, 19*(1), 347. https://doi.org/10.1186/s12888-019-2344-8

Mahato, P. K., van Teijlingen, E., Simkhada, P., Angell, C., Ireland, J., van Teijlingen, E., Simkhada, P., Mahato, P., Devkota, B., Fanning, P., Ireland, J., Simkhada, B., Sherchan, L., Silwal, R. C., Maharjan, S. K., Maharjan, R. K., Angell, C., & Douglas, F. (2018). Qualitative evaluation of mental health training of auxiliary nurse midwives in rural Nepal. *Nurse Education Today, 66*, 44–50. https://doi.org/10.1016/j.nedt.2018.03.025

Ministry of Health and Population Nepal & ICF. (2023). Nepal demographic and health survey 2022. Ministry of Health and Population [Nepal]. https://www.dhsprogram.com/pubs/pdf/FR379/FR379.pdf

National Population and Housing Census 2021 Results. (2021). Retrieved February 19, 2025, from https://censusnepal.cbs.gov.np/results/population

Nepal Law Commission |The Labour Act. (2017). Retrieved January 21, 2025, from https://lawcommission.gov.np/content/13309/labor-act-2017/

Nepal, UNFPA. (2017). Population situation analysis of Nepal. Kathmandu: UNFPA Nepal. Retrieved February 19, 2025, from https://nepal.unfpa.org/sites/default/files/pub-pdf/Nepal%20Population%20Situation%20Analysis.pdf

Neupane, M., Bartaula, M., Pradhan, S., Adhikari, H. P., Shrestha, L., Sharma, P., & Devkota, N. (2024). Postpartum depression among mothers in a maternity hospital Kathmandu, Nepal: A mixed method approach. *JNMA: Journal of the Nepal Medical Association, 62*(277), 575–581. https://doi.org/10.31729/jnma.8746

Niroula, S., Paudel, S., Chalise, A., Acharya, S., & Marasine, N. R. (2025). Menstruation experiences and its association with psychological distress among school-going adolescent girls of Nepal: A cross-sectional study. *British Journal of Developmental Psychology, 43*(1), 161–173. https://doi.org/10.1111/bjdp.12531

Paudel, R., Lee, K., Singh, J. K., Yoo, S.-J., Acharya, D., Kadel, R., Adhikari, S., Paudel, M., & Mahotra, N. (2018). Prevalence of behavioral risk factors of cardiovascular diseases and associated socio-economic factors among pregnant women in a rural area in southern Nepal. *BMC Pregnancy and Childbirth, 18*(1), 484. https://doi.org/10.1186/s12884-018-2122-5

Paudel, R., Paudyal, S., & Shrestha, S. (2020). Prevalence & factors associated with anxiety among pregnant women attending antenatal clinic of a hospital. *Journal of Psychiatrists' Association of Nepal, 9*(2) Article 2. https://doi.org/10.3126/jpan.v9i2.36285

Pokharel, A., Philip, S., Pokharel, A., Acharya, N., Dahal, S., & Ransing, R. (2023). Perinatal depression among teenage mothers in a tertiary care teaching hospital of Nepal: A cross-sectional study. *Asian Journal of Psychiatry, 90*, 103810. https://doi.org/10.1016/j.ajp.2023.103810

Pradhananga, P., Mali, P., Poudel, L., & Gurung, M. (2020). Prevalence of postpartum depression in a tertiary health care. *JNMA: Journal of the Nepal Medical Association, 58*(223), 137–140. https://doi.org/10.31729/jnma.4805

Rimal, S. P., Thapa, K., & Shrestha, R. (2022). Psychological distress and coping among pregnant women during the COVID 19 pandemic. *Journal of Nepal Health Research Council, 20*(1), 234–240. https://doi.org/10.33314/jnhrc.v20i01.4063

Rishal, P., Pun, K. D., Darj, E., Joshi, S. K., Bjørngaard, J. H., Swahnberg, K., Schei, B., Lukasse, M., Schei, B., Bjørngaard, J. H., Darj, E., Infanti, J. J., Lund, R., Lukasse, M., Swahnberg, K., Campbell, J. C., Joshi, S. K., Koju, R., Pun, K. D., et al. (2018). Prevalence and associated factors of domestic violence among pregnant women attending routine antenatal care in Nepal. *Scandinavian Journal of Public Health, 46*(8), 785–793. https://doi.org/10.1177/1403494817723195

Sah, L. K., Hatzidimitriadou, E., Wier, J., & Sah, R. K. (2024). Social determinants of the mental health of pregnant women in Nepal: Stakeholder perspectives. *PLoS One, 19*(12), e0314736. https://doi.org/10.1371/journal.pone.0314736

Sapkota, D., Anderson, D., Saito, A., & Baird, K. (2021). Domestic and family violence and its association with mental health among pregnant women attending antenatal care in a tertiary hospital of eastern Nepal. *Journal of Nepal Health Research Council, 19*(50), pp. 115–121.

Sharma, P., Gautam, K., & Marahatta, K. (2024). Access to mental health care in Nepal: Current status, potential challenges, and ways out. In S. M. Y. Arafat & S. K. Kar (Eds.), *Access to mental health care in South Asia: Current status, potential challenges, and ways out* (pp. 91–111). Springer Nature. https://doi.org/10.1007/978-981-99-9153-2_6

Sharma, S., Adhikari, L., Karmacharya, I., & Kaphle, M. (2021). Menopausal symptoms among postmenopausal women of a selected municipality: A cross-sectional survey. *JNMA: Journal of the Nepal Medical Association, 59*(243), 1155–1160. https://doi.org/10.31729/jnma.7052

Sharma, S. K., Sawangdee, Y., & Sirirassamee, B. (2007). Access to health: Women's status and utilization of maternal health services in Nepal. *Journal of Biosocial Science, 39*(5), 671–692. https://doi.org/10.1017/S0021932007001952

Shawon, M. S. R., Hossain, F. B., Hasan, M., & Rahman, M. R. (2024). Gender differences in the prevalence of anxiety and depression and care seeking for mental health problems in Nepal: Analysis of nationally representative survey data. *Cambridge Prisms: Global Mental Health, 11*, e46. https://doi.org/10.1017/gmh.2024.37

Shrestha, D., Saha, R., Manandhar, N., Adhikari, A., & Dahal, J. (2021a). Anxiety among pregnant women about Corona virus infections during COVID-19 pandemic at a Tertiary Care Center in Nepal: A descriptive cross-sectional study. *JNMA: Journal of the Nepal Medical Association, 59*(234), 152–155. https://doi.org/10.31729/jnma.5377

Shrestha, P., Mahato, V., Subedi, A., & Shrestha, S. (2021b). Anxiety and depression in pregnant women amid COVID-19 pandemic. *Asian Journal of Medical Sciences, 12*(9) Article 9. https://nepjol.info/index.php/AJMS/article/view/37229

Shrestha, S., & Pun, K. D. (2018). Anxiety on Primigravid women attending antenatal care: A hospital based cross-sectional study. *Kathmandu University Medical Journal, 16*(61), 23–27. https://doi.org/10.3102/0034654310362998

Singh, D. R., Sunuwar, D. R., Adhikari, S., Singh, S., & Karki, K. (2021). Determining factors for the prevalence of depressive symptoms among postpartum mothers in lowland region in southern Nepal. *PLoS One, 16*(1), e0245199. https://doi.org/10.1371/journal.pone.0245199

Singh, J. K., Evans-Lacko, S., Acharya, D., Kadel, R., & Gautam, S. (2018). Intimate partner violence during pregnancy and use of antenatal care among rural women in southern Terai of Nepal. *Women and Birth: Journal of the Australian College of Midwives, 31*(2), 96–102. https://doi.org/10.1016/j.wombi.2017.07.009

Subba, P., Petersen Williams, P., Luitel, N. P., Jordans, M. J. D., & Breuer, E. (2024). A qualitative study on the adaptation of community programmes for the promotion of early detection and health-seeking of perinatal depression in Nepal. *BMC Women's Health, 24*(1), 273. https://doi.org/10.1186/s12905-024-03122-y

Suvedi, B., Pradhan, A., Barnett, S., Puri, M., Chitrakar, S., & Poudel, P. (2009). *Nepal maternal mortality and morbidity study 2008/09: Summary of preliminary findings*. Health Division, Department of Health Services.

Thapa, N., Aryal, K. K., Puri, R., Shrestha, S., Shrestha, S., Thapa, P., Mehata, S., Thapa, P., Banjara, M. R., & Stray-Pedersen, B. (2016). Alcohol consumption practices among married women of reproductive age in Nepal: A population based household survey. *PLoS One, 11*(4), e0152535. https://doi.org/10.1371/journal.pone.0152535

Tohan, M. M., Saha, B. R., Moon, M. I., Howlader, M. H., & Rahman, M. A. (2025). Predictors of anxiety among women of reproductive age in Nepal: A comprehensive nationwide analysis. *Social Psychiatry and Psychiatric Epidemiology, 60*(2), 475–486. https://doi.org/10.1007/s00127-024-02791-2

van Teijlingen, E., Simkhada, P., Devkota, B., Fanning, P., Ireland, J., Simkhada, B., Sherchan, L., Silwal, R. C., Pradhan, S., Maharjan, S. K., & Maharjan, R. K. (2015). Mental health issues in pregnant women in Nepal. *Nepal Journal of Epidemiology, 5*(3), 499–501. https://doi.org/10.3126/nje.v5i3.13607

WHO. (2024). *Breaking ground in maternal mental health care in Nepal*. Retrieved March 21, 2025, from https://www.who.int/nepal/news/detail/24-12-2024-breaking-ground-in-maternal-mental-health-care-in-nepal

Chapter 7
Women's Reproductive Mental Health in Pakistan

Tamkeen Saleem and Shemaila Saleem

1 Introduction

Reproductive psychiatry is a sub-specialized field of psychiatry that focuses on the complex interactions between reproductive stages and mental health across a woman's lifespan. Reproductive life stages such as menstruation, pregnancy, postpartum, infertility, and menopause have profound effects on women's mental health, influenced by hormonal changes and social pressures. However, reproductive mental health remains a low priority in Pakistan, where cultural, societal, and systemic barriers hamper open discussion on women's reproductive and mental health subjects. The intersection of biological vulnerability and sociocultural pressures significantly influences Pakistani women's mental health during reproductive events (Mirza & Jenkins, 2004).

Deeply ingrained gender roles and stigma surrounding reproductive health contribute to poor mental health outcomes among women. Patriarchal norms often deprioritize women's mental well-being, and reproductive events are frequently medicalized or moralized without adequate psychological support (Alvi et al., 2024). Women facing infertility, for example, are often blamed and ostracized, leading to increased rates of depression and anxiety (Qadir et al., 2013).

Cultural factors in Pakistan, such as son preference, early marriage, and lack of autonomy in reproductive decisions, exacerbate women's psychological distress. The expectation to bear children soon after marriage can lead to heightened anxiety and depression, especially in cases of infertility or multiple miscarriages. Women

T. Saleem (✉)
Department of Clinical Psychology, Shifa Tameer-e-Millat University, Islamabad, Pakistan
e-mail: tamkeen.dcp@stmu.edu.pk

S. Saleem
Department of Physiology, Federal Medical College, Islamabad, Pakistan

P. Kukreti et al. (eds.), *Women's Reproductive Mental Health in South Asia*, South Asian Perspectives in Mental Health and Psychology,
https://doi.org/10.1007/978-981-96-9219-4_7

who give birth to daughters are more likely to experience depressive symptoms due to social devaluation and familial disappointment (Qadir et al., 2011). Furthermore, many Pakistani women are reluctant to discuss reproductive, sexual, or mental health issues due to fear of social exclusion, leading to delays in seeking help (Punjani et al., 2023; Causier et al., 2024).

Gender-based violence in terms of physical abuse is a major predictor of anxiety/depression (Fikree & Bhatti, 1999). Reproductive coercion is a significant public health concern, as it has been linked to adverse mental health outcomes (Muñoz et al., 2023). Women who experience reproductive coercion in the form of forced pregnancies or denial of contraception often exhibit mental health problems, specifically symptoms of depression and posttraumatic stress disorder (PTSD), as observed in both clinical and college populations (Ali et al., 2009; Ghayur et al., 2023).

2 Prevalence of Mental Health Disorders during Reproductive Phases

2.1 Menstruation

The menstrual cycle starts at menarche, continues throughout the reproductive years, and concludes at menopause. Typically, it begins between the ages of 11 and 15. In healthy women, menstrual bleeding lasts up to 8 days, with an average blood loss ranging from 37 to 43 milliliters and a maximum limit of 80 milliliters (Kilby & Luesley, 2016). In Pakistan, menstrual problems are quite common (Farhan et al., 2020). The intersection of menstruation and mental health is influenced by cultural taboos, limited awareness, and inadequate healthcare access. These factors contribute to the underdiagnosis and undertreatment of menstrual-related mental health disorders. The family served as the primary support system, providing access and addressing the needs of individuals in this age group. This support was both time-specific and based on immediate needs—information was typically shared only after a girl experienced her first menstrual cycle, offering limited guidance on the physical and emotional changes she would face and how to manage them. Discussing topics related to sexuality remained a sensitive and often avoided issue. Menstruation remains a taboo subject in many parts of Pakistan (Aflaq & Jami, 2012), leading to misinformation and stigma. A cross-sectional study in Karachi universities revealed that only 19% of female students were aware of PMDD, highlighting the country's lack of awareness and the taboo associated with menstruation in Pakistan's conservative society (Mohib et al., 2018; Waseem et al., 2025). The following are common menstrual problems and their connection to mental health in Pakistan.

2.1.1 Premenstrual Dysphoric Disorder (PMDD)

A study involving 635 female medical students in Pakistan found that 12.1% met the criteria for PMDD. Those affected reported significantly lower scores in both physical and psychological domains of quality of life compared to their peers without PMDD (Mahmood et al., 2023).

2.1.2 Premenstrual Syndrome (PMS)

PMS is prevalent among Pakistani women, with symptoms such as anxiety, depression, fatigue, and anger being commonly reported. The study found that 12.9% of females were unaware of menstruation, while 38.7% lacked awareness of premenstrual syndrome (PMS). PMS was present in 27.1% of the participants, yet only 16.8% sought medical help during emergencies. Significant associations were identified between PMS and various anthropometric and physiological factors, including weight, parity, blood group, marital status, monthly income, daily routines, emotional impact, communication about PMS, medical consultations, as well as pain and autonomic symptoms. These findings highlight a substantial gap in awareness about menstruation and PMS among women in Azad Kashmir and Pakistan. There is an urgent need for targeted awareness campaigns to educate women about PMS, improve health literacy, and promote overall well-being (Zahid et al., 2023).

2.1.3 Psychological Stress and Menstrual Disorders

A study reported that women presenting with new-onset menstrual disorders exhibited elevated psychological stress levels (Tufail et al., 2022). Another study reported that the most prevalent menstrual problems were dysmenorrhea and premenstrual symptoms, which were strongly associated with stress among students (Rafique & Al-Sheikh, 2018).

2.2 Pregnancy and Post-Natal Period

Depression and anxiety during pregnancy are highly prevalent, with postpartum depression (PPD) emerging as a significant public health issue. A study reported that around 36% of women in the postnatal period experience depression in comparison to global estimates of around 13% (Husain et al., 2006). Another study reported that the prevalence of PPD is estimated between 28% and 63%, much higher than in high-income countries (Rahman et al., 2008). These high rates are linked with factors like poverty, lack of emotional, social, and medical support, domestic violenceDomestic violence, and unplanned pregnancies.

2.3 Abortion

Abortion remains a highly sensitive issue, with legal restrictions and strong social stigma creating significant psychological burdens for women (Shah & Ahman, 2009). Despite the fact that abortion is legally restricted in Pakistan except to save the life of the mother, many women rely on abortion when they experience an unintended pregnancy. However, due to restrictions, many women are compelled to seek unsafe procedures that carry not only physical risks but also long-term emotional trauma (Sathar et al., 2014, 2025). Research has shown that the fear of legal repercussions and the lack of accessible, safe abortion options contribute to a cycle of anxiety and depression among women in these regions (Rajkumar, 2022). In Pakistan, restrictive abortion laws and cultural taboos often result in feelings of guilt, trauma, and anxiety, particularly when women seek abortions outside the legal or prescribed medical channels.

2.4 Infertility

Infertility remains a deeply stigmatized condition across South Asia, often resulting in significant psychological distress for women. Cultural expectations surrounding motherhood, particularly the high value placed on childbearing within marriage, intensify emotional burdens such as depression, anxiety, and social isolation (Unisa, 2010). Similar patterns have been observed in Pakistan, where infertility can severely compromise a woman's social status and quality of life (Ali et al., 2011).

2.5 Menopause

During the phase of menopause, predominantly the perimenopausal period, women tend to get vulnerable to experiencing mood disturbances. Globally, women are found to be 30% more likely to experience major depressive disorder and over twice as likely to develop mania in the years following menopause (Woods et al., 2008). A study found a higher prevalence of depression and anxiety among postmenopausal women (Malik et al., 2021). Another study reported that women tend to experience greater levels of depression during menopause. The findings further revealed that women not taking hormone replacement therapy reported severe symptoms of menopause and climacteric depression in comparison to women taking hormone replacement therapy (Saleem et al., 2017).

2.6 *Polycystic Ovarian Syndrome*

Women with polycystic ovary syndrome (PCOS) are reported to have higher levels of depression, anxiety, and body image dissatisfaction in comparison to women without PCOS. In a cross-sectional study in Pakistan, 61% of women with PCOS testified to experiencing moderate to severe depressive symptoms, which are linked to hormonal imbalance and infertility-related concerns (Hussain & Tabassum, 2023).

Mostly disorders like Premenstrual dysphoric disorder (PMDD), perinatal depression, and postpartum psychosis are underdiagnosed due to stigma and limited access to mental health professionals trained in reproductive psychiatry.

3 Barriers to Reproductive Psychiatric Care

Several systemic and socio-cultural barriers hinder the growth of reproductive psychiatry in Pakistan. Stigma surrounding both mental health and reproductive issues discourages women from seeking help (Mirza & Jenkins, 2004).

Furthermore, a severe shortage of trained psychiatrists and mental health professionals—approximately 0.2 psychiatrists per 100,000 population—exacerbates the treatment gap (Ahmad, 2007). Most available services are urban-centered, leaving rural populations significantly underserved. Current findings from consultations and literature indicate that around 51% of psychiatrists in Pakistan practice in private settings, predominantly located in urban areas, while 45% are employed in the public sector, and the remaining 4% work across both sectors. The majority are based in tertiary-level provincial hospitals, whereas public hospital positions at the district level remain largely unfilled. Additionally, only 72% of trained psychologists are actively practicing in the country, with contributing factors including limited career opportunities, household responsibilities, and a lack of advanced educational options. Among non-specialized healthcare providers, although social workers are involved in community services, only 0.005 per 100,000 population have received mental health training (Bhugra et al., 2015).

Gender norms and lack of autonomy also impact women's mental health. Many women face marital pressures, early and repeated pregnancies, and limited support systems, all contributing to psychological distress (Ali et al., 2009). Additionally, obstetricians and gynecologists often lack formal training in recognizing and managing psychiatric symptoms related to reproductive events, creating a critical gap in integrated care (Mazhar, 2017).

4 Current Initiatives and Opportunities for Reproductive Psychiatry

In Pakistan, reproductive psychiatry remains an emerging field, though significant strides have been made through various initiatives aimed at improving mental health services for women during reproductive phases. These initiatives focus on addressing mental health concerns associated with pregnancy, postpartum depression, infertility, and other reproductive health challenges.

The *Thinking Healthy Programme*, developed by Rahman et al. (2008), is a notable mental health initiative in Pakistan that integrates cognitive behavioral therapy (CBT) techniques into maternal and child health care. Implemented within the existing health system in a rural sub-district, the intervention equips community health workers—particularly those in the Lady Health Worker Program—with skills such as active listening, family collaboration, guided discovery (a method of gentle questioning to explore beliefs and introduce alternative perspectives), and the assignment of homework tasks to help mothers apply learned strategies between sessions. These techniques are incorporated into their routine maternal and child health education. These pilot studies revealed that both health workers and mothers with perinatal depression found the program highly relevant and beneficial. Overall, such initiatives have demonstrated promising outcomes in reducing depressive symptoms and improving maternal mental health at the community level in rural Pakistan (Rahman, 2007).

The Government of Pakistan has established the Lady Health Worker Program (LHW-P), which holds significant potential for delivering basic mental health services at the community level. However, the current training curriculum for Lady Health Workers does not include mental health as a core subject. To address this gap, the World Health Organization's Mental Health Gap Intervention Guide (mhGAP-IG), Version 2.0—designed for managing mental, neurological, and substance use disorders in non-specialist settings—could be adapted and integrated into the LHW-P curriculum. This adaptation would enhance the capacity of community health workers to identify and address mental health issues effectively at the grassroots level (Rabbani et al., 2023).

Telepsychiatry and digital mental health interventions offer new opportunities, especially for women in remote areas or who feel limited access due to stigmatization to visit a health care center for psychiatric care. Culturally adapted tools, community-based interventions, and collaboration between psychiatric and gynecological services can further enhance the reach of reproductive psychiatric care.

Women in Pakistan are disproportionately impacted by the increasing prevalence of depression and anxiety. Telepsychiatry presents a promising solution to address this growing mental health burden. As an innovative and accessible mode of care, telepsychiatry has the potential to transform mental health service delivery. It offers policymakers and mental health professionals a valuable tool for designing cost-effective, scalable mental health interventions, particularly suited for low-income and underserved populations (Aga et al., 2023; Ishtiaq & Shah, 2024).

Similarly, telehealth applications are expanding within obstetrics and gynecology, offering innovative platforms that allow obstetricians, gynecologists, and other healthcare providers to enhance prenatal, intrapartum, and postpartum care. Through maternal-fetal medicine telehealth, specialists and subspecialists can collaborate in a team-based approach, improving the quality and safety of obstetric care, particularly in fragmented healthcare systems, such as those found in rural areas with limited access to high-quality services. In this context, telepsychiatric services could be integrated to provide reproductive psychiatric care for women, further enhancing the overall healthcare experience (Bilal et al., 2022).

5 Recommendations for Advancing Reproductive Psychiatry in Pakistan

5.1 Integration of Reproductive Psychiatric Care in General Healthcare for Women

There is a growing recognition of the importance of integrating reproductive mental health into existing maternal healthcare services. Initiatives such as perinatal mental health screening during antenatal visits could be integrated into routine care in public hospitals. This would provide early identification of mental health issues, ensuring timely intervention and support for women.

5.2 Telepsychiatric Services

Given Pakistan's vast rural areas with limited access to mental health professionals, telepsychiatry offers a promising solution. The rise of telehealth services presents an opportunity to extend reproductive psychiatric care to remote regions. Telepsychiatry can help address the growing mental health needs of women by offering counseling and psychiatric support, particularly for conditions like postpartum depression and perinatal anxiety.

5.3 Research and Policy Development

There is an increasing need for research related to reproductive psychiatric care in Pakistan. Research studies examining the mental health implications of reproductive events, such as pregnancy, the postpartum period, and menopause, are slowly gaining momentum. However, more research is needed to understand the unique mental health challenges faced by women in Pakistan. Policymakers also need to recognize the need for addressing women's reproductive mental health in national health policies.

5.4 Curriculum for Lady Health Worker Program (LHW-P)

The LHW-P is an established initiative aimed at providing basic healthcare services, including maternal and child health, at the community level. However, there is a need for integrating mental health care into this program to address issues like perinatal depression and other mental health problems experienced at various reproductive stages. Current training for Lady Health Workers does not cover mental health, but there are opportunities to adapt and integrate the World Health Organization's Mental Health Gap Action Programme (mhGAP-IG) into their curriculum, which could enable health workers to address common mental health issues in reproductive women at the grassroots level.

5.5 Training Healthcare Providers

Integrating reproductive mental health education into the curricula of medical and nursing schools is essential for equipping healthcare providers with the necessary knowledge and skills to address the mental health needs of women during reproductive stages. Also, launching fellowship programs for reproductive psychiatry will lead to the availability of trained personnel.

5.6 Education and Awareness

Mental health issues related to reproductive health are often stigmatized, with many women feeling reluctant to seek help due to cultural norms and taboos surrounding reproductive health. Educating via seminars and media about reproductive mental health can help reduce this stigma and normalize the conversation around mental health, making it easier for women to seek help without fear of judgment. Developing campaigns that are sensitive to the diverse cultural contexts within a country is essential.

5.7 *Access to Counseling Services*

Counseling services must be made more accessible, particularly in rural and underserved areas. Establishing community-based mental health services and incorporating counseling into prenatal, postnatal, and fertility treatments will provide much-needed psychological support for women.

5.8 *Early Treatment and Easy Therapies*

Menstrual problems are common in Pakistani women. These disorders are a significant source of morbidity. Awareness should be given for early treatment and management within the available reproductive health resources and programs, including educational packages and easy therapies like hormonal contraceptives.

6 Conclusion

Women's reproductive psychiatric care in Pakistan remains a critical yet underaddressed aspect of public health, exacerbated by sociocultural norms, limited access to specialized services, and a lack of awareness about the mental health challenges women face during various reproductive stages. From menstruation and pregnancy to postpartum depression, infertility, and menopause, reproductive transitions are deeply intertwined with mental health, yet they are often overlooked in healthcare policies and services.

Several challenges contribute to this gap, including a lack of trained mental health professionals in rural areas, insufficient mental health education in healthcare curricula, and the persistent stigma surrounding mental health issues. These challenges are compounded by gender-based violence, reproductive coercion, and deeply ingrained cultural norms that discourage women from seeking help for mental health concerns related to reproduction.

References

Aflaq, F., & Jami, H. (2012). Experiences and attitudes related to menstruation among female students. *Pakistan Journal of Psychological Research, 27*(2) .

Aga, I. Z., Khurram, S. S., Karim, M., Muzzamil, M., Hashmi, S., & Shafique, K. (2023). Employing telepsychiatry services to assess the prevalence and identify mental health disorders using the PHQ-9 and GAD-7 in resource-constrained regions of Dadar Mansehra, Pakistan: An observational cross-sectional study. *BMJ Open, 13*(12), e078976. https://doi.org/10.1136/bmjopen-2023-078976

Ahmad, K. (2007). Shortage of psychiatrists a problem in Pakistan. *The Lancet, 370*(9590), 817–818. https://doi.org/10.1016/S0140-6736(07)61397-X

Ali, S., Sophie, R., Imam, A. M., Khan, F. I., Ali, S. F., Shaikh, A., & Farid-ul-Hasnain, S. (2011). Knowledge, perceptions and myths regarding infertility among selected adult population in Pakistan: A cross-sectional study. *BMC Public Health, 11*, 760. https://doi.org/10.1186/1471-2458-11-760

Ali, F. A., Israr, S. M., Ali, B. S., & Janjua, N. Z. (2009). Association of various reproductive rights, domestic violence and marital rape with depression among Pakistani women. *BMC Psychiatry, 9*, 1–13. https://doi.org/10.1186/1471-244X-9-77

Alvi, M. H., Ashraf, T., Naz, F., Sardar, A., Ullah, A., Patel, A., et al. (2024). Burden of mental disorders by gender in Pakistan: Analysis of global burden of disease study data for 1990–2019. *BJPsych Bulletin, 48*(6), 333–340. https://doi.org/10.1192/bjb.2023.76

Bhugra, S. D., Roger, N., & Takei, N. (2015). *Routledge handbook of psychiatry in Asia*. Abingdon: Routledge.

Bilal, W., Qamar, K., Siddiqui, A., Kumar, P., & Essar, M. Y. (2022). Digital health and telemedicine in Pakistan: Improving maternal healthcare. *Annals of Medicine and Surgery, 81*. https://doi.org/10.1016/j.amsu.2022.104425

Bhugra, S. D., Roger, N., & Takei, N. (2015). *Routledge handbook of psychiatry in Asia*. Routledge.

Causier, C., Johns, L., Radez, J., Hassan, H., Maughan, D., & Waite, F. (2024). Experiences of help-seeking for severe mental health problems in young Pakistani women: A preliminary qualitative study. *Journal of Cross-Cultural Psychology, 55*(4), 429–443. https://doi.org/10.1177/00220221241236944

Farhan, I., Akhtar, M., & Abid, R. (2020). Prevalence of menstrual disorders in woman of reproductive age group. *Education, 30*(40), 249. https://pjmhsonline.com/2020/jan_march/pdf/194.pdf

Fikree, F. F., & Bhatti, L. I. (1999). Domestic violence and health of Pakistani women. *International Journal of Gynecology & Obstetrics, 65*(2), 195–201. https://doi.org/10.1016/s0020-7292(99)00035-1

Ghayur, M. S., Jamil, J., Sadia, H., Jamil, M., Adeeb, H., Nadir, S., & Iftikhar, B. (2023). Reproductive coercion and its effects on women's reproductive health outcomes-a cross-sectional study. *Journal of Medical Sciences, 31*(3), 173–177. https://doi.org/10.52764/jms.23.31.3.1

Husain, N., Bevc, I., Husain, M., Chaudhry, I. B., Atif, N., & Rahman, A. (2006). Prevalence and social correlates of postnatal depression in a low income country. *Archives of women's mental health, 9*(4), 197–202.

Hussain, A., & Tabassum, A. (2023). Descriptive investigation of depression and anxiety: Emphasis on women with polycystic ovary syndrome. *Journal of Asian Development Studies, 12*(3), 860–868.

Ishtiaq, K., & Shah, W. S. (2024). Commentary: Transforming mental health care in Pakistan through telemedicine. *The Professional Medical Journal, 31*(12), 1635–1637. https://doi.org/10.29309/TPMJ/2024.31.12.8393

Kilby, M. D., & Luesley, D. M. (Eds.). (2016). *Obstetrics & gynaecology: An evidence-based text for MRCOG*. CRC Press.

Mahmood, Z., Butt, A., & Cheema, M. A. (2023). Frequency of premenstrual dysphoric disorder (PMDD) and comparison of quality of life between female medical students with and without premenstrual dysphoric disorder. *Journal of the College of Physicians and Surgeons–Pakistan, 69*, 56–100. https://doi.org/10.29271/jcpsp.2023.06.638

Malik, M., Mahjabeen, M., Rana, S., Hussain, A., & Hashmi, A. (2021). Quality of life and depression among postmenopausal women in Pakistan. *Archives of Pharmacy Practice, 12*(3), 29–33. https://doi.org/10.51847/MAPShK83EB

Mazhar, S. B. (2017). The Obstetrician and Gynecologist and Unmet Mental Health Needs. *Journal of The Society of Obstetricians and Gynaecologists of Pakistan, 7*(3), 112–113.

Mirza, I., & Jenkins, R. (2004). Risk factors, prevalence, and treatment of anxiety and depressive disorders in Pakistan: Systematic review. *BMJ, 328*(7443), 794. https://doi.org/10.51847/MAPShK83EB

Mohib, A., Zafar, A., Najam, A., Tanveer, H., & Rehman, R. (2018). Premenstrual syndrome: Existence, knowledge, and attitude among female university students in Karachi. *Cureus, 10*(3). https://doi.org/10.7759/cureus.2290

Muñoz, E. A., Shorey, R. C., & Temple, J. R. (2023). Reproductive coercion victimization and associated mental health outcomes among female-identifying young adults. *Journal of Trauma & Dissociation, 24*(4), 538–554. https://doi.org/10.1080/15299732.2023.2212407

Punjani, N. S., Papathanassoglou, E., Hegadoren, K., Hirani, S., Mumtaz, Z., & Jackson, M. (2023). Sexuality and mental health of Pakistani-descent adolescent girls living in Canada: Perceptions and recommendations. *Adolescents, 3*(3), 564–580. https://doi.org/10.3390/adolescents3030040

Rabbani, F., Akhtar, S., Nafis, J., Khan, S., Siddiqi, S., & Merali, Z. (2023). Addition of mental health to the lady health worker curriculum in Pakistan: Now or never. *Human Resources for Health, 21*(1), 29. https://doi.org/10.1186/s12960-023-00814-8

Rafique, N., & Al-Sheikh, M. H. (2018). Prevalence of menstrual problems and their association with psychological stress in young female students studying health sciences. *Saudi Medical Journal, 39*(1), 67. https://doi.org/10.15537/smj.2018.1.21438

Rahman, A. (2007). Challenges and opportunities in developing a psychological intervention for perinatal depression in rural Pakistan—a multi-method study. *Archives of Women's Mental Health, 10*, 211–219. https://doi.org/10.1007/s00737-007-0193-9

Rahman, A., Malik, A., Sikander, S., Roberts, C., & Creed, F. (2008). Cognitive behaviour therapy-based intervention by community health workers for mothers with depression and their infants in rural Pakistan: A cluster-randomised controlled trial. *The Lancet, 372*(9642), 902–909. https://doi.org/10.1016/S0140-6736(08)61400-2

Rajkumar, R. P. (2022). The relationship between access to abortion and mental health in women of childbearing age: Analyses of data from the global burden of disease studies. *Cureus, 14*(11). https://doi.org/10.7759/cureus.31433

Saleem, T., Ishfaq, W., & Saleem, S. (2017). Menopause symptoms and climacteric depression in women with and without hormone replacement therapy. *Pakistan Journal of Physiology, 13*(1), 43–45. https://doi.org/10.69656/pjp.v13i1.266

Sathar, Z., Singh, S., Shah, I. H., Niazi, M. R., Parveen, T., Mulhern, O., & Mir, A. M. (2025). Abortion and unintended pregnancy in Pakistan: New evidence for 2023 and trends over the past decade. *BMJ Globalization and Health, 10*(1). https://doi.org/10.1136/bmjgh-2024-017239

Sathar, Z., Singh, S., Rashida, G., Shah, Z., & Niazi, R. (2014). Induced abortions and unintended pregnancies in Pakistan. *Studies in Family Planning, 45*(4), 471–491. https://doi.org/10.1111/j.1728-4465.2014.00004.x

Shah, I. H., & Ahman, E. (2009). *Unsafe abortion: The global public health challenge. Management of unintended and abnormal pregnancy* (pp. 10–23). Wiley-Blackwell. https://doi.org/10.1002/9781444313031.ch2

Tufail, A., Mustafa, R., Munaver, S. A., & Nawaz, B. (2022). Frequency of psychological stress among women with new onset menstrual disorders amid corona pandemic lockdown. *Pakistan Journal of Medical Sciences, 38*(5), 1159. https://doi.org/10.12669/pjms.38.5.4606

Unisa, S. (2010). Infertility and treatment seeking in India: Findings from district level household survey. *Facts, Views & Vision in ObGyn, 2*(2), 59–65.

Qadir, F., Khan, M. M., Medhin, G., & Prince, M. (2011). Male gender preference, female gender disadvantage as risk factors for psychological morbidity in Pakistani women of childbearing age-a life course perspective. *BMC Public Health, 11*, 1–13. https://doi.org/10.1186/1471-2458-11-745

Qadir, F., Khalid, A., Haqqani, S., & Medhin, G. (2013). The association of marital relationship and perceived social support with mental health of women in Pakistan. *BMC Public Health, 13*, 1–13. https://doi.org/10.1186/1471-2458-13-1150

Waseem, H., Sohail, M., & Rab, S. (2025). Overlooked consequences of undiagnosed premenstrual dysphoric disorder in Pakistani women. *The Journal of the Pakistan Medical Association, 75*(1), 174–175. https://doi.org/10.47391/JPMA.20522

Woods, N. F., Smith-DiJulio, K., Percival, D. B., Tao, E. Y., Mariella, A., & Mitchell, E. S. (2008). Depressed mood during the menopausal transition and early postmenopause: Observations from the Seattle midlife women's health study. *Menopause, 15*(2), 223–232. https://doi.org/10.1097/gme.0b013e3181450fc2

Zahid, K., Aijaz, D., Tariq, Z., Qadeer, M. I., Alam, N., Hisham, K., ... & Ali, Z. (2023). Prevalence of premenstrual syndrome among the females of Azad Kashmir and Pakistan and its explicating factors. https://doi.org/10.21203/rs.3.rs-3194711/v1

Chapter 8
Women's Reproductive Mental Health in Sri Lanka

Dulshika Waas and Thilini Rajapakse

1 Introduction

Sri Lanka is a small island in the Indian Ocean, a lower-middle-income country (LMIC) with a total population of 22.3 million in mid-2023. There is a slight female preponderance, with the total female population amounting to approximately 11.4 million. The number of women in the reproductive age group between 15 and 49 years in Sri Lanka is approximately 6.7 million, which equals 67.2% of the total female population. The literacy rate for those aged 15 and above is 91.7% for females and 90.8% for males (Department of Census and statistics, 2024). Government-funded mental health services in Sri Lanka have developed considerably over the last four decades. Mental health clinics are available in all districts of the country, and psychiatry inpatient units are available in many regions. *Government-funded* mental health services are provided free of charge to the public. However, specific services for females, such as psychiatry mother and baby units, remain limited and restricted to urban areas.

D. Waas
Department of Psychiatry, Faculty of Medical Sciences, University of Sri Jayewardenepura, Nugegoda, Sri Lanka

T. Rajapakse (✉)
Department of Psychiatry, Faculty of Medicine, University of Peradeniya, Kandy, Sri Lanka
e-mail: trajapakse@pdn.ac.lk

P. Kukreti et al. (eds.), *Women's Reproductive Mental Health in South Asia*, South Asian Perspectives in Mental Health and Psychology,
https://doi.org/10.1007/978-981-96-9219-4_8

2 Perinatal Mental Health Disorders

Motherhood is often a much-look-forward-to and positive experience for women. However, this transitional period could also be stressful for the mother because of the associated physiological, cognitive, emotional and social changes. The World Health Organization (WHO) reports that 7% of the global burden of disease in women is due to mental health problems in the reproductive age groups (WHO, 2017). This highlights the importance of good mental health for women in this age group and especially for pregnant and peripartum women.

In Sri Lankan culture, expectant mothers are often revered as symbols of prosperity and are known in the Sinhala language as 'Gabbara Asiriya' (Dalupotha, 2003). From ancient times, there exists a local culture of traditions and rituals which are performed for the mental and physical well-being of the pregnant mother during the perinatal period, which varies between different ethnic communities (Fargnoli and Seneviratne, 2022).

It is reported that in LMICs, overall perinatal mental health problems affect 18–25% of women (Gelaye et al., 2016). The Family Health Bureau of the Ministry of Health, Sri Lanka, in its annual report states that in the years 2019 and 2020, there were 27 cases of post-partum psychiatric disorders diagnosed for every 10,000 deliveries in Sri Lanka. Although studies are limited, available data shows that a significant prevalence of perinatal depressive and anxiety disorders are present among women in Sri Lanka too. These are described in more detail below.

2.1 Perinatal Depression

A systematic review and meta-analysis conducted in 2023 found that the pooled point prevalence of depression among the perinatal mothers was 16.9% (Alwis et al., 2024). Regarding antenatal depression, there is a range of prevalence reported, and data are limited by possible differences of study methodology and geographical variation. A study on antenatal depression conducted in a large district in the North Central Province reported a rate of 16.2% (Agampodi & Agampodi, 2013), whereas a study in a district in the North Western Province reported 25.6% (Rowel, 2004). In the capital city of Colombo, data from antenatal clinics of two tertiary care maternity hospitals found that 33.6% of mothers were experiencing depression (Suraweera et al., 2021). Having a history of depression, suicidal ideation (Agampodi & Agampodi, 2013; Palfreyman, 2021), lack of support from the spouse and intimate partner violence were associated with increased risk of depression (Palfreyman, 2021).

As expected, the reported prevalence of post-partum depression seems higher than antenatal depression, though again there is no national level data. A large descriptive cross-sectional study on post-partum depression in a district in the North Central Province of Sri Lanka reported the prevalence of post-partum depression to be 27.1%, during 2 weeks to 12 months of post-partum (Agampodi et al., 2011). The reported prevalence was 32.1% in a district in the Northwestern province (Rowel, 2004). Another study from a suburb in the Colombo district reported a 4-week post-partum prevalence of 7.1% (Gankanda, 2021), and similar rates of 7.8–9.5% were reported from a district in the Southern province (Roystead-Solas, 2022; Fan, 2020).

When considered overall, evidence indicates varying rates of antenatal and post-partum depression from different parts of the country, which may reflect differences in study methodology. These findings are broadly in keeping from findings in South Asia which report the prevalence of post-partum depression to be between 5% and 49% (Hahn-Holbrook et al., 2018). The challenges in interpreting these findings are that studies are often limited to certain areas of the country.

2.2 *Perinatal Anxiety Disorders*

Publications regarding perinatal anxiety disorders in Sri Lanka are scarce compared with studies published on depressive disorders. One study assessed a random sample of 221 antenatal women attending routine antenatal clinics at a teaching hospital in Colombo and reported that antenatal anxiety disorders (AADs) were diagnosed in 81 (37%) of women (Priyadarshanie et al., 2023). A community study in the Badulla district using the Depression, Anxiety and Stress Scale (DASS 21) screening tool found that 20.7% of primigravida mothers were suffering from anxiety (Nishshanka et al., 2023). Another study done in a major maternity hospital in Colombo reported that 42.6% of attendees have anxiety, out of which 4.6% were reported to have severe anxiety (Anjalika et al., 2023).

Antenatal anxiety in LMICs ranges from 10% to 41%, which is comparable with the rates reported from Sri Lanka (WHO, 2022). The correlates that were significantly associated with antenatal anxiety in Sri Lanka included younger age of mother, lower educational level, pregnancy-related medical conditions and younger age of partner (Anjalika et al., 2023). Antenatal comorbidities such as pregnancy-induced hypertension (OR 6.1; 95% CI 1.2–31.9) and gestational diabetes mellitus (OR 12.6; 95% CI 1.5–107.2) were also associated with antenatal anxiety disorders (Priyadarshanie et al., 2023). Delivery-associated outcomes linked to AADs were preterm labour (OR 4.3; 95% CI 1.4–13.0), prolonged labour (OR 19.0; 95% CI 7.1–51.1) and lower segment caesarean section (LSCS) (OR 4.7; 95% CI 2.5–8.7) (Priyadarshanie et al., 2023). AADs were also associated with low birth weight in the neonate (OR 11.2; 95% CI 4.8–26.3) (Priyadarshanie et al., 2023).

Local research regarding interventions for perinatal anxiety is sparse, but one randomized control trial reported that progressive muscle relaxation therapy was effective in improving pregnancy outcomes in primigravida mothers with anxiety (Nishshanka et al., 2023).

3 Psychological Impact of Miscarriage and Medical Termination of Pregnancy

Miscarriage is defined as a pregnancy loss before the viability of an embryo or foetus, i.e. occurring at 20 weeks of gestation or less (American College of Obstetricians and gynaecologists 2009). A study conducted in a tertiary care hospital in Colombo among 405 women admitted after miscarriage found that 55.7% met the cut-off scores for depression, 66.6% for anxiety and 50.2% for stress (this study used the locally validated DASS-21 scale) (Pathiraja et al., 2018). The symptoms of depression, anxiety and stress were severe in 14%, 40% and 18% of the patients, respectively. The scores for depression and anxiety were significantly higher in women who had undergone treatment for subfertility (Pathiraja et al., 2018).

A cohort study carried out to explore psychological morbidity following miscarriage at a tertiary care hospital in Colombo North found that rates of psychological morbidity were as high as 40% in the initial stage, and this persisted in up to 25% after 6–8 weeks (Wijesooriya et al., 2015). Women were more likely to experience higher levels of psychological morbidity at the end of 12 weeks if they were more than 30 years of age and had a history of infertility preceding the miscarriage, a history of previous miscarriage or a nulliparity or a gestation period of >12 weeks (Wijesooriya et al., 2015).

Induced abortion (IA) is illegal in Sri Lanka except when it is performed to save the mother's life. Despite this, it is estimated that over 500 illegal induced abortions occur daily in Sri Lanka (Ban, 2002). It is reported that in Sri Lanka, 5–6% of all maternal deaths occur in the context of abortion (Department of Census and Statistics, 2008). Despite the availability of statistics on women who have undergone induced abortions, we were not able to find any local studies on the psychological morbidity of the woman after this procedure.

4 Menopause

Sri Lankan women are known to experience menopause between 49 and 51 years of age on average. Approximately three decades of a woman's life is in the postmenopausal period, given the approximate life expectancy of a woman to be 78 years. There are very few studies on quality of life among pre- and postmenopausal women in Sri Lanka (Waidyasekera, 2009) and even fewer studies on their psychological morbidity. Most available Sri Lankan studies in this field have used the culturally adapted Menopause Rating Scale. A cross-sectional study done in the South of Sri Lanka reported that among premenopausal women, the most frequently reported psychological symptoms were mental exhaustion (49.5%) and irritability (41.3%), and postmenopausal women reported a slightly higher rate of physical and mental exhaustion (53%) and irritability (48.2%), in addition to a depressive mood (43.4%) (Rathnayake et al., 2019).

A community-based case-control study conducted in the district of Colombo reported that risk factors specific for depression among menopausal women were related to reproductive factors (presence of premenstrual symptoms in the past and presence of menopausal symptoms) and social and psychological factors such as the nuclear family structure, the social support available and stressful life events (Dheerasinghe, 2019). No published studies were found on interventions for this condition.

5 Maternal Suicide and Suicide Among Females in the Reproductive Age Group in Sri Lanka

When considering suicide among women overall, in 2022 in Sri Lanka, the rate of suicide was highest among young females in the reproductive age group, aged between 17 and 25 years, mostly by hanging (Bandara et al., 2024a). This contrasts with data from the Western world, where the highest proportion of suicides are among older people (above 50 years), in both genders—but this is similar to findings from other South Asian countries, such as India (Arya et al., 2019; Patel et al., 2012).

The number and rate of maternal suicides (women who died by suicide during pregnancy or up to 1 year post-partum) in Sri Lanka increased from 0.8 per 100,000 live births in 2002 to a peak of 12.1 in 2010—an increase that is of significant concern. The rate of maternal suicides showed a slight decline to 8.4 in 2017 (Jayaratne et al., 2018), but rates were 9.8 and 8.7 per 100,000 live births in 2020 and 2021, respectively (Family Health Bureau, 2020). In the review by Jayaratne et al. of the suicides between years 2002 and 2017, 42.3% of women committed suicide during pregnancy and 31.4% post-partum (Jayaratne et al., 2018).

Regarding methods of suicide, Jayaratne et al. in 2018 reported that the common methods used were self-poisoning (36.8%) and hanging (31.6%). A shift in the trend was seen in 2020 with suicide by hanging becoming the most common method (54.5%), followed by suicide by self-immolation (22.7%)—based on analysis of 22 of 29 suicides in 2020 (Bureau, 2020). This may reflect changes of methods of suicide in Sri Lanka as a whole, since from 2015 onwards, the most common method of suicide overall in the country among males and females has been by hanging, with pesticide ingestion taking the second place.

5.1 Non-fatal Self-Harm

Trends of non-fatal self-harm in Sri Lanka are in keeping with international patterns—again rates are higher among young females in the reproductive age group (Rajapakse et al., 2013; De Silva & Ratnayake, 2008; Rajapakse et al., 2013). With regard to self-harm during pregnancy and the post-partum period, data on intentional self-harm (ISH) interpolated from a cohort study of 1295 mothers conducted in 2023 showed that the calculated incidence density of ISH and attempted suicide was 11.6 and 7.6 per 1000 pregnant women, respectively (Agampodi et al., 2023).

5.2 Factors Associated with Maternal Suicide, Suicide and Self-Harm Among Females in the Reproductive Age Group in Sri Lanka

5.2.1 Domestic Violence

Experience of domestic violence repeatedly emerges as a key factor linked with suicidal behaviour among young females in the reproductive age group, in Sri Lanka and South Asia (Bandara et al., 2024b). Analysis of data gathered during the government-conducted nationwide Sri Lanka 2016 Demographic and Health Survey reveals that exposure to interpersonal violence (IPV) in the previous year was associated with 3.8 times increase of non-fatal self-harm (Bandara et al., 2024b). Similar associations between exposure to domestic violence and suicidal behaviour is reported from other LMICs as well (Vijayakumar et al., 2021). The national prevalence survey on violence against women, conducted in 2019 by the Department of Census and Statistics, Sri Lanka, reports that one in five (20.4%) ever-married women in the country has experienced physical or sexual violence from a partner, during their lifetime (*Women's Wellbeing Survey 2019 Sri Lanka*, 2019). The experience of violence by women was not limited to partners—the same survey found that 7.2% of women had experienced non-partner violence during their lifetime. Women who had experienced physical violence were much more likely to have had suicidal ideation (35.7%), compared to their counterparts who had never experienced violence from a partner (6.8%) (Department of Census and Statistics, 2019).

5.2.2 Poverty, Reduced Social Capital, Childhood Adversity and Psychiatric Morbidity

Work in Sri Lanka shows that non-fatal self-poisoning is associated with the experience of significant childhood adversity and having lower levels of education and social capital (Rajapakse et al., 2020). These findings have been with regard to males and females both, but the study populations included a greater proportion of young females. Being single was found to reduce the risk of self-poisoning, compared to being married/divorced/separated or widowed, and having a young child was linked to increased risk (Rajapakse et al., 2020). These latter findings go against the more conventional wisdom based on Western data, where marriage and having a young child are considered protective against self-harm (Nock et al., 2008; Qin et al., 2003). However marriage has been described as increasing the risk of self-harm and suicide in other South Asian countries (Shahid & Hyder, 2008). These findings may reflect the complex dynamics associated with self-harm that play out in LMICs, especially if marriage and having children occur at a young age, against a background of socio-economic deprivation and limited social capital (Shahid & Hyder, 2008). In the context of gender inequality and poverty, these may contribute to non-fatal self-harm and suicide among young females in the reproductive age group, in Sri Lanka and other South Asian countries (Marecek, 1998; Marecek & Senadheera, 2012). Domestic violence and substance misuse in the partner would further exacerbate these stressors.

Psychiatric morbidities, particularly depression, would be further contributory factors to suicide attempts and suicide. While these findings are with regard to suicide in among Sri Lankan females in the reproductive age group in general, it is likely that these factors have a significant impact on the psychological status of women in the perinatal period. In keeping with this, lack of support from the partner, domestic violence, having multiparity over three pregnancies and socio-economic difficulties have been reported to be associated with increased risk of depression (Alwis et al., 2024).

5.3 Exploration of Factors Associated with Maternal Suicides in Sri Lanka Via Maternal Psychological Autopsies

In the context of these concerning rates of maternal suicide, the Family Health Bureau (FHB) in collaboration with the Sri Lanka College of Psychiatrists in 2015 started the process of conducting psychological autopsies after every maternal suicide in the country. The process was structured to gather comprehensive medical and psychosocial information on each maternal suicide, so that the findings could be used to guide development of intervention strategies. It is conducted using the Psychological Autopsy Tool for Maternal Suicides (PAMS). Each maternal psychological autopsy is conducted confidentially and in a sensitive manner by a trained team, consisting of a psychiatrist, a medical officer of health (MOH), a family health worker and a social worker (Jayaratne et al., 2018).

Preliminary findings indicate that more than 70% of the suicides occurred after a recent interpersonal conflict, involving the woman and a close other. Together with this, underlying mental illness was identified in more than 25% of the deceased mothers, most often depression (Jayaratne et al., 2018). Depression had been present in 36.8% of women who died, and a family history of suicide was seen in 15.8% of women (Jayaratne et al., 2018). Of the maternal suicides analysed, 27.3% of women had a previously diagnosed mental illness (Bureau, 2020).

6 Mental Health Services for Women in Sri Lanka

6.1 Perinatal Mental Healthcare Services

Sri Lanka boasts of having a good antenatal and postnatal care and coverage since the 1920s in the South Asian region. There has been a huge decline in the maternal mortality ratio (MMR) in Sri Lanka, from 92 per 100,000 live births in 1990 to 36 per 100,000 in 2017. It was further reduced to 25 per 100,000 live births in 2023. This decline is attributed to the improved quality of obstetric care and timely referrals to hospitals by the teams in the primary healthcare setting (Wijesinghe et al., 2019; Family Health Bureau, 2020). Despite improvement of maternal healthcare services in general and the relatively low overall MMR in Sri Lanka, maternal *mental health* services have received relatively less attention until recently (Agampodi and Agampodi, 2013).

Community-level maternal healthcare services are provided through the medical officers of health (MOH) at a divisional level in the public health system in Sri Lanka. The team comprises the MOH, public health nursing sisters and public health midwives (PHM) who provide domiciliary and clinical care for pregnant and post-partum women (Agampodi et al., 2023). These services are coordinated by the Ministry of Health, Sri Lanka, and are provided free of charge to the public.

Antenatal care services cover 100% of the population, of which 95% of expectant females are registered for antenatal care before 12 weeks of pregnancy. About 85% of postnatal mothers are reported to receive at least one postnatal visit from a public health midwife during the first 10 days after their delivery (World Health Organization, 2017).

During the first booking visit, if there is a diagnosed history of a mental disorder in the mother, the pregnancy is categorized as high risk in the maternal record. Women who are found to have mental health problems during pregnancy (Fig. 8.1) or post-partum are generally referred by an MOH, medical officer of mental health (MOMH) obstetrician or paediatrician to psychiatry services in either the state or private sector, depending on the severity of the problem and the preference of the woman and/or her family, and are referred to the nearest psychiatric unit for further assessments (Hapangama & Kuruppuarachchi, 2021). The midwife also screens for depression using the validated Sinhala translation of the Edinburgh Postnatal Depression Scale (EPDS) during the first 6 weeks post-partum (Agampod et al.,

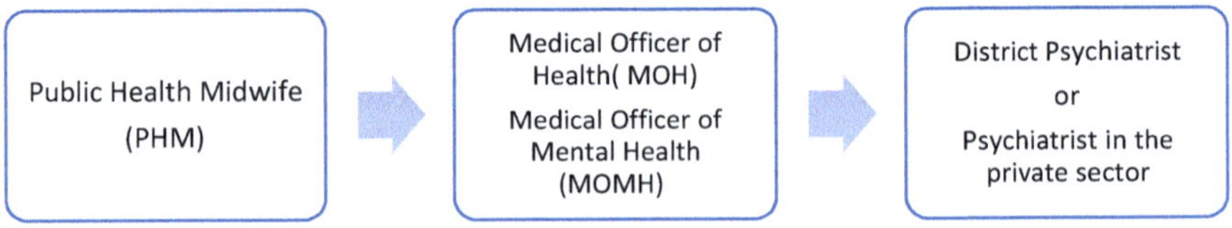

Fig. 8.1 Referral system for accessing perinatal mental health services, within the government healthcare system of Sri Lanka

2011), and if the woman screens positive, she is referred for further assessment and care to the MOH. Field healthcare staff are also instructed to conduct antenatal classes in the three trimesters to the pregnant woman and her partner. Mental health during pregnancy is a topic that is supposed to be discussed with couples during these classes, but the focus on psychological health is comparatively less during these sessions, which is a limitation in service provision.

6.2 Mental Healthcare Facilities for Antenatal and Postnatal Women

Specialized mother-baby units have been established at two tertiary care hospitals in the Colombo District. In addition, several secondary and tertiary care hospitals in the country have designated mother-baby beds within the ward (Kathriarachchi et al., 2024). In areas where such facilities are not available, when needed, the mother may be admitted to a general adult psychiatry ward to receive treatment, while the newborn is often either admitted to a paediatric ward with a family member or sent home (Hapangama & Kuruppuarachchi, 2021).

6.3 Well Woman Clinics

Well woman clinics (WWC) were started by the Family Health Bureau in 1996 and have been developed since. The objective of the Well Woman Program was to screen women between the ages of 35 and 45 years for selected health conditions, namely, diabetes, hypertension, breast cancer and cervical cancer, for early detection and to reduce mortality and morbidity. Health education on menopause, nutrition and appropriate family planning services is also delivered. Screening for domestic violence was initiated in 2023. Women who need further help are referred to the appropriate places. This clinic is run under the supervision of the Medical Office of Health with a team comprising a medical officer, public health nursing sister and public health midwives with or without a supervisory public health midwife. The WWC is conducted under the supervision of the MOH (Family Health Bureau, 2020).

6.4 Support for Women Facing Domestic Violence

The Family Health Bureau of Sri Lanka initially established first-contact points for women experiencing domestic violence, in the form of gender-based violence desks (GBV desks) at hospitals and clinics throughout the country, at the turn of the century (Guruge et al., 2015). This has now been replaced by the *Mithuru Piyasa*

(Friendly Abode) services, again established by the Family Health Bureau of the Ministry of Health, Sri Lanka (Guruge et al., 2015). These are easily accessible, first contact points for women experiencing domestic violence, situated in hospitals throughout the country. A woman can walk in or be referred by another healthcare provider. These *Mithuru Piyasa* centres are manned by a trained nurse or doctor, who greets the woman and serves as a befriender, to listen and discuss her concerns in a friendly and confidential manner. There could be ongoing contact, and the woman may also be referred to other relevant services, hospital based or out of hospital (Guruge et al., 2015). The *Mithuru Piyasa* services have now developed to provide support for woman in all districts of the country. However, residential support or 'safe houses' for women experiencing domestic violence are still limited. Another initiative by the Family Health Bureau in December 2023 was a telephone helpline to report domestic violence.

7 Current Challenges in Reproductive Mental Health Among Women

Lack of public awareness about disorders such as depression and stigma around these topics is a significant stumbling block. Research shows that only approximately one-third of pregnant women recognize depressive symptoms and are open to seeking help for maternal depression. Cultural stigma and lack of awareness also lead to challenges in referral and follow-up of women with psychiatric morbidity, even when the condition is initially recognized at primary care level (Amarasinghe and Agampodi, 2022).

While primary care staff are doing an exemplary job regarding maternal healthcare in the context of limited resources, there is room to improve services regarding maternal mental health, including screening and early detection of perinatal psychiatric morbidity at primary care level. Primary care health workers, and especially PHMs, are burdened with multiple tasks, and there is an urgent need for ongoing education and raising of skills and awareness among these and other healthcare workers, regarding mental health issues in mothers (Agampodi, 2017). Thus, programmes need to be ongoing rather than 'one off', to ensure efficacy, and provision of clear guidelines and referral pathways will also be beneficial (Patabendige, 2020). Further support could be given to primary healthcare workers by using telepsychiatry as an alternative method of communication with mental health professionals for prompt guidance.

The gap in the evidence, especially for effective screening methods and interventions, is an area which has to be dealt with. Planning research to bridge this gap in evidence is important.

Ongoing and improved collaboration between the Family Health Bureau and Professional Colleges such as the College of Psychiatrists, Obstetricians, Community

Physicians and the Department of Social Services with regard to policy planning is also a way forward to improve services.

8 Conclusions

Despite advances in psychiatric services, many gaps remain in addressing the specific mental health needs of women, especially expectant mothers. Evidence regarding mental health disorders in women of the reproductive age group are limited. For perinatal depression, rates range from 7.1% to 31.6%, with a meta-analysis reporting a pooled prevalence of 16.9%. Maternal suicide and suicide among young women in the reproductive age group are important areas of concern.

Complex factors are associated with maternal mental health disorders and suicide, including psychosocial factors such as low socio-economic status, domestic violence, childhood adversity, and psychiatric factors such as depression. Socio-economic factors such as poverty, low mental health literacy and cultural stigma surrounding mental illness further prevent access to mental health services and widens the mental health gap.

Thus, initiatives aimed at enhancing mental health services for maternal and female mental health, building collaboration between different service providers and improving mental health literacy in the community are important to bridge this gap. More research is also needed regarding mental disorders in women in the reproductive age group and possible interventions. Interventions need to be guided by evidence but also need to be incorporated into existing systems with the collaboration of the stakeholders and women themselves, to ensure relevance and sustainability.

References

Agampodi, S. B., & Agampodi, T. C. (2013). Antenatal depression in Anuradhapura, Sri Lanka and the factor structure of the Sinhalese version of Edinburgh postpartum depression scale among pregnant women. *PLoS One, 8*(7), e69708. https://doi.org/10.1371/journal.pone.0069708

Agampodi, T. C., Agampodi, S. B., Wickramasinghe, W. A., Adhikari, A. M., & Chathurani, H. K. (2011). Postpartum depression – A problem that needs early intervention. *Ceylon Medical Journal, 56*(4), 183–184. https://doi.org/10.4038/cmj.v56i4.3907

Agampodi, T. C., Rheinländer, T., Agampodi, S. B. et al. (2017). Social capital and health during pregnancy; an in-depth exploration from rural Sri Lanka. *Reproductive Health, 14*, 89. https://doi.org/10.1186/s12978-017-0349-7

Agampodi, T., Amarasinghe, G., Wickramasinghe, A., Wickramasinghe, N., Warnasekara, J., Jayasinghe, I., Hettiarachchi, A., Nimesha, D., Dilshani, T., Senadheera, S., & Agampodi, S. (2023). Incorporating early pregnancy mental health screening and management into routine maternal care: Experience from the Rajarata Pregnancy Cohort (RaPCo), Sri Lanka. *BMJ Global Health, 8*(9). https://doi.org/10.1136/bmjgh-2023-012852

Alwis, I., Baminiwatta, A., & Chandradasa, M. (2024). Prevalence and associated factors of depression in Sri Lanka: A systematic review and meta-analysis. *Social Psychiatry and Psychiatric Epidemiology, 59*(2), 353–373. https://doi.org/10.1007/s00127-023-02495-z

Amarasinghe, G. S., & Agampodi, S. B. (2022). Help-seeking intention for depression and suicidal ideation during pregnancy and postpartum in rural Sri Lanka; a cross sectional study. *Rural and Remote Health, 22*(3), 72–73. https://doi.org/10.22605/RRH7273

American College of Obstetricians and Gynecologists. (2009). Washington, DC: Repeated miscarriages, Educational Pamphlet AP100

Anjalika, T., Arachchi, H. E., Anpuchselvam, A., & de Zoysa, P. (2023). The burden of antenatal anxiety: A cross-sectional study of prevalence and selected risk factors among antenatal women in a government hospital in the Colombo district. *Ceylon Medical Journal, 68*, 101–107. https://doi.org/10.4038/cmj.v68i3.9856

Arya, V., Page, A., Gunnell, D., Dandona, R., Mannan, H., Eddleston, M., & Armstrong, G. (2019). Suicide by hanging is a priority for suicide prevention: Method specific suicide in India (2001–2014). *Journal of Affective Disorders, 257*, 1–9. https://doi.org/10.1016/j.jad.2019.07.005

Ban D. J., K. J. D. S. W. (2002). Induced abortion in Sri Lanka: Who goes to the providers for pregnancy termination. *Journal of Biosocial Science, 34*, 303–315.

Bandara, P., Page, A., Rajapakse, T., & Knipe, D. (2024b). Intimate partner violence, suicide and self-harm in Sri Lanka: Analysis of national data. *PLoS One, 19*(3), e0298413. https://doi.org/10.1371/journal.pone.0298413

Bandara, P., Wickrama, P., Sivayokan, S., Knipe, D., & Rajapakse, T. (2024a). Reflections on the trends of suicide in Sri Lanka, 1997–2022: The need for continued vigilance. *PLOS Global Public Health, 4*(4), e0003054. https://doi.org/10.1371/journal.pgph.0003054

Dalupotha, M. K. (2003). *Upathe Vagathuga*. Godage Publishers.

De Silva, V., & Ratnayake, A. (2008). Increased use of medicinal drugs in self-harm in urban areas in Sri Lanka. *Archives of Suicide Research, 12*(4), 366–369. https://doi.org/10.1080/13811110802325265

Department of Census and Statistics. (2008). *Sri Lanka demographic and health survey 2006/07: Preliminary report (draft)*. Department of Census and Statistics. http://www.statistics.gov.lk/social/DHS%20Sri%20Lanka%20Preliminary%20Report.pdf

Department of Census and Statistics, S. L. (2019). Women's wellbeing survey 2019, Sri Lanka.

Dheerasinghe D. S. A. A. F., Kathriarachchi S. S. H. R. C. M. F. P. (2019). Risk factors of depression among menopausal women in Sri Lanka: A case control study. *Transactions of the Royal Society of Tropical Medicine and Hygiene*, 199–245.

Fan Q, L. Q. D. S. V. V. et al. (2020). Prevalence and risk factors for postpartum depression in Sri Lanka: A population-based study. *Asian Journal of Psychiatry, 47*, 101855. https://doi.org/10.1016/j.ajp.2019.101855

Family Health Bureau. (2020). *Maternal desk review*.

Fargnoli, A., & Seneviratne, D. (2022). Exploring Rata Yakuma: Weaving Dance/movement therapy and a Sri Lankan healing ritual. https://doi.org/10.15212/CAET/2021/7/23.

Gankanda WI, G. I. K. N. R. A. (2021). Prevalence and associated factors of posttraumatic stress disorder (PTSD) among a cohort of Srilankan post-partum mothers: a crosssectional study. *BMC Pregnancy Childbirth, 21*(1), 1–7.

Gelaye, B. (2016). Epidemiology of maternal depression, risk factors, and child outcomes in low-income and middle-income countries. *Lancet Psychiatry, 3*(10), 973–982. https://doi.org/10.1016/S2215-0366(16)30284-X

Guruge, S., Jayasuriya-Illesinghe, V., & Gunawardena, N. (2015). A review of the Sri Lankan health-sector response to intimate partner violence: Looking back, moving forward. *WHO South-East Asia Journal of Public Health, 4*(1), 6–11. https://doi.org/10.4103/2224-3151.206622

Hahn-Holbrook, J., Cornwell-Hinrichs, T., & Anaya, I. (2018). Economic and Health Predictors of National Postpartum Depression Prevalence: A Systematic Review, Meta-analysis, and

Meta-Regression of 291 Studies from 56 Countries. *Frontiers in Psychiatry, 8*, 248. https://doi.org/10.3389/fpsyt.2017.00248

Hapangama, A., & Kuruppuarachchi, K. A. L. A. (2021). Maternal mental health services in Sri Lanka: challenges and solutions. *BJPsych International, 18*(4), 100–102. https://doi.org/10.1192/bji.2020.52

Jayaratne, K., Karunasena, C., Rajapakse, T., Kathriarachchi, S., & Ranatunga, R. (2018). Counting and reviewing maternal suicides in resource limited settings: Lessons from Sri Lanka. India.

Kathriarachchi, S. T., Suraweera, C., & Batakandage, P. M. (2024). Maternal suicides, a tip of an iceberg. *Sri Lanka Journal of Perinatal Medicine, 5*(1), 4–14.

Marecek, J. (1998). Culture, gender, and suicidal behavior in Sri Lanka. *Suicide & Life-Threatening Behavior, 28*(1), 69–81. https://doi.org/10.1111/j.1943-278X.1998.tb00627.x

Marecek, J., & Senadheera, C. (2012). 'I drank it to put an end to me': Narrating girls' suicide and self-harm in Sri Lanka. *Contributions to Indian Sociology, 46*(1–2), 53–82. https://doi.org/10.1177/006996671104600204

Nishshanka, N. M. C. L., Goonewardena, C. S. E., Kasturiarachchi, S. K., Waas, M. D. I. A., Kulathunga, K. A. C. J. R., & Gamagedara, N. S. (2023). Effectiveness of progressive muscle relaxation therapy on pregnancy outcomes among stressed and anxious Primigravida antenatal mothers: A randomized controlled trial. *Sri Lanka Journal of Perinatal Medicine, 4*(1), 9–18. https://doi.org/10.4038/sljpm.v4i1.63

Nock, M. K., Borges, G., Bromet, E. J., Alonso, J., Angermeyer, M., Beautrais, A., Bruffaerts, R., Chiu, W. T., De Girolamo, G., Gluzman, S., De Graaf, R., Gureje, O., Haro, J. M., Huang, Y., Karam, E., Kessler, R. C., Lepine, J. P., Levinson, D., Medina-Mora, M. E., et al. (2008). Cross-national prevalence and risk factors for suicidal ideation, plans and attempts. *The British Journal of Psychiatry, 192*(2), 98–105. https://doi.org/10.1192/bjp.bp.107.040113

Palfreyman, A. (2021). Addressing Psychosocial Vulnerabilities Through Antenatal Care—Depression, Suicidal Ideation, and Behavior: A Study Among Urban Sri Lankan Women. *Frontiers in Psychiatry, 12*. https://doi.org/10.3389/fpsyt.2021.554808

Patabendige, M., Athulathmudali, S. R., Chandrasinghe, S. K. (2020). Mental Health Problems during Pregnancy and the Postpartum Period: A Multicenter Knowledge Assessment Survey among Healthcare Providers. *Journal of Pregnancy*, 2020, 4926702. https://doi.org/10.1155/2020/4926702

Patel, V., Ramasundarahettige, C., Vijayakumar, L., Thakur, J. S., Gajalakshmi, V., Gururaj, G., Suraweera, W., Jha, P., & Million Death Study, C. (2012). Suicide mortality in India: A nationally representative survey. *Lancet, 379*(9834), 2343–2351. https://doi.org/10.1016/S0140-6736(12)60606-0

Pathiraja, R. P., Rohanachandra, Y. M., Kathriarachchi, S. T., & Nishadd, A. A. N. (2018). A descriptive cross sectional study on mental health outcome and perceived care needs following miscarriage in a tertiary care hospital in Sri Lanka. *Sri Lanka Journal of Obstetrics and Gynaecology, 40*(4), 71–71. https://doi.org/10.4038/sljog.v40i4.7868

Priyadarshanie, M. N., Waas, D. A., Goonewardena, S., Senaratna, C. V., & Fernando, S. (2023). Association of antenatal anxiety disorders with antenatal comorbidities and adverse pregnancy outcomes among clinic attendees at a tertiary-care hospital in Sri Lanka. *Heliyon, 9*(3), e13900. https://doi.org/10.1016/j.heliyon.2023.e13900

Qin, P., Agerbo, E., & Mortensen, P. B. (2003). Suicide risk in relation to socioeconomic, demographic, psychiatric, and familial factors: A national register-based study of all suicides in Denmark, 1981–1997. *American Journal of Psychiatry, 160*(4), 765. https://doi.org/10.1176/appi.ajp.160.4.765

Rajapakse, T., Griffiths, K. M., & Christensen, H. (2013). Characteristics of non-fatal self-poisoning in Sri Lanka: A systematic review. *BMC Public Health, 13*, 331. https://doi.org/10.1186/1471-2458-13-331

Rajapakse, T., Russell, A. E., Kidger, J., Bandara, P., López-López, J. A., Senarathna, L., Metcalfe, C., Gunnell, D., & Knipe, D. (2020). Childhood adversity and self-poisoning: A hospital case control study in Sri Lanka. *PLoS One, 15*(11), e0242437. https://doi.org/10.1371/journal.pone.0242437

Rathnayake, N., Lenora, J., Alwis, G., & Lekamwasam, S. (2019). Prevalence and Severity of Menopausal Symptoms and the Quality of Life in Middle-aged Women: A Study from Sri Lanka. *Nursing Research and Practice*, 1–9. https://doi.org/10.1155/2019/2081507

Rowel, D. (2004). Prevalence, incidence and correlates of postpartum depression in the Puttalam district. In U. o. Post Graduate Institute of Medicine & C. (Eds.).

Roystead-Solas T, H. S. U. L. D. S. V. (2022). Mothers at risk of postpartum depression in Sri Lanka: A population based study using a validated tool. *Plos One, 17*(5), e0268748. https://doi.org/10.1371/journal.pone.0268748

Shahid, M., & Hyder, A. A. (2008). Deliberate self-harm and suicide: A review from Pakistan. *International Journal of Injury Control and Safety Promotion, 15*(4), 233–241. https://doi.org/10.1080/17457300802149811

Suraweera, C., Perera, I., Isuru, L. A., & Galhenage, J. (2021). Prevalence and associated factors of antenatal depression of women attending antenatal clinics in two tertiary care hospitals in Sri Lanka. *BJPsych Open, 18*(7 suppl 1), s292–s293. https://doi.org/10.1192/bjo.2021.776

Vijayakumar, L., Ray, S., Fernandes, T. N., & Pathare, S. (2021). A descriptive mapping review of suicide in vulnerable populations in low and middle countries. *Asia-Pacific Psychiatry, 13*(3), e12472. https://doi.org/10.1111/appy.12472

Waidyasekera, H., Wijewardena, K., Lindmark, G., Naessen, T. (2009). Menopausal symptoms and quality of life during the menopausal transition in Sri Lankan women. *Menopause, 16*(1), 164–170. https://doi.org/10.1097/gme.0b013e31817a8abd

WHO. (2017). *World Health Organization report.*

WHO. (2022). *WHO guide for integration of perinatal mental health in maternal and child health services.* World Health Organization. Retrieved from https://www.who.int/publications/i/item/9789240057142

Wijesooriya, L. R. A., Palihawadana, T. S., & Rajapaksha, R. N. G. (2015). A study of psychological impact on women undergoing miscarriage at a Sri Lankan hospital setting. *Sri Lanka Journal of Obstetrics and Gynaecology, 37*(2), 10.

Wijesinghe, P. S., Jayaratne, K., & Peiris, D. (2019). National Maternal Death surveillance and Response: Sri Lankan scenario. *Ceylon Medical Journal, 64*(1), 1. https://doi.org/10.4038/cmj.v64i1.8822

Women's Wellbeing Survey 2019 *Sri Lanka*. (2019). S. L. Department of Census and Statistics.

Chapter 9
Public Mental Health Aspects of Women's Reproductive Mental Health in South Asia

Russell Kabir

1 Introduction

Mental health is essential for individual and public health (Min et al., 2013). Public mental health plays a crucial role in promoting mental well-being, preventing mental disorders, and reducing suicide rates. It addresses mental health's social and economic determinants, emphasising that it is integral to overall public health (Wahlbeck, 2015). By adopting a population-based approach, public mental health encourages cross-sectoral collaboration to tackle issues related to education, housing, and employment (World Health Organization, 2013). This field promotes awareness and reduces the stigma associated with mental disorders, aiming to empower individuals through inclusive policies and accessible services (Anderson et al., 2011; Norman et al., 2012; Nyqvist et al., 2013). Ultimately, it seeks to improve community mental health outcomes and enhance overall societal well-being (Wahlbeck, 2015).

Integrating mental health services into primary care, including reproductive health settings, is essential (Hossain & Purohit, 2019). This integration can improve the early detection and management of mental health conditions, such as postpartum depression (Johansen et al., 2020). Intimate partner violence (IPV) is a significant public health concern that disproportionately affects women and is closely linked to reproductive health and mental well-being (Sweeney et al., 2013). Public health interventions should include universal screening for IPV in primary care and reproductive health settings, comprehensive responses, and coordinated support services (Sweeney et al., 2013). History of trauma, including sexual abuse and

R. Kabir (✉)
School of Allied Health and Social Care, Faculty of Health, Medicine and Social Care, Anglia Ruskin University, Chelmsford, UK
e-mail: russell.kabir@aru.ac.uk

P. Kukreti et al. (eds.), *Women's Reproductive Mental Health in South Asia*, South Asian Perspectives in Mental Health and Psychology,
https://doi.org/10.1007/978-981-96-9219-4_9

intimate partner violence, can increase the risk of mental health problems during the reproductive years (Seng et al., 2005).

These services can include social work, legal assistance, and mental health treatment, addressing both the immediate and long-term consequences of IPV. Maternal mental health is a critical area of focus for public health, encompassing mental well-being during pregnancy, childbirth, and the post-partum period (Kendig et al., 2017). Public health initiatives should prioritise screening for mood and anxiety disorders during these periods, using validated tools and providing access to appropriate treatment and support (Johansen et al., 2020). Adolescents and young adults face unique challenges related to reproductive health and mental well-being, including navigating relationships, making decisions about contraception, and experiencing unintended pregnancies (Lindberg, 2020). Anxiety disorders are common during pregnancy and the post-partum period, often co-occurring with depression (Kendig et al., 2017).

Public health programmes promoting sexual and reproductive health should integrate mental health considerations to ensure a holistic approach to well-being (Wellings & Johnson, 2013). Individuals with intellectual and developmental disabilities may experience significant mental health challenges, often compounded by social stigma and lack of access to appropriate services (Narayan & John, 2017). Social determinants of health, such as poverty, discrimination, and lack of access to education and employment, can significantly impact mental health outcomes in reproductive psychiatry (Gregory et al., 2022). Early intervention and prevention strategies are essential for addressing mental health issues in reproductive psychiatry (Patton & Temmerman, 2016). Implementing routine screening for mental health conditions in reproductive healthcare settings can help identify individuals who may benefit from early intervention (Johansen et al., 2020). Identifying risk factors such as prior diagnoses is crucial for early detection and intervention (Johansen et al., 2020). Routine screening using validated tools is recommended post-partum (Johansen e al., 2020).

Promotive approaches focus on enhancing mental well-being and resilience, empowering individuals to cope with stress and adversity, and fostering positive mental health throughout the reproductive lifespan (FusarPoli et al., 2019). Increasing mental health literacy among individuals and communities can reduce stigma, promote help-seeking behaviour, and empower individuals to care for their mental health (Jenkins et al., 2010). Social support and community engagement can give individuals a sense of belonging, connection, and purpose, promoting mental well-being and resilience (Kohrt & Song, 2018). The purpose of this chapter is to evaluate the role of public mental health interventions in addressing psychiatric issues during women's reproductive period.

2 Prevalence and Burden of Reproductive Mental Health Issues in South Asia

Public mental health in South Asia faces several challenges due to a range of socio-economic and cultural factors. In this region, mental health is stigmatised and often not considered a priority health issue. One of the biggest challenges in South Asia is the lack of awareness and understanding of mental health issues (Kabir et al., 2024). Pregnancy is often viewed as a time of joy, but for many women in South Asia, it can be a stressful experience associated with cultural stigmas, gender discrimination, and concerns about abnormal births (Waqas et al., 2015). A systematic review and meta-analysis by Insan et al. (2022) revealed that antenatal depression and anxiety are significantly associated with intimate partner violence, unplanned pregnancy, male gender preference, and poor relationships with in-laws (Insan et al., 2022).

Post-partum depression (PPD) is a major public health concern due to its adverse effects on the cognitive and social development of infants (Ali et al., 2009). Studies in India have estimated the overall pooled prevalence of PPD to be 22% (Upadhyay et al., 2017). Risk factors include financial difficulties, domestic violence, a history of psychiatric illness, marital conflict, and lack of support from the husband after the birth of a female baby (Upadhyay et al., 2017). In Pakistan, the prevalence rates of PPD have been reported to be even higher, ranging from 28% to 63% (Aliani & Khuwaja, 2017). Infertility and its treatment can significantly impact the emotional health of women in South Asia (Hassan et al., 2022). A study by Hassan et al. (2022) in Pakistan found that treatment tolerability and the quality of the treatment environment are associated with women's coping mechanisms and emotional well-being. High treatment tolerability was linked to positive reframing, while a better treatment environment enabled women to use problem-focused coping mechanisms (Hassan et al., 2022).

A qualitative study in Pakistan by Rowther et al. (2020) highlighted that gender norms constrain women's agency and contribute to anxiety during pregnancy (Rowther et al., 2020). Women's avenues for self-advocacy are often limited, and their mental health is heavily influenced by their levels of autonomy in decision-making and the availability of social support (Rowther et al., 2020). Social support, particularly from husbands and extended family, is crucial for women's mental well-being during pregnancy and post-partum (Jones, 2012). In many South Asian cultures, the extended family plays a significant role in women's lives, and conflicts within these relationships can contribute to mental distress (Takegata et al., 2017). Stigma surrounding mental health issues is a major barrier to seeking care in South Asia (Insan et al., 2022). Women may be reluctant to discuss their mental health problems due to fear of judgement, discrimination, or social isolation (Ahmed & Mao, 2023). This stigma is often compounded by a lack of awareness and understanding of mental health conditions, leading to delays in seeking help and exacerbation of symptoms (Insan et al., 2022). Kabir et al. (2017) identified the relationship between education and employment are related to decision-making power of women of reproductive age group in Bangladesh.

Lack of education can also limit women's access to employment opportunities and economic independence, further increasing their vulnerability to mental health problems (Sheikh & Loney, 2018). Even when mental health services are available, the quality of care may be inadequate. Lack of training among healthcare providers, limited resources, and a focus on biomedical interventions can result in suboptimal care for women with reproductive mental health problems (Thara & Padmavati, 2013). Culturally sensitive and evidence-based interventions are needed to address the specific needs of women in South Asia (Bright et al., 2018).

Poverty, low education, and social exclusion are significant determinants of mental disorders in low- and middle-income countries (LAMCs) (Patel, 2007). Women in South Asia face systemic disadvantages that increase their risk of common mental disorders (Rowther et al., 2020; Gailits et al., 2019). Rapid urbanisation in South Asia is associated with a range of mental disorders and deviancies, including psychoses, depression, substance abuse, and family disintegration (Trivedi et al., 2008). Women in South and Southeast Asia have a higher prevalence of adverse mental health outcomes following natural disasters (Fatema et al., 2021). Factors such as socio-demographics, disaster exposure, and pre-existing vulnerabilities significantly influence women's mental health in these contexts (Fatema et al., 2021).

Maternal mental health is closely linked to both maternal and child health outcomes (Patel et al., 2004). Antenatal and post-partum depression and anxiety can lead to adverse outcomes such as low birth weight, preterm birth, and impaired foetal development (Insan et al., 2022). Studies have also shown that maternal mental health problems can negatively impact infant growth and development (Patel et al., 2003). Reproductive mental health issues can strain family and social relationships, leading to conflict, isolation, and reduced social support (Jones, 2012). Women with depression and anxiety may struggle to fulfil their roles as wives, mothers, and caregivers, which can have a ripple effect on the entire family (Waqas et al., 2015). This can exacerbate poverty and financial strain, further compounding the challenges faced by women and their families (Ferreira & Ravallion, 2008).

Mental health's crucial role in overall wellness is widely acknowledged, yet obstacles to accessing mental healthcare persist. This challenge is especially pronounced in Southeast Asian nations, where additional stigma further complicates seeking mental health support (Andray et al., 2023). South Asia also faces a significant shortage of mental healthcare, leaving many without needed treatment. The region is also vulnerable to mental health crises during substantial disasters. The COVID-19 pandemic clearly showed this problem, with depression rates climbing to 34% and anxiety reaching 40% across South Asia (Hossain et al., 2021). The stigma associated with mental illness is a significant barrier to seeking help in South Asia (Kallivayalil, 2012; Ng et al., 2009). Traditional beliefs about the causes and treatment of mental illness can also hinder access to care (Ito et al., 2012). Many people in South Asia seek help from traditional healers or religious leaders rather than mental health professionals (Prajapati & Liebling, 2022). Gender norms and power imbalances can affect women's mental health and their access to care. Women in South Asia often face discrimination, limited autonomy, and high levels of stress, increasing their risk of mental disorders (Niaz and Hassan, 2006). While family support can be beneficial, family dynamics can also create barriers to care. In some cases, families may be reluctant to acknowledge or seek help for mental health problems due to stigma or cultural beliefs (Ito et al., 2012). Mental health services are often underfunded and understaffed in South Asia, mainly rural areas. This lack of resources limits access to care and service quality (Thara & Padmavati, 2013). Poverty is a significant determinant of mental health in South Asia (McDaid et al., 2008). Mental healthcare is often poorly integrated into the broader health system in South Asia (Ng et al., 2009). This lack of integration can lead to fragmented care and difficulty accessing services. There is a severe shortage of trained mental health professionals in South Asia, including psychiatrists, psychologists, and psychiatric nurses (Thara & Padmavati, 2013).

Mental disorders are a leading cause of disability worldwide, and South Asia is no exception. Depression is a major contributor to disability as measured by years lived with disability (YLDs) (Reddy, 2010). Mental illnesses affect an individual's ability to function, be productive, establish and maintain positive relationships, and experience a state of well-being (Kallivayalil, 2012). In India, it is estimated that 3–4% of the population suffers from major mental disorders, and about 7–10% suffers from minor depressive disorders (Reddy, 2010). In Southeast Asia, neuropsychiatric diseases account for 11% of disability-adjusted life years (DALYs) and 27% of YLDs (Reddy, 2010). These statistics highlight the substantial impact of mental disorders on the overall burden of disease in South Asia. The economic costs associated with mental disorders are significant, including direct healthcare expenses and indirect costs related to lost productivity and reduced workforce participation. In India, the financial burden of mental disorders is considerable, with a significant impact on the country's overall economic development. The cost of depression, particularly in lost workdays, is as great as or greater than the cost of many other common medical illnesses (Reddy, 2010). Mental health stigma is prevalent in Asian nations and low- and middle-income countries (Vaishnav et al., 2023). This stigma can lead to reduced access to mental healthcare, poor adherence to treatment, and unfavourable outcomes (Vaishnav et al., 2023). Stigma can manifest at the structural or organisational level, the societal level (interpersonal stigma), and the individual level (internalised stigma) (Vaishnav et al., 2023). Vulnerable populations, such as gender minorities, children, adolescents, and geriatric populations, are more prone to stigma (Vaishnav et al., 2023). Depression is strongly associated with suicidality (Reddy, 2010). Women in Southeast Asia face a disproportionately high suicide burden. The region has a female age-standardised suicide rate of 11.5 per 100,000 compared to the global average of 7.5 per 100,000 (Fastenau et al., 2024). A meta-analysis found the pooled prevalence of suicidal ideation among South Asian women was 17%, while suicide attempt was 5% (Mazumder et al., 2022). Approximately 50% of individuals who died by suicide have a primary diagnosis of depression (Reddy, 2010). In India, a significant percentage of people who die due to suicide (37.8%) are below 30 years of age, and the majority of those suicide suffer from depression or other mental disorders (Reddy, 2010). Suicide trends in Asia and the Pacific differ from those in Europe and North America, with a proportionately higher number of female suicides in China, India, and Pacific Island countries (Milner & Leo, 2010). A study from India shows that suicides among pregnant women occur predominantly in the first and second trimesters, with third-trimester suicide deaths being less common (Behera & Sikary, 2022). Notably, the most affected age group was 21–25 years, and hanging was the predominant method. An intriguing finding suggested that being pregnant with male foetuses might be a risk factor compared to female foetuses, though this requires further investigation (Behera & Sikary, 2022).

3 Reproductive Mental Health Programs in South Asia: International Collaborations, Regional Programmes, and Challenges

Reproductive mental health is a critical area of concern, particularly in South Asia, where cultural, economic, and health system-related barriers can significantly impact access to care. This response examines international collaborations and regional programmes aimed at promoting reproductive mental health in South Asia, successful regional models or pilot programs, the integration of technology for mental health promotion and increased access, and challenges and barriers to preventive and promotive approaches, including cultural, economic, and health system-related factors. Several international collaborations and regional programmes focus on improving mental health in LMICs, including South Asia. The WHO sets guidelines and provides technical support for mental health programmes globally. The WHO's Mental Health Gap Action Programme (mhGAP) offers evidence-based guidance for integrating mental healthcare into primary care settings, particularly relevant for LMICs with limited resources (Liu et al., 2011). The World Psychiatric Association (WPA) has actively promoted community mental healthcare through task forces and action plans (Thara & Padmavati, 2013; Ito et al., 2012).

Collaborative research between high-income countries and South Asian institutions is essential for evidence generation and local capacity building in reproductive mental health. These partnerships adapt interventions to specific cultural contexts while developing training programmes for mental health professionals (Kallivayalil, 2012). NGOs implement community-based programmes and advocate for those with mental disorders, with international organisations partnering with local groups to deliver services and promote mental health literacy (Thara & padmavati, 2013). The "SHARE" study exemplifies this approach, evaluating the Thinking Healthy Programme for perinatal depression in Pakistan and India (Sikander et al., 2015). Several South Asian countries have successfully integrated mental health into primary care (Thara & Padmavati, 2013). Community-based rehabilitation programmes empower local communities to support individuals with mental disorders (Ng et al., 2009). Regional NGOs have developed various programmes addressing mental health through advocacy, promotion, prevention, rehabilitation, and direct service provision focused on reproductive health needs (Thara & Padmavati, 2013).

4 Preventive Strategies

South Asia is characterised by unique sociocultural factors that significantly influence women's mental health. Addressing these requires multifaceted interventions that challenge traditional norms and promote gender equality (Decker et al., 2013; Jayachandran, 2015). For instance, initiatives promoting women's education and economic empowerment can indirectly improve their mental well-being by enhancing their social standing and decision-making power (Decker et al., 2013). Raising public awareness is crucial in reducing stigma and encouraging early help-seeking behaviours. Campaigns should utilise culturally appropriate channels and messaging to effectively reach and engage target populations (Hossain & Puohit, 2019; Thara & Padmavati, 2013). This includes using local media—print, audio (community radio), and visual (local TV channels)—and organising classes in schools and other educational institutions (Thara & Padmavati, 2013). The content should focus on dispelling myths, promoting understanding of mental illness, and encouraging help-seeking without fear of judgement or discrimination (Vaishnav et al., 2023).

Gender-based violence (GBV), including IPV and sexual violence, is a significant risk factor for mental health disorders among women (Decker et al., 2013; Stewart et al., 2015). Primary prevention strategies should focus on addressing the root causes of GBV, such as gender inequality and harmful norms (Decker et al., 2013), and implementing effective prevention programmes (Hossain & Purohit, 2019). This includes promoting healthy relationships, challenging patriarchal attitudes, and strengthening legal frameworks to protect women from violence (Decker et al., 2013). The effectiveness of such interventions has been demonstrated in various settings (Decker et al., 2013), but their implementation in South Asia requires careful consideration of local contexts and cultural nuances. Furthermore, the role of religion and caste systems in perpetuating GBV needs cautious assessment and integration into prevention strategies (Kamin & Marusic, 2005). Certain groups of women in South Asia are at a higher risk of developing mental health disorders during the reproductive period. These include adolescents (Thara & Padmavati, 2013; Weiss & Ferrand, 2019), those from marginalised communities (Stewart et al., 2015), and victims of GBV (Decker et al., 2013). Targeted interventions should focus on providing tailored support and resources to address the unique challenges faced by these groups (Hossain & Purohit, 2019). For example, school-based adolescent programmes could promote mental well-being, resilience, and healthy coping mechanisms (Hossain & Purohit, 2019; Weiss & Ferrand, 2019). Similarly, community-based programmes for women facing poverty could provide access to mental health services, economic support, and social networks (Thara & Padmavati, 2013). However, the design and implementation of such programmes must be tailored to the specific context of each country (Hossain & Purohit, 2019), considering factors such as literacy levels, cultural beliefs, and access to healthcare services (Kohrt & Song, 2018). Screening tools must be culturally adapted and validated to ensure accuracy and acceptability (Kohrt & Song, 2018).

Furthermore, integrating mental health screening into routine reproductive healthcare visits could significantly improve early detection rates (Trang et al., 2024). Effective secondary prevention requires strong collaboration between reproductive health and mental health providers (Trang et al., 2024). This collaboration should involve joint training programmes, shared protocols, and referral pathways to ensure seamless access to appropriate care (Hossain & Purohit, 2019). Joint training programmes could improve providers' knowledge and skills in identifying, assessing, and managing perinatal mental health disorders (Trang e al., 2024). Shared protocols could standardise screening and referral procedures across healthcare settings (Kohrt & Song, 2018). Referral pathways should ensure timely access to specialised mental healthcare when needed (Hossain & Purohit, 2019).

The status of health systems in South Asia poses significant challenges to providing reproductive psychiatry services (Thara & Padmaati, 2013; Liu et al., 2011). Many countries lack comprehensive mental health policies and programmes (Hossain & Purohit, 2019), resulting in inadequate resources, limited access to specialised care, and significant treatment gaps (Trang et al., 2024). Many individuals suffering from mental health disorders do not receive evidence-based care, leading to chronicity, increased suffering, and substantial costs (Patel, 2007). Strengthening existing services and integrating mental healthcare into primary healthcare settings are crucial steps in improving access to treatment (Patel, 2007; Thara & Padmavati, 2013). Mental health disorders can lead to significant disability, impacting women's ability to participate fully in society (van Brakel et al., 2012). Addressing this requires interventions aimed at reducing disability and improving functional outcomes (Liu et al., 2011). This includes providing psychosocial rehabilitation, vocational training, and support services to help women regain their independence and quality of life (Thara & Padmaati, 2013). The significant unmet needs in reproductive psychiatry in South Asia, including the lack of access to appropriate care, are underscored by several studies (Patel, 2007; Thara & Padmaati, 2013; Liu et al., 2011).

Promotive interventions should be tailored to the specific cultural context of South Asia (Hossain & Purohit, 2019; Thara & Padmaati, 2013). This includes incorporating traditional practices and beliefs into interventions where appropriate and using culturally sensitive language and communication styles (Kohrt & song, 2018). For example, interventions could incorporate yoga, meditation, or other traditional practices that promote mental well-being in South Asian cultures (Hossain & Purohit, 2019). Furthermore, community-based programmes emphasising social and peer support could help reduce stigma and encourage help-seeking behaviours (Thara & Padmaati, 2013). Many South Asian countries have made progress in developing national mental health policies and programmes (Liu et al., 2011; Hossain & Purohit, 2019), but implementation remains a significant challenge (Thara & Padmaati, 2013). Integrating mental health services into existing reproductive health programmes can improve access to care and reduce stigma (Hossain

& Purohit, 2019). This requires inter-sectoral collaboration, adequate resource allocation, and capacity building for healthcare providers (Liu et al., 2011). Gender-responsive health policies are critical for addressing the unique mental health needs of women in South Asia (Decker et al., 2013). These policies should address gender inequality, promote women's empowerment, and ensure equitable access to healthcare services (Decker et al., 2013; Jayachandran, 2015). This requires addressing discriminatory practices, promoting gender equality in healthcare settings, and involving women in the design and implementation of health programmes (Stewart et al., 2015). The lack of comprehensive gender-responsive policies in many South Asian countries is a significant impediment to improving women's mental health (Decker et al., 2013).

5 Conclusion and Recommendations

Despite progress, significant research gaps persist in women's reproductive psychiatry across South Asia, impeding effective interventions and policy development. Current studies often have methodological limitations, including small samples, cross-sectional designs, and self-report measures. Robust longitudinal studies with mixed-method approaches are needed to understand mental health determinants among South Asian women comprehensively.

Research must better address cultural contexts that shape mental health experiences, including local idioms of distress and cultural influences on help-seeking behaviours. The scarcity of high-quality, nationally representative data remains a critical barrier to evidence-based policy creation. Future research should employ intersectional approaches examining the combined effects of gender, socioeconomic status, caste, and religion. Rigorous programme evaluations with standardised outcome measures are essential to identify best practices. Additionally, more investigation is needed regarding barriers to mental health service utilisation, including stigma, cost, distance, and cultural appropriateness of care. Addressing these gaps requires integrating mental health into existing healthcare systems with culturally sensitive approaches and supportive policy frameworks.

References

Ahmed, R., & Mao, Y. (2023). An intersectional approach to understanding beliefs and attitudes toward mental health issues among Muslim immigrant women in Canada. *Health Communication, 39*(10), 2014–2025. https://doi.org/10.1080/10410236.2023.2252644

Ali, N. S., Ali, B. S., & Azam, I. S. (2009). Post partum anxiety and depression in peri-urban communities of Karachi, Pakistan: A quasi-experimental study. *BMC Public Health, 9*, 384. https://doi.org/10.1186/1471-2458-9-384

Aliani, R., & Khuwaja, B. (2017). Epidemiology of postpartum depression in Pakistan: A review of literature. *National Journal of Health Sciences, 2*(1), 24–30. https://doi.org/10.21089/njhs.21.0024

Andary, S., Bassani, J., Burrell, G., Cole, E., Evans, R., Redman, E., & Kumar, S. (2023). Barriers and enablers to accessing and utilising mental health care services across Southeast Asia: A preliminary scoping review. *Asia-Pacific Psychiatry, 15*(4), e12549. https://doi.org/10.1111/appy.12549

Anderson, P., Jané-Llopis, E., & Hosman, C. (2011). Reducing the silent burden of impaired mental health. *Health Promotion International, 26*(Suppl 1), i4–i9. https://doi.org/10.1093/heapro/dar051

Behera, C., & Sikary, A. K. (2022). Suicidal deaths in pregnancy at an apex institute in India: A retrospective analysis of autopsy cases. *Asian Journal of Psychiatry, 68*, 102979. https://doi.org/10.1016/j.ajp.2021.102979

Bright, K. S., Norris, J. M., Letourneau, N. L., King Rosario, M., & Premji, S. S. (2018). Prenatal maternal anxiety in South Asia: A rapid best-fit framework synthesis. *Frontiers in Psychiatry, 9*, 467. https://doi.org/10.3389/fpsyt.2018.00467

Decker, M. R., Miller, E., Illangasekare, S., & Silverman, J. G. (2013). Understanding gender-based violence perpetration to create a safer future for women and girls. *The Lancet. Global Health, 1*(4), e170–e171. https://doi.org/10.1016/S2214-109X(13)70085-8

Fastenau, A., Chahal, P., Shaheen, A., & Basak, M. (2024). Risk factors for suicide among South-East Asian women: A public health crisis in need of gender-specific solutions. *PLOS Mental Health, 1*(6), e0000183. https://doi.org/10.1371/journal.pmen.0000183

Fatema, S. R., East, L., Islam, M., & Usher, K. (2021). Health impact and risk factors affecting south and southeast Asian women following natural disasters: A systematic review. *International Journal of Environmental Research and Public Health, 18*(21), 11068. https://doi.org/10.3390/ijerph182111068

Ferreira, F. H. G., & Ravallion, M. (2008). Global poverty and inequality: A review of the evidence. World Bank Policy Research Working Paper No. 4623. https://ssrn.com/abstract=1149126

FusarPoli, P., Pablo, G. S. D., Micheli, A. D., Nieman, D. H., Correll, C. U., Kessing, L. V., Pfennig, A., Bechdolf, A., Borgwardt, S., Arango, C., & Amelsvoort, T. V. (2019). What is good mental health? A scoping review. *European Neuropsychopharmacology, 31*, 33–46. https://doi.org/10.1016/j.euroneuro.2019.12.105

Gailits, N., Mathias, K., Nouvet, L., Pillai, P., & Schwartz, L. (2019). Women's freedom of movement and participation in psychosocial support groups: a qualitative study in Northern India. *BioMed Central Public Health, 19*(1), 725. https://doi.org/10.1186/s12889-019-7019-3

Gregory, J. W., Cameron, F., Joshi, K., Eiswirth, M. E., Garrett, C., Garvey, K. C., Agarwal, S., & Codner, E. (2022). Clinical practice consensus guidelines 2022: Diabetes in adolescence. *Pediatric Diabetes, 23*(7), 857. https://doi.org/10.1111/pedi.13408

Hassan, S. U., Zahra, A., Parveen, N., Iqbal, N., Mumtaz, S., & Batool, A. (2022). Quality of infertility care services and emotional health of south Asian women. *Psychology Research and Behavior Management, 15*, 1131–1146. https://doi.org/10.2147/PRBM.S357301

Hossain, M., & Purohit, N. (2019). Improving child and adolescent mental health in India: Status, services, policies, and way forward. *Indian Journal of Psychiatry, 61*(4), 415–419. https://doi.org/10.4103/psychiatry.indianjpsychiatry_217_18

Hossain, M. M., Rahman, M., Trisha, N. F., Tasnim, S., Nuzhath, T., Hasan, N. T., Clark, H., Das, A., McKyer, E. L. J., Ahmed, H. U., & Ma, P. (2021). Prevalence of anxiety and depression in South Asia during COVID-19: A systematic review and meta-analysis. *Heliyon, 7*(4), e06677. https://doi.org/10.1016/j.heliyon.2021.e06677

Insan, N., Weke, A., Forrest, S., & Rankin, J. (2022). Social determinants of antenatal depression and anxiety among women in South Asia: A systematic review & meta-analysis. *PLoS One, 17*(2), e0263760. https://doi.org/10.1371/journal.pone.0263760

Ito, H., Setoya, Y., & Suzuki, Y. (2012). *Lessons learned in developing community mental health care in East and South East Asia. World Psychiatry, 11*(3), 186–190. https://doi.org/10.1002/j.2051-5545.2012.tb00129.x

Jayachandran, S. (2015). The roots of gender inequality in developing countries. *Annual Review of Economics, 7*(1), 63–88. https://doi.org/10.1146/annurev-economics-080614-115404

Jenkins, R., Kiima, D., Njenga, F., Okonji, M., Kingora, J., Kathuku, D., & Lock, S. (2010). *Integration of mental health into primary care in Kenya.* Wiley. https://doi.org/10.1002/j.2051-5545.2010.tb00289.x

Johansen, S. L., Stenhaug, B. A., Robakis, T., Williams, K. E., & Cullen, M. R. (2020). Past Psychiatric Conditions as Risk Factors for Postpartum Depression: A Nationwide Cohort Study. *The Journal of Clinical Psychiatry, 81*(1), 19m12929. https://doi.org/10.4088/jcp.19m12929

Jones, C. J., Creedy, D. K., & Gamble, J. A. (2012). Australian midwives' awareness and management of antenatal and postpartum depression. *Women and Birth, 25*(1), 23–28.

Kabir, R., Isigi, S. S., & Candussi, C. (2024). Public mental health and access to mental health Services in South Asia. In S. M. Y. Arafat & S. K. Kar (Eds.), *Access to mental health Care in South Asia.* Springer. https://doi.org/10.1007/978-981-99-9153-2_11

Kabir, R., Rahman, S., Monte-Serrat, D. M., & Arafat, S. Y. (2017). Exploring the decision-making power of Bangladeshi women of reproductive age: Results from a national survey. *South East Asia Journal of Medical Sciences, 1*(1), 4–8. https://doi.org/10.5281/zenodo.2530400

Kallivayalil, R. A. (2012). The importance of psychiatry in undergraduate medical education in India. *Indian Journal of Psychiatry, 54*(3), 208–216. https://doi.org/10.4103/0019-5545.102336

Kamin, T., & Marusic, A. (2005). Book review of culture and self-harm: Attempted suicide in South Asians in London Dinesh Bhugra, Psychology Press, Taylor and Francis Group, 2004, 295 pp., ISBN 1-84169-521-1 (HB). *International Review of Psychiatry, 17*(5), 433–434. https://doi.org/10.1080/09540260500195027

Kendig, S., Keats, J. P., Hoffman, M. C., Kay, L. B., Miller, E. S., Simas, T. A. M., Frieder, A., Hackley, B., Indman, P., Raines, C., Semenuk, K., Wisner, K. L., & Lemieux, L. A. (2017). Consensus Bundle on Maternal Mental Health Perinatal Depression and Anxiety. *Obstetrics & Gynecology, 129*(3), 422–430. https://doi.org/10.1097/aog.0000000000001902

Kohrt, B. A., & Song, S. J. (2018). Who benefits from psychosocial support interventions in humanitarian settings?. *The Lancet. Global Health, 6*(4), e354–e356. Elsevier BV. https://doi.org/10.1016/s2214-109x(18)30102-5

Lindberg, L. D., Bell, D. L. & Kantor, L. M. (2020), The Sexual and Reproductive Health of Adolescents and Young Adults During the COVID-19 Pandemic. *Perspectives on Sexual and Reproductive Health, 52*, 75–79. https://doi.org/10.1363/psrh.12151

Liu, J., Ma, H., He, Y., Xie, B., Xu, Y., Tang, H., Li, M., Hao, W., Wang, X., Zhang, M., Ng, C. H., Goding, M., Fraser, J., Herrman, H., Chiu, H., Chan, S. S. M., Chiu, E., & Yu, X. (2011). Mental health system in China: History, recent service reform and future challenges. *World Psychiatry, 10*(3), 210–216. https://doi.org/10.1002/j.2051-5545.2011.tb00059.x

Mazumder, H., Lugemwa, T., Shimul, M. M. H., Gain, E. P., Hossain, M. M., & Ward, K. D. (2022). Prevalence of suicidal ideation and attempted suicide amongst women and girls in South Asia: A systematic review and meta-analysis. *Psychiatry Research Communications, 2*(4), 100083. https://doi.org/10.1016/j.psycom.2022.100083

McDaid, D., Knapp, M., & Raja, S. (2008). *Barriers in the mind: Promoting an economic case for mental health in low and middle-income countries*. Wiley. https://doi.org/10.1002/j.2051-5545.2008.tb00160.x

Milner, A., & Leo, D. D. (2010). Suicide research and prevention in developing countries in Asia and the Pacific. *Bulletin of the World Health Organization, 88*, 795–796. https://doi.org/10.2471/BLT.09.070821

Min, J. A., Lee, C. U., & Lee, C. (2013). Mental health promotion and illness prevention: A challenge for psychiatrists. *Psychiatry Investigation, 10*(4), 307–316. https://doi.org/10.4306/pi.2013.10.4.307

Narayan, C., & John, T. (2017). TRightshts of persons with disabilities act, 2016: Does it address the needs of persons with mental illness and their families? *Indian Journal of Psychiatry, 59*(1), 17–20. https://doi.org/10.4103/psychiatry.indianjpsychiatry_75_17
Ng, C. H., Herrman, H., Chiu, E., & Singh, B. (2009). Community mental health care in the Asia-Pacific region: Using current best-practice models to inform future policy. *World Psychiatry, 8*(1), 49–55. Wiley. https://doi.org/10.1002/j.2051-5545.2009.tb00211.x
Niaz, U., & Hassan, S. (2006). Culture and mental health of women in Southeast Asia. *World Psychiatry, 5*(2), 118–120.
Norman, R. E., Byambaa, M., De, R., et al. (2012). The long-term health consequences of child physical abuse, emotional abuse, and neglect: A systematic review and meta-analysis. *PLoS Medicine, 9*(5), e1001349. https://doi.org/10.1371/journal.pmed.1001349
Nyqvist, F., Forsman, A. K., Giuntoli, G., et al. (2013). Social capital as a resource for mental Well-being in older people: A systematic review. *Aging & Mental Health, 17*(4), 394–410. https://doi.org/10.1080/13607863.2012.742490
Patel, V. (2007). *Mental health in low- and middle-income countries*. Oxford University Press. https://doi.org/10.1093/bmb/ldm010
Patel, V., DeSouza, N., & Rodrigues, M. (2003). Postnatal depression and infant growth and development in low income countries: A cohort study from Goa, India. *Archives of Disease in Childhood, 88*(1), 34–37. https://doi.org/10.1136/adc.88.1.34
Patel, V., Rahman, A., Jacob, K. S., & Hughes, M. (2004). Effect of maternal mental health on infant growth in low income countries: New evidence from South Asia. *BMJ (Clinical Research ed.), 328*(7443), 820–823. https://doi.org/10.1136/bmj.328.7443.820
Patton, G. C., & Temmerman, M. (2016). Evidence and Evidence Gaps in Adolescent Health. *The Journal of Adolescent Health, 59*(4S), S1–S3. https://doi.org/10.1016/j.jadohealth.2016.08.001
Prajapati, R., & Liebling, H. (2022). Accessing mental health services: A systematic review and meta-ethnography of the experiences of south Asian service users in the UK. *Journal of Racial and Ethnic Health Disparities, 9*(2), 598–619. https://doi.org/10.1007/s40615-021-00993-x
Reddy, M. (2010). Depression: The disorder and the burden. *Indian Journal of Psychological Medicine, 32*(1), 1–2. https://doi.org/10.4103/0253-7176.70510
Rowther, A. A., Kazi, A. K., Nazir, H., Atiq, M., Atif, N., Rauf, N., Malik, A., & Surkan, P. J. (2020). "A Woman Is a Puppet." Women's Disempowerment and Prenatal Anxiety in Pakistan: A Qualitative Study of Sources, Mitigators, and Coping Strategies for Anxiety in Pregnancy. *International Journal of Environmental Research and Public Health, 17*(14), 4926. https://doi.org/10.3390/ijerph17144926
Seng, J., Graham-Bermann, S., Clark, M. K., McCarthy, A., & Ronis, D. (2005). Posttraumatic stress disorder and physical comorbidity among female children and adolescents: Results from service-use data. *Paediatrics, 116*(6), e767–e776. https://doi.org/10.1542/peds.2005-0608
Sheikh, S. M., & Loney, T. (2018). Is educating girls the best investment for South Asia? Association between female education and fertility choices in South Asia: A systematic review of the literature. *Frontiers in Public Health, 6*, 172. https://doi.org/10.3389/fpubh.2018.00172
Sikander, S., Lazarus, A., Bangash, O., Fuhr, D. C., Weobong, B., Krishna, R. N., Ahmad, I., Weiss, H. A., Price, L. N., Rahman, A., & Patel, V. (2015). The effectiveness and cost-effectiveness of the peer-delivered Thinking Healthy Programme for perinatal depression in Pakistan and India: The SHARE study protocol for randomised controlled trials. *Trials, 16*, 534. https://doi.org/10.1186/s13063-015-1063-9
Stewart, D. E., Aviles, R., Guedes, A., Riazantseva, E., & Mac Millan, H. (2015). Latin American and Caribbean countries' baseline clinical and policy guidelines for responding to intimate partner violence and sexual violence against women. *BMC Public Health, 15*, 665. https://doi.org/10.1186/s12889-015-1994-9
Sweeney, A., Weitlauf, J. C., Manning, E. A., Sze, J., Waldrop, A. E., & Hasser, C. (2013). Intimate partner violence: Perspectives on universal screening for women in VHA primary care. *Women's Health Issues, 23*(2), e73–e76. https://doi.org/10.1016/j.whi.2012.12.004

Takegata, M., Ohashi, Y., Lazarus, A., & Kitamura, T. (2017). Cross-national differences in psychosocial factors of perinatal depression: A systematic review of India and Japan. *Healthcare (Basel, Switzerland), 5*(4), 91. https://doi.org/10.3390/healthcare5040091

Thara, R., & Padmavati, R. (2013). Community mental health care in South Asia. *World Psychiatry, 12*(2), 176. https://doi.org/10.1002/wps.20042

Trang, D. T. H., Ha, B. T. T., Vui, L. T., Chi, N. T. Q., Thi, L. M., Duong, D. T. T., Hung, D. T., Cronin de Chavez, A., Manzano, A., Lakin, K., Kane, S., & Mirzoev, T. (2024). Understanding the barriers to integrating maternal and mental health at primary health care in Vietnam. *Health Policy and Planning, 39*(6), 541–551. https://doi.org/10.1093/heapol/czae027

Trivedi, J., Sareen, H., & Dhyani, M. (2008). Rapid urbanisation – Its impact on mental health: A south Asian perspective. *Indian Journal of Psychiatry, 50*(3), 161–165. https://doi.org/10.4103/0019-5545.43623

Upadhyay, R. P., Chowdhury, R., Salehi, A., Sarkar, K., Singh, S. K., Sinha, B., Pawar, A., Rajalakshmi, A. K., & Kumar, A. (2017). Postpartum depression in India: A systematic review and meta-analysis. *Bulletin of the World Health Organization, 95*(10), 706–717C. https://doi.org/10.2471/BLT.17.192237

Vaishnav, M., Javed, A., Gupta, S., Kumar, V., Vaishnav, P., Kumar, A., Salih, H., Levounis, P., Ng, B., Alkhoori, S., Luguercho, C., Soghoyan, A., Moore, E., Lakra, V., Aigner, M., Wancata, J., Ismayilova, J., Islam, M. A., Silva, A. G. D., et al. (2023). Stigma towards mental illness in Asian nations and low-and-middle-income countries, and comparison with high-income countries: A literature review and practice implications. *Indian Journal of Psychiatry, 65*(10), 995–1011. https://doi.org/10.4103/indianjpsychiatry.indianjpsychiatry_667_23

van Brakel, W. H., Sihombing, B., Djarir, H., Beise, K., Kusumawardhani, L., Yulihane, R., Kurniasari, I., Kasim, M., Kesumaningsih, K. I., & Wilder-Smith, A. (2012). Disability in people affected by leprosy: The role of impairment, activity, social participation, stigma and discrimination. *Global Health Action, 5*, 18394. https://doi.org/10.3402/gha.v5i0.18394

Wahlbeck, K. (2015). Public mental health: The time is ripe for translation of evidence into practice. *World Psychiatry, 14*(1), 36–42. https://doi.org/10.1002/wps.20178

Waqas, A., Raza, N., Lodhi, H. W., Muhammad, Z., Jamal, M., & Rehman, A. (2015). Psychosocial factors of antenatal anxiety and depression in Pakistan: Is social support a mediator? *PLoS One, 10*(1), e0116510. https://doi.org/10.1371/journal.pone.0116510

Weiss, H. A., & Ferrand, R. A. (2019). Improving adolescent health: An evidence-based call to action. *Lancet (London, England), 393*(10176), 1073–1075. https://doi.org/10.1016/S0140-6736(18)32996-9

Wellings, K., & Johnson, M. (2013). *Framing sexual health research: Adopting a broader perspective*. Elsevier BV. https://doi.org/10.1016/s0140-6736(13)62378-8

World Health Organization. (2013). *Comprehensive mental health action plan 2013–2020*. World Health Organization.

Chapter 10
Substance Use Among Women in the Perinatal Period in South Asia

Shalini Singh and New fight Seth

1 Introduction

Perinatal substance use is deleterious for both mother and child. This delicate phase is also linked to a higher incidence of sleep difficulties, pain, and peri-partum psychiatric disorders that make abstinence a challenging prospect. In South Asia, sociocultural norms, strict gender roles, poorer awareness, and healthcare disparities shape women's health experiences (Goyal & Mohan, 2025). Perinatal substance use remains an under recognized and often stigmatized problem. This also reflects in the widespread lack of data on incidence of perinatal substance use (abuse) in the South Asian region. The problem is further compounded by underreporting, lack of systematic data collection, and strong cultural taboos associated with female substance use. This chapter explores the epidemiology, risk factors, health consequences, management nuances, and policy landscape related to perinatal substance use in South Asia.

2 Epidemiology

South Asia demonstrates distinct perinatal substance use patterns shaped by traditional practices and modernization. Traditional substance use persists through indigenous medicinal practices and ritualistic consumption. For example, many women in the rural parts of South Asia use opium and gul (a form of chewable tobacco) as remedy for pregnancy-associated nausea (Singh et al., 2024). In Bengali *paan* ceremonies, a high rate of perinatal tobacco use is witnessed. In the

S. Singh (✉) · N. f. Seth
National Drug Dependence Treatment Centre, AIIMS, New Delhi, India

P. Kukreti et al. (eds.), *Women's Reproductive Mental Health in South Asia*, South Asian Perspectives in Mental Health and Psychology,
https://doi.org/10.1007/978-981-96-9219-4_10

pre-conception stage, around 4.3% of Indian women report alcohol and tobacco use according to a nationwide survey done in 2014–2015 (Biradar & Halli, 2023). One of the risk factors linked to substance use in this phase was already having children. The pooled prevalence of tobacco use from studies on pregnant women in India (n = 69,552) was found to be 8.4%, while the prevalence rate for alcohol use was found to be 20.9% (n = 755) (Dhir et al., 2025). Qualitative report (n = 39) on unchecked alcohol intake by pregnant women in the India's tribal belt indicates that cultural acceptability, easy accessibility, erroneously false perception of the health benefits of home brewed liquor, and poor alcohol literacy are the major contributing factors (Pati et al., 2018). Besides this data there is no systematic analysis of prevalence of perinatal substance use in South Asia.

3 Comparison with Other Regions

When comparing South Asia to other regions, particularly sub-Saharan Africa and Western countries, distinct differences emerge:

- **Sub-Saharan Africa**: This region also reports high rates of perinatal mental health issues, with studies showing prevalence rates for perinatal depressive symptoms ranging from 41.6% to 70% across various countries. However, the specific data on substance use during pregnancy is less comprehensive than in South Asia (Palfreyman & Gazeley, 2022).
- **Western Countries**: In contrast, Western nations generally report lower prevalence rates of perinatal substance use. Studies indicate that postnatal depression rates hover around 13%, significantly lower than those observed in South Asian contexts. The lower cultural stigma surrounding substance use and mental health issues may contribute to these differences (Panolan & Thomas, 2024).

4 Key Risk Factors for Perinatal Substance Use in South Asian Women

Drug use experiences in the perinatal period are linked to a complex interplay between biological, psychosocial, cultural, and systemic factors. Some of these factors are unique to the South Asian region, while some are linked to gender disparities which are common across societies. Table 10.1 highlights the regional risk amplifiers for substance use in the South Asian region. We have refrained from listing risk factors unique to the region because of sparse epidemiological literature. Below is a 'theoretical' classification of the risk factors where the South Asian amplifiers have been highlighted.

Table 10.1 Regional risk amplifiers in South Asia

Factor	Regional context	Impact
Polysubstance use	Concurrent tobacco and opioid use in pregnancy	Higher preterm birth rates
Economic inequality	Poverty in informal settlements	Higher substance use in low-income groups
Post-partum relapse	Postnatal social isolation and pressure to resume household duties	Nearly half women relapse within 6 months post-partum

4.1 Socioeconomic and Demographic Factors

- *Women are especially vulnerable to fewer education opportunities and higher rates of unemployment* (UN Women, 2024). Limited education correlates with reduced awareness of substance-related foetal risks, while unemployment exacerbates stress and financial instability (Lal et al., 2015). Microdata from developing countries indicates that women are more likely to find themselves in vulnerable forms of labour such as jobs with no security, lacking legal protection, and working in precarious conditions (Lo Bue et al., 2022). These setbacks are more pronounced in developed countries with lower fertility rates indicating that the perinatal period makes the women more vulnerable to these socio-demographic risk factors. Unintended pregnancy is linked to delayed prenatal care and unhealthy coping behaviours. This leads to increased risk of substance use (Forray & Foster, 2015). In South Asia, stigma around unplanned pregnancies further limits healthcare access precluding adequate screening for drug use (Lal et al., 2015). The growing urbanization in the south Asian region and migration due to economic and climate related stressors have led to isolation from protective family networks and greater exposure to substance use across genders (Morgan & Mall, 2019).

4.2 Psychosocial and Mental Health Factors

- *The perinatal period is linked to higher rates of psychiatric comorbidities* such as depression, anxiety, sleep disturbances, and adjustment disorder. Overall prevalence of post-partum depression and anxiety in India ranges between 5.6% and 22% (Upadhyay et al., 2017). Depression and anxiety are strongly associated with substance use and can be considered as key indicator for screening for drug use (Vyas et al., 2023). Besides this, intimate partner violence is prevalent in the South Asian region. This perpetuates cycles of trauma and substance dependence. Adverse childhood experiences increase vulnerability to addiction, particularly in cultures with high rates of gender-based violence.

4.3 Cultural and Behavioural Factors

- Use of culturally normalized substances like gul, *paan* (betel quid), and *gutkha* (tobacco mixtures) persists among nearly 4.6% of Indian women during pregnancy with smokeless tobacco forms being the predominant route of use. They use it during pregnancy for nausea relief. Being from a lower socio-economic class is the predominant risk factor (Pasupuleti et al., 2021). In most countries in the South Asian region, use of drugs is criminalized. This is compounded by the feelings of fear and shame related to continued drug use during pregnancy. This leads to missed reporting drug use and absent treatment seeking for the problem (Stone, 2015).

4.4 Systemic and Healthcare Barriers

- **Limited prenatal care access**: Nearly half of South Asian women do not get access to quality antenatal care, with substance users facing additional barriers like transportation costs and childcare gaps (Al-Zubayer et al., 2024). Healthcare workers often stigmatize substance-using women, reducing trust and engagement (Vythilingum et al., 2012). Nearly a third of pregnant women avoid treatment due to child custody concerns (Stone, 2015). This is linked to criminalization of drug use.

5 Physiological and Developmental Consequences of Perinatal Substance Use in South Asian Women

Perinatal substance use in South Asia poses significant risks to both maternal and child health, with consequences that extend across generations. The region's unique cultural practices, such as the use of betel nut (*supari*), tobacco mixtures (*gutkha*), home-brewed liquor, and traditional opioid remedies, compound these risks, creating distinct physiological and developmental challenges.

5.1 Maternal Health Outcomes

Substance use during pregnancy exacerbates maternal health risks, particularly in resource-limited settings. *Tobacco and betel nut*, widely consumed in South Asia, are linked to anaemia (prevalence: 52% in users vs. 33% in non-users) and gestational hypertension (OR = 2.1) due to vasoconstrictive effects (Lange et al., 2018). *Opioid use*, prevalent in rural India and Pakistan, increases risks of obstetric complications such as preterm labour (18% higher incidence) and postpartum haemorrhage (Singh et al., 2024). Additionally, polysubstance use—common among urban populations—amplifies maternal malnutrition, as stimulants like tobacco suppress appetite and impair nutrient absorption. These factors might contribute to South Asia's maternal mortality rate (138 deaths/100,000 live births) (*World Bank Open Data*, 2025).

5.2 *Foetal and Neonatal Effects*

Prenatal exposure to substances disrupts foetal development through multiple pathways:

- **Traditional tobacco and areca nut use**: Betel nut's arecoline alkaloid crosses the placenta, correlating with 2.5x higher rates of cleft palate and intrauterine growth restriction (García-Algar et al., 2005). Smokeless tobacco use reduces placental blood flow, increasing low birth weight (LBW) rates by 40% (adjusted OR = 1.4) (Duko et al., 2021).
- **Opioids**: Heroin and prescription opioid use are linked to neonatal abstinence syndrome (NAS), growth restriction, and increased rate of preterm births (McQueen & Murphy-Oikonen, 2016).

Long-term neurodevelopmental deficits are pronounced, with children exposed to opioids showing *12.3-point lower IQ scores* at age 6 compared to controls (Nygaard et al., 2015). Prenatal alcohol exposure, though underreported due to stigma, is associated with impaired executive functioning and 3x higher rates of attention deficit hyperactivity disorder (ADHD) in cohort studies (Akison et al., 2024).

5.3 *Transgenerational Impacts*

The consequences of perinatal substance use cascade across generations through biological and socio-economic pathways:

- **Epigenetic modifications**: Tobacco use alters DNA methylation patterns in genes regulating stress responses (e.g. *NR3C1*), predisposing offspring to anxiety disorders (Knopik et al., 2012).
- **Socio-economic cycles**: Women with substance use disorders (SUDs) often face employment discrimination, perpetuating poverty. In India, children born to mothers with substance use disorders drop out of school by adolescence, citing caregiving responsibilities for younger siblings (Sarkar et al., 2016).

- **Family dynamics**: Stigma isolates affected families, reducing access to community support. Many relatives disengage from households where maternal substance use is disclosed, exacerbating child neglect risks (Monari et al., 2024).

6 Regional Vulnerabilities

South Asia's distinct challenges include:

1. **Cultural normalization** of stimulants like *paan* (betel quid), used by 41% of pregnant women for morning sickness relief (Islam et al., 2024).
2. **Genetic factors**: Polymorphisms in *CYP2A6* genes slow nicotine metabolism in 23% of South Asians, prolonging foetal exposure (López-Flores et al., 2017).
3. **Healthcare gaps**: Virtually none of the rurally situated clinics provide NAS treatment, and mental health services for affected mothers are virtually non-existent (Patrick et al., 2019).

7 Management

The physiological and developmental consequences of perinatal substance use in South Asia demand urgent, culturally tailored interventions.

Community health workers (CHWs) play a vital role in addressing perinatal substance use in South Asia, particularly through their engagement in maternal and child health initiatives (Thomas et al., 2018). Their integration into healthcare systems has been crucial for enhancing access to care, providing education, and supporting women during the perinatal period. Here are the key aspects of their role.

7.1 Screening and Identification

One feature unique to healthcare delivery in South Asian region is the community health workers (CHWs), such as Accredited Social Health Activists (ASHAs) in India, who are often the first point of contact for pregnant women in rural communities. They conduct home visits and community outreach programmes that can facilitate the early identification of substance use among expectant mothers. For instance, ASHAs have been trained to use screening tools like the Edinburgh Postnatal Depression Scale (EPDS) to identify mental health issues, including those related to substance use (Szajna et al., 2024). This proactive approach allows for timely interventions and referrals to appropriate healthcare services. Programmes that enhance their knowledge about mental health issues, substance use disorders, and culturally sensitive intervention strategies are critical for improving their effectiveness.

Training initiatives should also focus on equipping CHWs with skills to handle sensitive discussions around substance use without reinforcing stigma.

Table 10.2 outlines the screening tools available for perinatal substance use. However, it should be pointed out that none of these tools have yet been culturally adapted for south Asian countries.

7.2 Gender-Sensitized Professional Care

Women are less likely to enter treatment as compared to men. Their comorbid psychiatric disorders and trauma histories often complicate drug abuse treatment outcomes and add to psychosocial risk. This is further complicated by additional clinical considerations during the perinatal period. At the same time, many women consider pregnancy as a window when they seriously consider sobriety and a healthier lifestyle. Treatment-seeking women should be offered gender-sensitized care, i.e. care of women by women in women-only settings has better outcomes, that is trauma informed and family centred. This results in higher treatment retention and better outcomes (Polak et al., 2015). Family-centred care would mean allocating for a case manager to look after the intensive psychosocial needs, providing childcare services, allowing children to accompany the mother during in-patient care, arranging transportation, interdisciplinary collaboration, provision of mental health services, specialized prenatal care, and reproductive counselling. Motivation counselling and contingency management are the most effective psychosocial treatments. Group therapy designed exclusively for mothers with substance use disorders has better outcome than when they are mixed with men (Evans et al., 2013). A study assessing recidivism rates reported that women in gender-sensitive treatment

Table 10.2 Screening tools for identifying perinatal substance use

Tool	Purpose	Substances assessed	Format	Time required	Best for
4P's Plus (*The 4P's Plus*, 2025)	Screening	Alcohol, drugs	Five-item questionnaire	<5 min	Prenatal care settings, primary care
TWEAK (Treatment, 1997)	Screening	Alcohol	Five questions	<5 min	Detecting risky drinking in pregnancy
T-ACE (Chang et al., 2010)	Screening	Alcohol	Four questions	<5 min	Quick screening for alcohol use
CRAFFT (*CRAFFT*, 2018)	Screening	Alcohol, drugs	Six questions	<5 min	Pregnant adolescents and young women
Substance Use Risk Profile Pregnancy Scale (SURP-P) (Yonkers et al., 2010)	Screening	Alcohol, drugs	Four domains (risk assessment)	5–10 min	Identifying risk factors for substance use

had better outcomes (Kissin et al., 2014). Besides this, the following are some of the special considerations for pregnant women:

1. NRT is still rarely prescribed during pregnancy, due to concerns over foetal safety. One recent study found similar rates of major congenital anomalies for pregnant women prescribed NRT and those who continued to smoke (35% and 27%, respectively) (Dhalwani et al., 2015).
2. Although the effects of marijuana on neonatal outcome are inconclusive, infant growth restriction and low birth weight have been associated with prenatal use, particularly in mid-to-late pregnancy (Marroun et al., 2009).
3. Prescription opioid use among pregnant women has increased substantially over the past two decades, with a parallel rise in neonatal opioid exposure and neonatal abstinence syndrome (NAS) (Whiteman et al., 2014).
4. Buprenorphine in combination with naloxone, a partial opioid agonist and antagonist, respectively, is emerging as the gold standard in opioid substitution therapy for pregnant opioid-dependent women. Methadone is linked to higher incidence of neonatal abstinence syndrome (CDC, 2025).
5. At present, there is no FDA-approved medication for infants with NAS; oral morphine and methadone are often used, and buprenorphine shows potential but is in need of further research. NAS severity is not related to maternal opioid dose, and infants with NAS often require care in the NICU and extended hospital stays. Variants in the OPRM1 and COMT genes were associated with shorter hospital stays and less need for treatment among infants with NAS (Wachman et al., 2013).
6. Recent studies on prenatal use of methamphetamines found high rates of medical and psychiatric comorbidity, including low birth weight, preterm delivery, intrauterine foetal death, and abruption, and longitudinal studies report cognitive problems in children with in utero exposure to methamphetamines (Diaz et al., 2014).
7. Family support is integral to managing perinatal substance use in South Asian communities, highlighting the need for family-centred approaches in treatment strategies (Sarkar et al., 2016).

7.3 Education and Awareness

The local public health departments must provide essential education about the risks associated with substance use during pregnancy. They can conduct awareness programmes that inform women about the potential impacts of substances on both maternal and foetal health. This educational role is crucial, especially in regions where traditional practices may normalize certain substance uses, such as betel nut or alcohol consumption.

8 Policy Considerations for Preventing and Managing Perinatal Substance Use in South Asia

Addressing perinatal substance use in South Asia requires a nuanced approach that balances the need for treatment with the complexities of cultural, legal, and healthcare systems. Policymakers must consider the implications of punitive versus supportive policies, focusing on maximizing treatment access, enhancing provider training, and involving child welfare and law enforcement judiciously. Below are certain unique policy considerations.

8.1 Maximizing Treatment Access

Policies should prioritize access to substance use disorder (SUD) treatment for pregnant women (Lester et al., 2004). Current punitive approaches that criminalize prenatal substance use or classify prenatal exposure as child maltreatment can deter women from seeking necessary care due to fear of legal repercussions. Instead, supportive policies should facilitate priority access to treatment programmes tailored for pregnant women. Such programmes can include comprehensive services that integrate prenatal care with substance use treatment, mental health support, and social services. Evidence suggests that collaborative care models improve outcomes, reducing prenatal substance use and enhancing maternal health (Kissin et al., 2014).

8.2 Focus on Providers

Training healthcare providers to adopt a non-punitive, supportive approach is essential. Many providers hold stigmatizing views towards pregnant women who use substances, which can hinder effective communication and care (Lester et al., 2004). Policies should mandate training programmes that educate providers on the physiological impacts of substance use during pregnancy and the importance of compassionate care. Implementing universal screening for substance use at the first antenatal visit and regularly thereafter can help identify at-risk women early and facilitate timely interventions.

8.3 *Involvement of Child Welfare and Law Enforcement*

While child welfare policies are crucial for protecting children from harm, they must be designed to support rather than punish mothers. Policies that threaten child custody based on substance use can create significant barriers to seeking help. Instead, collaborative frameworks involving child welfare agencies should focus on providing resources and support for families rather than punitive measures. This approach not only protects children but also encourages mothers to engage in treatment without fear of losing their parental rights.

8.4 *Addressing Unintended Consequences of Punitive Policies*

Research indicates that punitive approaches may lead to unintended adverse pregnancy outcomes, including increased rates of preterm birth and low birth weight (Lester et al., 2004). Punishing mothers for substance use can exacerbate feelings of shame and isolation, further complicating their willingness to seek help. Supportive policies that emphasize treatment over punishment have been shown to improve perinatal health outcomes by fostering a more positive environment for recovery.

8.5 *Community Engagement and Public Awareness*

Engaging communities in public awareness campaigns about the risks associated with perinatal substance use is vital. These campaigns should aim to reduce stigma and promote understanding of SUD as a health issue rather than a moral failing. Involving community leaders can enhance the reach and effectiveness of these initiatives.

9 Conclusion

In conclusion, effective policy considerations regarding perinatal substance use in South Asia must prioritize treatment access, provider education, supportive child welfare practices, and community engagement. By shifting from punitive measures to supportive frameworks, policymakers can improve maternal and child health outcomes while addressing the complex challenges posed by substance use during pregnancy.

References

Akison, L. K., Hayes, N., Vanderpeet, C., Logan, J., Munn, Z., Middleton, P., Moritz, K. M., Reid, N., Anderson, S., Barnett, D., Crawford, A., Doney, R., Elliott, E., Friend, R., Goldsbury, S., Gullo, M., Harrington, S., Harris, K., Hewlett, N., & The Australian FASD Guidelines Development Group, on behalf of the A. F. G. C. (2024). Prenatal alcohol exposure and associations with physical size, dysmorphology and neurodevelopment: A systematic review and meta-analysis. *BMC Medicine, 22*(1), 467. https://doi.org/10.1186/s12916-024-03656-w

Al-Zubayer, M. A., Shanto, H. H., Kundu, S., Sarder, M. A., & Ahammed, B. (2024). The level of utilization and associated factors of WHO recommended antenatal care visits in South Asian countries. *Dialogues in Health, 4*, 100175. https://doi.org/10.1016/j.dialog.2024.100175

Biradar, R. A., & Halli, S. S. (2023). Alcohol and tobacco use among preconception women in India. *Journal of Substance Use, 28*(3), 320–324. https://doi.org/10.1080/14659891.2022.2043473

CDC. (2025, January 31). Treatment of opioid use disorder before, during, and after pregnancy. Opioid use during pregnancy. https://www.cdc.gov/opioid-use-during-pregnancy/treatment/index.html

Chang, G., Fisher, N. D. L., Hornstein, M. D., Jones, J. A., & Orav, E. J. (2010). Identification of risk drinking women: T-ACE screening tool or the medical record. *Journal of Women's Health, 19*(10), 1933–1939. https://doi.org/10.1089/jwh.2009.1911

CRAFFT. (2018). Retrieved April 7, 2025, from https://crafft.org/

Dhalwani, N. N., Szatkowski, L., Coleman, T., Fiaschi, L., & Tata, L. J. (2015). Nicotine replacement therapy in pregnancy and major congenital anomalies in offspring. *Pediatrics, 135*(5), 859–867. https://doi.org/10.1542/peds.2014-2560

Dhir, D., Kumari, S., Devi, V., Chaudhary, V., Murti, K., Dhingra, S., Yanadaiah, P., & Pal, B. (2025). Prevalence of tobacco and alcohol use among pregnant women in India: A systematic review and meta-analysis. *Journal of Substance Use, 0*(0), 1–9. https://doi.org/10.1080/14659891.2024.2448806

Diaz, S. D., Smith, L. M., LaGasse, L. L., Derauf, C., Newman, E., Shah, R., Arria, A., Huestis, M. A., Grotta, S. D., Dansereau, L. M., Neal, C., & Lester, B. M. (2014). Effects of prenatal methamphetamine exposure on Behavioral and cognitive findings at 7.5 years of age. *The Journal of Pediatrics, 164*(6), 1333–1338. https://doi.org/10.1016/j.jpeds.2014.01.053

Duko, B., Pereira, G., Tait, R. J., Nyadanu, S. D., Betts, K., & Alati, R. (2021). Prenatal tobacco exposure and the risk of tobacco smoking and dependence in offspring: A systematic review and meta-analysis. *Drug and Alcohol Dependence, 227*, 108993. https://doi.org/10.1016/j.drugalcdep.2021.108993

Evans, E., Li, L., Pierce, J., & Hser, Y.-I. (2013). Explaining long-term outcomes among drug dependent mothers treated in women-only versus mixed-gender programs. *Journal of Substance Abuse Treatment, 45*(3), 293–301. https://doi.org/10.1016/j.jsat.2013.04.003

Forray, A., & Foster, D. (2015). Substance use in the perinatal period. *Current Psychiatry Reports, 17*(11), 91. https://doi.org/10.1007/s11920-015-0626-5

García-Algar, O., Vall, O., Alameda, F., Puig, C., Pellegrini, M., Pacifici, R., & Pichini, S. (2005). Prenatal exposure to arecoline (areca nut alkaloid) and birth outcomes. *Archives of Disease in Childhood. Fetal and Neonatal Edition, 90*(3), F276–F277. https://doi.org/10.1136/adc.2004.061325

Goyal, R., & Mohan, M. (2025). *How gendered are healthcare systems in South Asia? Women's experiences of care-seeking*. IHP. https://www.internationalhealthpolicies.org/blogs/how-gendered-are-healthcare-systems-in-south-asia-womens-experiences-of-care-seeking/

Islam, M. R., Aktar, S., Pervin, J., Rahman, S. M., Rahman, M., Rahman, A., & Ekström, E.-C. (2024). Maternal betel quid use during pregnancy and child growth: A cohort study from rural Bangladesh. *Global Health Action, 17*(1), 2375829. https://doi.org/10.1080/16549716.2024.2375829

Kissin, W. B., Tang, Z., Campbell, K. M., Claus, R. E., & Orwin, R. G. (2014). Gender-sensitive substance abuse treatment and arrest outcomes for women. *Journal of Substance Abuse Treatment, 46*(3), 332–339. https://doi.org/10.1016/j.jsat.2013.09.005

Knopik, V. S., Maccani, M. A., Francazio, S., & McGeary, J. E. (2012). The epigenetics of maternal cigarette smoking during pregnancy and effects on child development. *Development and Psychopathology, 24*(4), 1377–1390. https://doi.org/10.1017/S0954579412000776

Lal, R., Deb, K. S., & Kedia, S. (2015). Substance use in women: Current status and future directions. *Indian Journal of Psychiatry, 57*(Suppl 2), S275. https://doi.org/10.4103/0019-5545.161491

Lange, S., Probst, C., Rehm, J., & Popova, S. (2018). National, regional, and global prevalence of smoking during pregnancy in the general population: A systematic review and meta-analysis. *The Lancet Global Health, 6*(7), e769–e776. https://doi.org/10.1016/S2214-109X(18)30223-7

Lester, B. M., Andreozzi, L., & Appiah, L. (2004). Substance use during pregnancy: Time for policy to catch up with research. *Harm Reduction Journal, 1*, 5. https://doi.org/10.1186/1477-7517-1-5

Lo Bue, M. C., Le, T. T. N., Santos Silva, M., & Sen, K. (2022). Gender and vulnerable employment in the developing world: Evidence from global microdata. *World Development, 159*, 106010. https://doi.org/10.1016/j.worlddev.2022.106010

López-Flores, L. A., Pérez-Rubio, G., & Falfán-Valencia, R. (2017). Distribution of polymorphic variants of CYP2A6 and their involvement in nicotine addiction. *EXCLI Journal, 16*, 174–196. https://doi.org/10.17179/excli2016-847

Marroun, H. E., Tiemeier, H., Steegers, E. A. P., Jaddoe, V. W. V., Hofman, A., Verhulst, F. C., van den Brink, W., & Huizink, A. C. (2009). Intrauterine cannabis exposure affects Fetal growth trajectories: The generation R study. *Journal of the American Academy of Child & Adolescent Psychiatry, 48*(12), 1173–1181. https://doi.org/10.1097/CHI.0b013e3181bfa8ee

McQueen, K., & Murphy-Oikonen, J. (2016). Neonatal abstinence syndrome. *New England Journal of Medicine, 375*(25), 2468–2479.

Monari, E. N., Booth, R., Forchuk, C., & Csiernik, R. (2024). Experience of family members of relatives with substance use disorders: An integrative literature review. *Creative Nursing, 30*(3), 232–244. https://doi.org/10.1177/10784535241252169

Morgan, N., & Mall, S. (2019). Pathways between urbanization and harmful substance use. *Current Opinion in Psychiatry, 32*(3), 218. https://doi.org/10.1097/YCO.0000000000000488

Nygaard, E., Moe, V., Slinning, K., & Walhovd, K. B. (2015). Longitudinal cognitive development of children born to mothers with opioid and polysubstance use. *Pediatric Research, 78*(3), 330–335. https://doi.org/10.1038/pr.2015.95

Palfreyman, A., & Gazeley, U. (2022). Adolescent perinatal mental health in South Asia and Sub-Saharan Africa: A systematic review of qualitative and quantitative evidence. *Social Science & Medicine, 313*, 115413. https://doi.org/10.1016/j.socscimed.2022.115413

Panolan, S., & Thomas, M. B. (2024). Prevalence and associated risk factors of postpartum depression in India: A comprehensive review. *Journal of Neurosciences in Rural Practice, 15*(1), 1–7. https://doi.org/10.25259/JNRP_584_2023

Pasupuleti, S. S. R., Mohan, P., & Babu, P. J. (2021). Prevalence and predictors of tobacco use among currently married pregnant women in India. *Population Medicine, 3*(April), 1–10. https://doi.org/10.18332/popmed/134755

Pati, S., Chauhan, A. S., Mahapatra, P., Hansdah, D., Sahoo, K. C., & Pati, S. (2018). Weaved into the cultural fabric: A qualitative exploration of alcohol consumption during pregnancy among tribal women in Odisha, India. *Substance Abuse Treatment, Prevention, and Policy, 13*(1), 9. https://doi.org/10.1186/s13011-018-0146-5

Patrick, S. W., Faherty, L. J., Dick, A. W., Scott, T. A., Dudley, J., & Stein, B. D. (2019). Association among county-level economic factors, clinician supply, metropolitan or rural location, and neonatal abstinence syndrome. *JAMA, 321*(4), 385–393. https://doi.org/10.1001/jama.2018.20851

Polak, K., Haug, N. A., Drachenberg, H. E., & Svikis, D. S. (2015). Gender considerations in addiction: Implications for treatment. *Current Treatment Options in Psychiatry, 2*(3), 326–338.

Sarkar, S., Patra, B. N., & Kattimani, S. (2016). Substance use disorder and the family: An Indian perspective. *Medical Journal of Dr. D.Y. Patil Vidyapeeth, 9*(1), 7. https://doi.org/10.4103/0975-2870.172413

Singh, A., Joshi, M., & Parmar, A. (2024). Substance use disorder among women and children in South Asia. In S. M. Y. Arafat & S. K. Kar (Eds.), *Current perspectives on substance use disorders in South Asia: Public mental health aspects* (pp. 279–303). Springer Nature. https://doi.org/10.1007/978-981-97-6619-2_14

Stone, R. (2015). Pregnant women and substance use: Fear, stigma, and barriers to care. *Health & Justice, 3*(1), 2. https://doi.org/10.1186/s40352-015-0015-5

Szajna, A., Tekkalaki, B., Nandagaon, V., Udapi, G., Sogalad, M., Dandagi, S., Kole, U., Patil, S., Raddi, S., Short, V., & Kelly, P. J. (2024). Feasibility and acceptability of a community health worker administered behavioral activation intervention for postpartum depression: A single arm pilot study from India. *Frontiers in Psychiatry, 15*, 1284674. https://doi.org/10.3389/fpsyt.2024.1284674

The 4P's Plus. (2025). NTI Upstream. Retrieved April 7, 2025, from https://www.ntiupstream.com/4psabout

Thomas, R., Pandian, R. D., & Murthy, P. (2018). Treatment service related needs and concerns of women with substance use disorders: A qualitative study. *International Journal of Culture and Mental Health, 11*(2), 123–133. https://doi.org/10.1080/17542863.2017.1334076

Treatment, C. For S. A. (1997). *[Table], TWEAK Test* [Text]. Substance Abuse and Mental Health Services Administration (US). https://www.ncbi.nlm.nih.gov/books/NBK64830/table/A46454/

UN Women. (2024). *Facts and figures: Economic empowerment*. UN Women—Headquarters. Retrieved April 24, 2025, from https://www.unwomen.org/en/what-we-do/economic-empowerment/facts-and-figures

Upadhyay, R. P., Chowdhury, R., Salehi, A., Sarkar, K., Singh, S. K., Sinha, B., Pawar, A., Rajalakshmi, A. K., & Kumar, A. (2017). Postpartum depression in India: A systematic review and meta-analysis. *Bulletin of the World Health Organization, 95*(10), 706–717C. https://doi.org/10.2471/BLT.17.192237

Vyas, S., Jansen, H. A. F. M., Gardner, J., Tuladhar, S., Hammond, K., & Diemer, K. (2023). An analysis of changes in the prevalence and patterns of intimate partner violence against women in seven Asian countries. *BMC Women's Health, 23*(1), 399. https://doi.org/10.1186/s12905-023-02534-6

Vythilingum, B., Roos, A., Faure, S. C., Geerts, L., & Stein, D. J. (2012). Risk factors for substance use in pregnant women in South Africa. *South African Medical Journal, 102*(11), 853–854.

Wachman, E. M., Hayes, M. J., Brown, M. S., Paul, J., Harvey-Wilkes, K., Terrin, N., Huggins, G. S., Aranda, J. V., & Davis, J. M. (2013). Association of OPRM1 and COMT single-nucleotide polymorphisms with hospital length of stay and treatment of neonatal abstinence syndrome. *JAMA, 309*(17), 1821–1827. https://doi.org/10.1001/jama.2013.3411

Whiteman, V. E., Salemi, J. L., Mogos, M. F., Cain, M. A., Aliyu, M. H., & Salihu, H. M. (2014). Maternal opioid drug use during pregnancy and its impact on perinatal morbidity, mortality, and the costs of medical Care in the United States. *Journal of Pregnancy, 2014*(1), 906723. https://doi.org/10.1155/2014/906723

World Bank Open Data. (2025). World Bank Open Data. Retrieved April 7, 2025, from https://data.worldbank.org

Yonkers, K. A., Gotman, N., Kershaw, T., Forray, A., Howell, H. B., & Rounsaville, B. J. (2010). Screening for prenatal substance use: Development of the substance use risk profile-pregnancy scale. *Obstetrics & Gynecology, 116*(4), 827. https://doi.org/10.1097/AOG.0b013e3181ed8290

Chapter 11
Suicidal Behavior and Self-Harm Among Women in Perinatal Period in South Asia

Syeda Ayat-e-Zainab Ali, Tamkeen Saleem, and S. M. Yasir Arafat

1 Introduction

A substantial global public health concern is suicide, which ranks as the third largest cause of death globally for females aged 15–29 and accounts for 70% of all intentional harm deaths among women (Fastenau et al., 2024; World Health Organization, 2014). An alarming combination of social, cultural, patriarchal, and psychological factors contributes to the disproportionate percentage of young women who die by suicide in the WHO South Asia Region (Fastenau et al., 2024). Suicide is one of the main causes of mortality for women, particularly in South Asia, where it accounts for over half of all female suicides globally (World Health Organization, 2019). The prevalence of suicidal behavior among South Asian women is significant, based on data particular to each nation. According to Chakrabarti and Devkota (2004) and Shah et al. (2019), approximately two-thirds of hospitalized cases of attempted suicide in Nepal include women. In India, young women under 30 have been reported to be more likely to die by suicide (Mazumder et al., 2022; Rane & Nadkarni, 2014). According to existing literature, young females in Bangladesh are more likely than males to attempt suicide (Shuvo et al., 2024). Suicidal thoughts have been reported in a Pakistani study conducted on women, particularly those who are young and married (Naveed et al., 2023). Compared to other South Asian nations, Sri Lanka has reported noticeably higher rates of prenatal self-harm, mostly as a result of its

S. A.-e-Z Ali (✉) · T. Saleem
Department of Clinical Psychology, Shifa Tameer-e-Millat University, Islamabad, Pakistan
e-mail: ayat.dcp@stmu.edu.pk; tamkeen.dcp@stmu.edu.pk

S. M. Y. Arafat
Department of Psychiatry, Bangladesh Specialized Hospital, Dhaka, Bangladesh

Department of Public and Community Health, Faculty of Medicine and Health Sciences, Frontier University Garowe, Garowe, Somalia

P. Kukreti et al. (eds.), *Women's Reproductive Mental Health in South Asia*, South Asian Perspectives in Mental Health and Psychology,
https://doi.org/10.1007/978-981-96-9219-4_11

routine screening procedures and comparatively sophisticated mental health treatment system. Postpartum depression (PPD) affects about 10% of women in Sri Lanka; mothers who have a history of mental illness or baby death are at the highest risk (Roysted-Solas et al., 2022). One of the main causes of maternal mortality in Sri Lanka has been shown to be suicide. According to a cross-sectional study conducted in a hospital in Anuradhapura, 0.8% of pregnant women have attempted intentional self-harm (ISH) (Agampodi et al., 2023; Arachchi et al., 2019).

According to estimates, suicide accounts for 2.2% of pregnancy-related deaths in Southeast Asia, despite the alarming rates of maternal suicide worldwide (Fellmeth et al., 2022; Fuhr et al., 2014). Because mental illness and suicide are stigmatized, many maternal suicide fatalities are categorized as accidental; as a result, official statistics are unlikely to accurately reflect the full burden (Fellmeth et al., 2022). According to Hossain et al. (2021), women in South Asia face a number of factors that can contribute to higher or distinct psychosocial stressors, including restricted autonomy, systemic discrimination, poor social status, gender inequity, financial dependency, gender-based violence, and a lack of education and opportunities. Risk factors for self-harm and suicidal behavior could be triggered by an underlying susceptibility, such as impulsivity, a family history of suicide, or past or present mental illnesses (Orsolini et al., 2016). In particular, women in the South Asian region may be at high risk for suicide due to major depressive disorder (MDD), psychosis, and other affective disorders. Additionally, two of the most prominent short- and long-term risk factors for suicide are suicidal ideation and a history of personal suicidal behavior (Ali et al., 2024a, 2024b; Orsolini et al., 2016).

Peripartum, which includes conception, pregnancy, and the postpartum period, is often linked to the beginning and/or recurrence of a psychiatric illness and can be a time of significant vulnerability to major depressive disorders and affective disorders (Jones et al., 2014). Hence, the perinatal period is a crucial time when mental health vulnerabilities can worsen and raise the risk of suicidal thoughts and behavior as well as self-harm (Howard et al., 2014). The psychological, physiological, and social stresses that women experience at this time make them especially vulnerable to mental health conditions, including anxiety and depression, which are closely associated with suicidal thoughts and actions (Jones et al., 2014). About 10–15% of women who give birth will have a major depressive episode overall, and 70% of women who have a family history of postpartum psychosis and 50% of women who have previously had a mood disorder will experience relapse and/or recrudescence after giving birth again (Healey et al., 2013; Orsolini et al., 2016). Therefore, an appropriate suicide screening evaluation is necessary to identify suicidal behavior and high-risk individuals, especially during the prenatal period (Orsolini et al., 2016).

2 Risk Factors for Suicidal Behavior and Self-Harm in Perinatal Period

In South Asia, the combination of biological, sociocultural, psychological, and economic pressures makes suicidal behavior during the perinatal period a serious problem. A number of significant risk factors are linked to suicidal thoughts and behavior as well as self-harm during the perinatal period:

2.1 Psychiatric Determinants

South Asian women are more likely to experience domestic violence during pregnancy and are at a higher risk of having suicidal ideation (Halim et al., 2018). Depression can develop or recur during the perinatal period, which can have long-term effects on the mother's and the child's health (Rao et al., 2021). According to a recent systematic review, a large number of pregnant South Asian women suffer from anxiety and depression, which increases their vulnerability to suicide. Compared to high-income nations, the prevalence is higher among women in Bangladesh, India, and Pakistan because of a lack of awareness and integration of mental health into prenatal care (Insan et al., 2022). Suicide is significantly predicted by depression and suicidal ideation. Suicidal ideation is common among LMIC perinatal women, with rates ranging from 5% to 23% (Mare et al., 2021; Orsolini et al., 2016). According to studies conducted in India, the prevalence of prenatal anxiety is 55.7% (Nath et al., 2019), and antenatal depression ranges widely between 9.8% and 36.7% (Ajinkya et al., 2013; George et al., 2016). Approximately 7.6% of pregnant Indian women suffer suicidal thoughts or behavior, and one in five of them suffers from a mental health illness during pregnancy (Kalra et al., 2021; Supraja et al., 2016). According to a recent review, in 2008–2009, the prevalence of postpartum depression prenatal anxiety ranged from 9% to 51.7%, and suicidal thought within 6 months of postpartum was 30.8% in Bangladesh (Arafat and Rajkumar, 2024). The prevalence of prenatal anxiety in Pakistan is roughly 34.5% (Ali et al., 2012), whereas the incidence of antenatal depression varies from 18% (Karmaliani et al., 2009) to 39.5% (Ayyub et al., 2018). According to an Indian study, untreated mental health issues, including anxiety and postpartum depression, do play a role in suicidality (Babu et al., 2008; Fastenau et al., 2024). Additionally, studies show that women who have a dysphoric-dysregulated temperament are more likely to experience a higher risk of postpartum suicide (Girardi et al., 2011). Abruptly stopping psychiatric medication during pregnancy has generally been associated with an increased risk of suicidality among mothers. A high risk of prenatal suicidality is associated with a history of prior suicide attempts (Orsolini et al., 2016).

Adverse childhood experiences or a history of trauma may make South Asian women particularly susceptible. The stigma associated with mental health in this area keeps many women from getting treatment. Furthermore, there is a dearth of research and mental health resources, particularly in rural areas where suicide rates are higher (Fastenau et al., 2024). The difficulties experienced by vulnerable South Asian women are made worse by a lack of easily accessible and culturally competent mental healthcare, as well as a decline in help-seeking behaviors.

2.2 *Socio-contextual and Economic Determinants*

According to research conducted in the South Asian region, socio-contextual factors can be just as significant as psychiatric risk factors (Fastenau et al., 2024). Rather than mental illness alone, external pressures, including marital conflicts, domestic violence, or financial difficulty, are more likely to trigger suicidal behavior in South Asia. Self-harm and suicidal behavior are associated with poverty, poor levels of education, unemployment, strained relationships, domestic abuse, isolation, and a lack of social support, regardless of mental health conditions (Fleischmann et al., 2016; Vijayakumar & Phillips, 2016). Young, married women from rural areas are particularly at risk of suicide, according to research conducted across South Asia (Fastenau et al., 2024). Suicidal behavior is significantly influenced by the lack of financial independence for women who are restricted to "traditional" housewife responsibilities. In the WHO Southeast Asin Region (SEAR), marriage, which is generally regarded as a protective factor for mental health, paradoxically raises the risk of suicide (Arafat et al., 2023; Vijayakumar & Lamech, 2020). Economic reliance on spouses or in-laws, together with the stress of marital disputes and domestic violence, can drive women into situations where suicide appears to be their only option, according to a Bangladeshi study (Feroz et al., 2012). According to Vijayakumar and Lamech (2020), poverty and economic dependence, along with cultural expectations like the necessity to have male offspring, make many women feel imprisoned, powerless, and ultimately suicidal. Additionally, women who are unable to fulfil these expectations frequently experience terrible abuse, which pushes many of them to take their own lives. These problems are made worse by the loneliness and lack of support that many women endure, especially in joint family structures. Suicidality in SEAR is also significantly influenced by gender-based violence, particularly intimate partner violence (IPV). According to Fastenau et al. (2024), women who experience physical, emotional, or sexual abuse are significantly more likely to attempt or died by suicide. Unplanned pregnancies, a lack of outside support networks, strained relationships with in-laws, and the widespread cultural acceptability of violence against women as a result of patriarchal norms in South Asia all contribute to the issue (Insan et al., 2022).

2.3 Biological Contributors

Numerous biological risk variables, including sleep, maternal age, lifestyle factors, genetics, and pregnancy-related problems, were found to be positively correlated with perinatal suicidality. Higher rates of suicidal ideation have been linked to sleep deprivation (Paris et al., 2009). Suicidal behaviors were 4.47 times more common in people with chronic medical illnesses than in people without such conditions (Molla et al., 2022). Postpartum depression (PPD) and suicidal behavior are significantly influenced by placental hormones such as estrogen, progesterone, and corticotropin-releasing hormone (CRH) (Glynn & Sandman, 2014). Rapid hormonal withdrawal following childbirth can alter brain chemistry, increasing the risk of depression and suicide, particularly in women who are already at risk (Payne & Maguire, 2019). Severe postpartum mental health problems may be avoided by early identification of placental hormone abnormalities. According to Achtyes et al. (2020), biological alterations like inflammation and low serotonin levels were also linked to suicidal behavior, which may indicate dysregulated immunity in postpartum depressive women. As a biological risk factor, younger maternal age was also linked to suicidal ideation (Gressier et al., 2017), while older maternal age was linked to lower odds of suicidality (Martini et al., 2019). An increased incidence of suicidal ideation during the perinatal period was also associated with physical pregnancy-related risk factors. Suicidal ideation was shown to be more common in women who had severe perineal lacerations, caesarean deliveries, severe hyperemesis gravidarum (3.2%), pregnancy-induced hypertension (9.7%), gestational diabetes mellitus (6.5%), and obesity (Bright et al., 2022). Additionally, it was noted that suicidal thoughts were linked to birth trauma, pregnancy and delivery problems, and newborn illness (Bodnar-Deren et al., 2016). Moreover, traumatic experiences associated with miscarriage were found to be a separate risk factor (Gressier et al., 2017; Tabb et al., 2019).

3 Prevention and Intervention Strategies for Suicide Prevention

Strategies that address the psychological and social elements that contribute to suicidality must be comprehensive and culturally appropriate in order to effectively address the perinatal suicide issue in South Asia. Below are key strategies.

3.1 Suicide Risk Assessment

The perinatal phase should include a thorough and preventive evaluation, screening, and detection for suicide ideation, self-harm, and suicidal behavior. According to Koslow et al. (2014), women who experience anxiety and depression should also be evaluated for suicide. It is imperative for clinicians to closely monitor and promptly detect potential risk factors, alarm signs, and related clinical manifestations associated with suicide. When a patient exhibits suicidal thoughts and self-harm, physicians should create a safety plan right away, refer them to a specific psychiatric evaluation, and follow up with them. In certain situations, hospitalization is also necessary (Orsolini et al., 2016). In general, perinatal screening—especially during pregnancy—is a crucial clinical strategy for identifying women who are more likely to experience perinatal suicidality (Koslow et al., 2014). The prevalence of late maternal fatalities may be reduced by identifying and supporting women who are particularly vulnerable to suicide within the first year after giving birth. In general, it should be suggested that medical professionals, especially gynecologists and primary care doctors, enquire about the family history and personal mental health history of every expectant mother. Women having a history of mental illness, especially bipolar disorder, major depressive disorder, and psychoses, should be offered a prenatal mental health evaluation and be under the supervision of a psychiatrist. A routine interview regarding lifetime suicidal behavior should also be conducted. Additionally, mothers should get consistent care and monitoring for at least a year after giving birth (Orsolini et al., 2016).

3.2 Legislative and Policy Reforms

Efforts to prevent suicide must be customized to meet the unique requirements of South Asian women. The leading causes of prenatal suicidality, such as marital conflict, domestic abuse, and psychological, social, and economic issues, should be the focus of policy. Laws that shield women from gender-based violence and make sure offenders are held responsible should be given top priority by governments. A gender-sensitive perspective should be incorporated into national suicide prevention initiatives, acknowledging that perinatal suicide experiences for women are distinct. The unique challenges faced by women in South Asia must be taken into consideration while creating mental health services, support systems, and legal protections. Domestic abusers must be convicted, and South Asian governments must guarantee that women have access to legal recourse. Additionally, legal protections have to enable women to leave violent marriages without worrying about social disgrace, stigma, and financial loss (Fastenau et al., 2024).

3.3 Strengthening Mental Health Services

In South Asia, especially in rural regions, mental health services are frequently inaccessible and underfunded. For women to have access to culturally competent and reasonably priced mental healthcare, governments must make investments in mental health infrastructure. It is also critical to work toward lowering the stigma associated with mental healthcare. Campaigns for public health should increase knowledge about mental health concerns and motivate women to get treatment when necessary. To reach vulnerable groups like young married women, community-based mental health services should be extended, particularly in rural regions (Fastenau et al., 2024). It is also essential to train healthcare professionals to identify the prevalent mental health issues that women in this area encounter, such as postpartum depression and psychosis. Preconception planning or counselling for women with preexisting mental health needs should be provided in the context of their mental health in order to address any medication-related concerns and to make sure that women are aware of symptoms associated with relapse and/or crisis, as this will enable a timely response. To ensure continuity of care within an established therapeutic relationship, the woman's mental health team should address this if she is currently receiving mental health services. Healthcare professionals need to recognize that pregnancy, childbirth, miscarriage, and perinatal loss can be stressful and that women should receive psychological support for these events (Bright et al., 2022). Furthermore, tele-psychiatric services provide a confidential and easily accessible way to support women with mental health problems specially in perinatal period, who frequently experience limited mobility, stigma, or a lack of knowledge about mental health issues (Malhotra et al., 2013). Depending on the patient's convenience and the severity of the mental health issue, programs such as Tele-MANAS in India would be useful in providing immediate mental healthcare to someone experiencing acute psychological distress. They would also help to ensure continuity of care by appropriately referring the patient to local specialized mental health services (Sagar & Singh, 2022). Early access to tele-psychiatric treatments aids in the detection of mood and anxiety disorders during perinatal period before they worsen and lead to serious consequences like suicide. Raising public awareness and incorporating teleconsultation helplines into standard obstetric care can improve the infrastructure for maternal mental health and ultimately save lives during the crucial perinatal period.

3.4 Education, Empowerment, and Community-Based Awareness Programs

One important way to reduce the causes that lead to suicide in South Asia is through education. Higher educated women are less likely to be victims of domestic violence, early marriage, or economic dependence—all of which are major risk factors for suicide. Education for women and girls should be a top priority for local governments, particularly in rural areas where dropout rates are greater. Reducing suicidality in South Asia requires empowerment initiatives that boost women's autonomy and sense of self (Fastenau et al., 2024). To provide women the skills they need to deal with crises without taking their own lives, these programs ought to be incorporated into community health and education systems. The financial strains that lead to suicidality can be lessened by expanding women's access to livelihood opportunities and enhancing their economic resilience. Additionally, educating the public on maternal mental health might lessen stigma and promote early help-seeking behaviors. Crisis intervention programs, healthcare practitioner training, and family-focused awareness campaigns are also essential. In South Asian nations, where traditional beliefs impact health decisions, programs engaging religious and community leaders can be particularly effective (Ali et al., 2024a, 2024b).

3.5 Means Restriction and Psychosocial Support Programs

Strategies for preventing suicide must take into account the particular vulnerabilities, such as the accessibility of lethal means. Priority should be given to initiatives that limit access to lethal means, such as insecticides, pesticides, firearms, rodenticides, and chemical agents, which are frequently used in suicides (WHO, 2019). By educating spouses and families on maternal mental health, suicide risks can be decreased by reducing domestic violence and boosting social support (Ogbe et al., 2020). Women in distress can receive urgent aid by setting up round-the-clock crisis helplines that offer mental health support (Chavan et al., 2012). Cognitive behavioral therapy (CBT)-based therapies, mother-infant bonding programs, and peer support groups have all demonstrated efficacy in lowering suicidal behavior, self-harm, and perinatal depression (Fastenau et al., 2024; Howard & Khalifeh, 2020).

4 Implications for Research

There is an urgent need for quantitative, qualitative, and mixed methods research to be conducted with women experiencing perinatal suicidal ideation in order to learn more about the correlated risk and protective factors and to gain a deeper understanding of women's experiences during the perinatal period, as there is a paucity of research on suicidal behavior and self-harm during this time in South Asia. Perinatal suicide prevention in South Asia requires a multifaceted, culturally specific strategy. Therefore, more experimental research is required in order to find evidence-based psychological interventions for women experiencing suicidal ideation, involving in self-harm and suicidal behavior during perinatal period. In order to improve screening instruments or tools for South Asian women, more investigation is required. Future studies based on systematic reviews ought to concentrate on the biological, psychological, financial, and familial risk factors for suicidal behavior and self-harm in the prenatal stage in the South Asian region. Moreover, systematic evaluations of the social and preventative antecedents of suicidal behavior may be useful in determining the ways in which these elements influence suicidality. Research should also focus on the effects of social policies, the availability and accessibility of healthcare, and protective variables including support from partners and family. By addressing these gaps, policymakers can work on the improvement of maternal mental health and lower perinatal suicide rates in South Asia.

5 Conclusion

South Asian women's perinatal suicidal behavior is a complicated public health issue that is caused by a number of factors, including poverty, low educational levels, domestic violence, gender disadvantage, social and mental health issues, patriarchal standards, and cultural expectations. There is an urgent need for comprehensive suicide prevention initiatives to meet the particular difficulties that pregnant women in South Asian region confront. In order to reduce suicidality among perinatal women, South Asian countries can make significant progress by bolstering their legal protections and healthcare systems, increasing and improving access to mental health services, and encouraging suicide risk screening, psychosocial support programs, education, cultural awareness, and economic empowerment. Action must be taken immediately to save more women from dying in a crisis that can be largely avoided with accurate interventions.

References

Achtyes, E., Keaton, S. A., Smart, L., Burmeister, A. R., Heilman, P. L., Krzyzanowski, S., & Brundin, L. (2020). Inflammation and kynurenine pathway dysregulation in post-partum women with severe and suicidal depression. *Brain, Behavior, and Immunity, 83*, 239–247. https://doi.org/10.1016/j.bbi.2019.10.017

Agampodi, T., Amarasinghe, G., Wickramasinghe, A., Wickramasinghe, N., Warnasekara, J., Jayasinghe, I., Hettiarachchi, A., Nimesha, D., Dilshani, T., Senadheera, S., & Agampodi, S. (2023). Incorporating early pregnancy mental health screening and management into routine maternal care: Experience from the Rajarata Pregnancy Cohort (RaPCo), Sri Lanka. *BMJ Global Health, 8*(9), e012852. https://doi.org/10.1136/bmjgh-2023-012852

Ajinkya, S., Jadhav, P. R., & Srivastava, N. N. (2013). Depression during pregnancy: Prevalence and obstetric risk factors among pregnant women attending a tertiary care hospital in Navi Mumbai. *Industrial Psychiatry Journal, 22*(1), 37–40. https://doi.org/10.4103/0972-6748.123615

Ali, S. A. E. Z., Arafat, S. Y., Rezaeian, M., & Khan, M. M. (2024a). Suicide prevention in muslim countries: Current status and way forward. In *Suicidal behavior in Muslim majority countries: Epidemiology, risk factors, and prevention* (pp. 343–352). Singapore. https://doi.org/10.1007/978-981-97-2519-9_22

Ali, N. S., Azam, I. S., Ali, B. S., Tabbusum, G., & Moin, S. S. (2012). Frequency and associated factors for anxiety and depression in pregnant women: A hospital-based cross-sectional study. *The Scientific World Journal, 2012*(1), 653098. https://doi.org/10.1100/2012/653098

Ali, S. A. E. Z., Saleem, T., & Arafat, S. Y. (2024b). Risk factors for suicide in Pakistan: A mixed methods study of psychological autopsies and perspectives of health professionals. *Archives of Suicide Research*, 1–20. https://doi.org/10.1080/13811118.2024.2436635

Arachchi, N. S. M., Ganegama, R., Husna, A. W. F., Chandima, D. L., Hettigama, N., Premadasa, J., et al. (2019). Suicidal ideation and intentional self-harm in pregnancy as a neglected agenda in maternal health; an experience from rural Sri Lanka. *Reproductive Health, 16*, 1–7. https://doi.org/10.1186/s12978-019-0823-5

Arafat, S. M. Y., Menon, V., Khan, M. A. S., Htay, M. N. N., Singh, R., Biyyala, D., Krishnamoorthy, Y., & Mynampally, K. (2023). Marital status and suicidal behavior in South Asia: A systematic review and meta-analysis. *Health Science Reports, 6*(12), e1781. https://doi.org/10.1002/hsr2.1781

Arafat, S. M. Y., & Rajkumar, R. P. (2024). Mental disorders during pregnancy and postpartum in Bangladesh: A narrative review. *Health Science Reports, 7*(9), e70027. https://doi.org/10.1002/hsr2.70027

Ayyub, H., Sarfraz, M., Mir, K., & tus Salam, F. (2018). Association of antenatal depression and household food insecurity among pregnant women: A cross-sectional study from slums of Lahore. *Journal of Ayub Medical College Abbottabad, 30*(3), 366–371.

Babu, G. N., Subbakrishna, D. K., & Chandra, P. S. (2008). Prevalence and correlates of suicidality among Indian women with post-partum psychosis in an inpatient setting. *Australian & New Zealand Journal of Psychiatry, 42*(11), 976–980. https://doi.org/10.1080/00048670802415384

Bodnar-Deren, S., Klipstein, K., Fersh, M., Shemesh, E., & Howell, E. A. (2016). Suicidal ideation during the postpartum period. *Journal of Women's Health, 25*(12), 1219–1224. https://doi.org/10.1089/jwh.2015.5346

Bright, A. M., Doody, O., & Tuohy, T. (2022). Women with perinatal suicidal ideation–A scoping review of the biopsychosocial risk factors to inform health service provision and research. *PLoS One, 17*(9), e0274862. https://doi.org/10.1371/journal.pone.0274862

Chakrabarti, K., & Devkota, K. C. (2004). Retrospective study of suicide cases admitted in Nepal medical college teaching hospital. *Nepal Medical College Journal, 6*(2), 116–118.

Chavan, B., Garg, R., & Bhargava, R. (2012). Role of 24 hour telephonic helpline in delivery of mental health services. *Indian Journal of Medical Sciences, 66*(5/6), 116–125.

Fastenau, A., Chahal, P., Shaheen, A., & Basak, M. (2024). Risk factors for suicide among southeast Asian women: A public health crisis in need of gender-specific solutions. *PLOS Mental Health, 1*(6), e0000183.

Fellmeth, G., Nosten, S., Khirikoekkong, N., Oo, M. M., Gilder, M. E., Plugge, E., Fazel, M., Fitzpatrick, R., & McGready, R. (2022). Suicidal ideation in the perinatal period: Findings from the Thailand-Myanmar border. *Journal of Public Health (Oxford, England), 44*(4), e514–e518. https://doi.org/10.1093/pubmed/fdab297

Feroz, A. H. M., Islam, S. N., Reza, S., Rahman, A. M., Sen, J., Mowla, M., & Rahman, M. R. (2012). A community survey on the prevalence of suicidal attempts and deaths in a selected rural area of Bangladesh. *Journal of Medicine, 13*(1), 3–9.

Fleischmann, A., Arensman, E., Berman, A., Carli, V., De Leo, D., Hadlaczky, G., & Saxena, S. (2016). Overview evidence on interventions for population suicide with an eye to identifying best-supported strategies for LMICs. *Global Mental Health, 3*, e5. https://doi.org/10.1017/gmh.2015.27

Fuhr, D. C., Calvert, C., Ronsmans, C., Chandra, P. S., Sikander, S., De Silva, M. J., & Patel, V. (2014). Contribution of suicide and injuries to pregnancy-related mortality in low-income and middle-income countries: A systematic review and meta-analysis. *The Lancet Psychiatry, 1*(3), 213–225. https://doi.org/10.1016/S2215-0366(14)70282-2

George, C., Lalitha, A. R., Antony, A., Kumar, A. V., & Jacob, K. (2016). Antenatal depression in coastal South India: Prevalence and risk factors in the community. *International Journal of Social Psychiatry, 62*(2), 141–147.

Girardi, P., Pompili, M., Innamorati, M., Serafini, G., Berrettoni, C., Angeletti, G., & Primiero, F. M. (2011). Temperament, post-partum depression, hopelessness, and suicide risk among women soon after delivering. *Women & Health, 51*(5), 511–524.

Glynn, L. M., & Sandman, C. A. (2014). Evaluation of the association between placental corticotrophin-releasing hormone and postpartum depressive symptoms. *Psychosomatic Medicine, 76*(5), 355–362. https://doi.org/10.1097/PSY.0000000000000066

Gressier, F., Guillard, V., Cazas, O., Falissard, B., Glangeaud-Freudenthal, N. M., & Sutter Dallay, A. L. (2017). Risk factors for suicide attempt in pregnancy and the post-partum period in women with serious mental illnesses. *Journal of Psychiatric Research, 84*, 284–291.

Halim, N., Beard, J., Mesic, A., Patel, A., Henderson, D., & Hibberd, P. (2018). Intimate partner violence during pregnancy and perinatal mental disorders in low and lower middle income countries: A systematic review of literature, 1990–2017. *Clinical Psychology Review, 66*, 117–135. https://doi.org/10.1016/j.cpr.2017.11.004

Healey, C., Morriss, R., Henshaw, C., Wadoo, O., Sajjad, A., Scholefield, H., & Kinderman, P. (2013). Self-harm in postpartum depression and referrals to a perinatal mental health team: An audit study. *Archives of Women's Mental Health, 16*, 237–245.

Hossain, M. M., Rahman, M., Trisha, N. F., Tasnim, S., Nuzhath, T., Hasan, N. T., Clark, H., Das, A., McKyer, E. L. J., Ahmed, H. U., & Ma, P. (2021). Prevalence of anxiety and depression in South Asia during COVID-19: A systematic review and meta-analysis. *Heliyon, 7*, e06677. https://doi.org/10.1016/j.heliyon.2021.e06677

Howard, L. M., & Khalifeh, H. (2020). Perinatal mental health: A review of progress and challenges. *World Psychiatry, 19*(3), 313–327.

Howard, L. M., Molyneaux, E., Dennis, C. L., Rochat, T., Stein, A., & Milgrom, J. (2014). Non-psychotic mental disorders in the perinatal period. *The Lancet, 384*(9956), 1775–1788.

Insan, N., Weke, A., Forrest, S., & Rankin, J. (2022). Social determinants of antenatal depression and anxiety among women in South Asia: A systematic review & meta-analysis. *PLoS One, 17*(2), e0263760. https://doi.org/10.1371/journal.pone.0263760

Jones, I., Chandra, P. S., Dazzan, P., & Howard, L. M. (2014). Bipolar disorder, affective psychosis, and schizophrenia in pregnancy and the post-partum period. *The Lancet, 384*(9956), 1789–1799.

Kalra, H., Tran, T. D., Romero, L., Chandra, P., & Fisher, J. (2021). Prevalence and determinants of antenatal common mental disorders among women in India: A systematic review and meta-analysis. *Archives of Women's Mental Health, 24*, 29–53.

Karmaliani, R., Asad, N., Bann, C. M., Moss, N., Mcclure, E. M., Pasha, O., & Goldenberg, R. L. (2009). Prevalence of anxiety, depression and associated factors among pregnant women of Hyderabad, Pakistan. *International Journal of Social Psychiatry, 55*(5), 414–424.

Koslow, S. H., Ruiz, P., & Nemeroff, C. B. (Eds.). (2014). *A concise guide to understanding suicide: Epidemiology, pathophysiology and prevention*. Cambridge University Press.

Malhotra, S., Chakrabarti, S., & Shah, R. (2013). Telepsychiatry: Promise, potential, and challenges. *Indian Journal of Psychiatry, 55*(1), 3–11. https://doi.org/10.4103/0019-5545.105499

Mare, K. T., Pellowski, J. A., Koopowitz, S.-M., Hoffman, N., van der Westhuizen, C., Workman, L., & Stein, D. J. (2021). Perinatal suicidality: Prevalence and correlates in a South African birth cohort. *Archives of Women's Mental Health, 24*(5), 737–748. https://doi.org/10.1007/s00737-021-01121-8

Martini, J., Bauer, M., Lewitzka, U., Voss, C., Pfennig, A., Ritter, D., & Wittchen, H. U. (2019). Predictors and outcomes of suicidal ideation during peripartum period. *Journal of Affective Disorders, 257*, 518–526.

Mazumder, H., Lugemwa, T., Shimul, M. M. H., Gain, E. P., Hossain, M. M., & Ward, K. D. (2022). Prevalence of suicidal ideation and attempted suicide amongst women and girls in South Asia: A systematic review and meta-analysis. *Psychiatry Research Communications, 2*(4), 100083.

Molla, A., Nigussie, J., & Girma, B. (2022). Prevalence and associated factors of suicidal behavior among pregnant mothers in Southern Ethiopia: A cross-sectional study. *BMC Public Health, 22*(1), 490. https://doi.org/10.1186/s12889-022-12957-9

Nath, A., Venkatesh, S., Balan, S., Metgud, C. S., Krishna, M., & Murthy, G. V. S. (2019). The prevalence and determinants of pregnancy-related anxiety amongst pregnant women at less than 24 weeks of pregnancy in Bangalore, Southern India. *International Journal of Women's Health, 11*, 241–248.

Naveed, S., Tahir, S. M., Imran, N., Rafiq, B., Ayub, M., Haider, I. I., & Khan, M. M. (2023). Sociodemographic characteristics and patterns of suicide in Pakistan: An analysis of current trends. *Community Mental Health Journal, 59*(6), 1064–1070. https://doi.org/10.1007/s10597-022-01086-7

Ogbe, E., Harmon, S., Van den Bergh, R., & Degomme, O. (2020). A systematic review of intimate partner violence interventions focused on improving social support and/mental health outcomes of survivors. *PLoS One, 15*(6), e0235177.

Orsolini, L., Valchera, A., Vecchiotti, R., Tomasetti, C., Iasevoli, F., Fornaro, M., De Berardis, D., Perna, G., Pompili, M., & Bellantuono, C. (2016). Suicide during perinatal period: Epidemiology, risk factors, and clinical correlates. *Frontiers in Psychiatry, 7*, 138. https://doi.org/10.3389/fpsyt.2016.00138

Paris, R., Bolton, R. E., & Weinberg, M. K. (2009). Postpartum depression, suicidality, and mother-infant interactions. *Archives of Women's Mental Health, 12*, 309–321.

Payne, J. L., & Maguire, J. (2019). Pathophysiological mechanisms implicated in postpartum depression. *Frontiers in Neuroendocrinology, 52*, 165–180. https://doi.org/10.1016/j.yfrne.2018.12.001

Rane, A., & Nadkarni, A. (2014). Suicide in India: A systematic review. *Shanghai Archives of Psychiatry, 26*(2), 69–80.

Rao, W.-W., Yang, Y., Ma, T.-J., Zhang, Q., Ungvari, G. S., Hall, B. J., & Xiang, Y.-T. (2021). Worldwide prevalence of suicide attempt in pregnant and postpartum women: A meta-analysis of observational studies. *Social Psychiatry and Psychiatric Epidemiology, 56*(5), 711–720. https://doi.org/10.1007/s00127-020-01975-w

Røysted-Solås, T., Hinderaker, S. G., Ubesekara, L., & De Silva, V. (2022). Mothers at risk of postpartum depression in Sri Lanka: A population-based study using a validated screening tool. *PLoS One, 17*(5), e0268748. https://doi.org/10.1371/journal.pone.0268748

Sagar, R., & Singh, S. (2022). National Tele-Mental Health Program in India: A step towards mental health care for all? *Indian Journal of Psychiatry, 64*(2), 117–119. https://doi.org/10.4103/indianjpsychiatry.indianjpsychiatry_145_22

Shah, B., Kuppili, P. P., Maiti, T., Joshi, S., & Shah, S. (2019). Profile and pattern of suicide attempts among admitted patients in a teaching hospital: A retrospective study from Nepal. *Acta Scientific Medical Sciences, 3*(12), 206–214.

Shuvo, T. A., Hossain, K., & Dey, D. R. (2024). Suicide attempts in Bangladesh: Prevalence, trends, and disparities. *Journal of Medicine, Surgery, and Public Health, 5*, 100170. https://doi.org/10.1016/j.glmedi.2024.100170

Supraja, T. A., Thennarasu, K., Satyanarayana, V. A., Seena, T. K., Desai, G., Jangam, K. V., & Chandra, P. S. (2016). Suicidality in early pregnancy among antepartum mothers in urban India. *Archives of Women's Mental Health, 19*, 1101–1108.

Tabb, K. M., Gavin, A. R., Faisal-Cury, A., Nidey, N., Chan, Y. F., Malinga, T., et al. (2019). Prevalence of antenatal suicidal ideation among racially and ethnically diverse WIC enrolled women receiving care in a Midwestern public health clinic. *Journal of Affective Disorders, 256*, 278–281.

Vijayakumar, L., & Lamech, N. (2020). Suicide and suicidal behavior in women. In P. Chandra, H. Herrman, J. Fisher, & A. Riecher-Rossler (Eds.), *Mental health and illness of women. Mental health and illness worldwide*. Springer.

Vijayakumar, L., & Phillips, M. (2016). Suicide prevention in low- and middle-income countries. In *The international handbook of suicide prevention* (2nd ed., pp. 507–523). Wiley & Sons.

World Health Organization. (2014). *Preventing suicide: A global imperative*. World Health Organization. Retrieved from https://www.who.int/publications/i/item/9789241564779

World Health Organization. (2019). *Suicide in the world: Global health estimates*. World Health Organization. Retrieved from https://www.who.int/publications/i/item/suicide-in-the-world

Chapter 12
Domestic Violence and Pregnancy

Anamika Das and Imon Paul

1 Introduction

Domestic violence (DV) is a pattern of abusive behaviour in any relationship within the domain of a home setting. It encompasses violence suffered by a person from any relative, but mostly it is used synonymously with spousal or intimate partner violence (IPV). Violence against women has been regarded as a serious condition as per the World Health Organization (WHO), and thus protection of women has been included in the Sustainable Development Goals too (*United Nations,* 2023). The menace of domestic violence in the South Asian subcontinent has been present for many decades with women being oppressed due to orthodox societal beliefs. History suggests that during the ancient period, males and females enjoyed equal status in major South Asian countries of current geography: India, Bangladesh, Pakistan, Nepal and Bhutan. However, it changed during the medieval period with evolving societal that led to degradation. In modern days even with empowerment of women, the menace still exists in its various forms, and thus women continue to be victimized till today. Pregnancy is a high-risk condition with increased vulnerability for all women. It also has a sociocultural impact on the role of the women in the family. Pregnancy and its biological underpinnings make women more exposed and threatened with higher impact caused by any stressful situation. Domestic violence in pregnancy thus is a double menace with the woman being exposed to a highly stressful situation during pregnancy. It thus has its aftermath in the form of detrimental impact to the mother, the foetus, newborn and childhood development in the long run. The mental health impact thus falls on all of the individuals across their lifespan. Majority of studies report physical violence during pregnancy, but

A. Das (✉) · I. Paul
Department of Psychiatry, IQ City Medical College and Hospital,
Durgapur, West Bengal, India

P. Kukreti et al. (eds.), *Women's Reproductive Mental Health in South Asia*,
South Asian Perspectives in Mental Health and Psychology,
https://doi.org/10.1007/978-981-96-9219-4_12

emotional and sexual abuse are also detrimental for the woman and the child (Agarwal et al., 2023). A special concern of physical violence is trauma to the abdomen of the women, thus not only injuring the woman but also posing a life-threatening risk for the baby. Physical violence by partners is quite high in Southeast Asia, and a meta-analysis done to find the prevalence of IPV in South Asia found out that overall prevalence from South Asian countries was 23.4% (physical violence 13.6%, emotional violence 20.2%, sexual violence 8.5%) (Nepal et al., 2022). This high prevalence has a major impact on social, health and economic consequences (Shrestha et al., 2022).

2 Domestic Violence (DV) and Intimate Partner Violence (IPV): Definition and Concept

Domestic violence can be defined as "as a pattern of behaviour in any relationship that is used to gain or maintain power and control" (*United Nations,* 2023). The violence can be inflicted on any woman in a home (domestic) setting by any family member which includes an intimate male partner, husband, cohabiting partner, sibling, parent or any other relative like in-laws (Ramalingappa et al., 2018). The majority of domestic violence and its impact occurs from intimate partner violence, and thus in many situations the terms are used interchangeably.

Domestic violence has been defined as harming, injuring or endangering "the health, safety, life, limb or well-being, whether mental or physical" and includes causing physical, sexual, verbal, emotional and/or economic abuse. Physical abuse encompasses any "bodily pain, harm, or danger to life, limb, or health or impair the health" and includes assault, criminal intimidation and criminal force. Sexual abuse includes "any conduct of a sexual nature that abuses, humiliates, degrades or otherwise violates the dignity of woman". Verbal and emotional abuse includes "insults, ridicule, humiliation, name calling and insults or ridicule especially with regard to not having a child or a male child". Economic abuse encompasses "deprivation of all or any economic or financial resources" including financial resources the person is entitled by virtue of the domestic relationship and is needed by the victim or her children or restricting the access to shared household facilities. It also includes marital rape and harassment due to unlawful dowry demand (India Code: Protection of Women from Domestic Violence Act, 2005; NFHS, 2022).

Violence inflicted by a partner or spouse can be categorized and measured in the form of physical, sexual and emotional violence as per National Family Health Survey-5 (NFHS-5) of India done in 2019–2020 and published in March 2022 (NFHS, 2022) as depicted in Table 12.1.

Table 12.1 Various forms of violence with descriptions

Type of violence	Description
Physical spousal violence	Push you, shake you or throw something at you; slap you; twist your arm or pull your hair; punch you with his fist or with something that could hurt you; kick you, drag you or beat you up; try to choke you or burn you on purpose; threaten or attack you with a knife, gun or any other weapon
Sexual spousal violence	Physically force you to have sexual intercourse with him even when you did not want to; physically force you to perform any other sexual acts you did not want to; force you with threats or in any other way to perform sexual acts you did not want to
Emotional spousal violence	Say or do something to humiliate you in front of others; threaten to hurt or harm you or someone close to you; insult you or make you feel bad about yourself

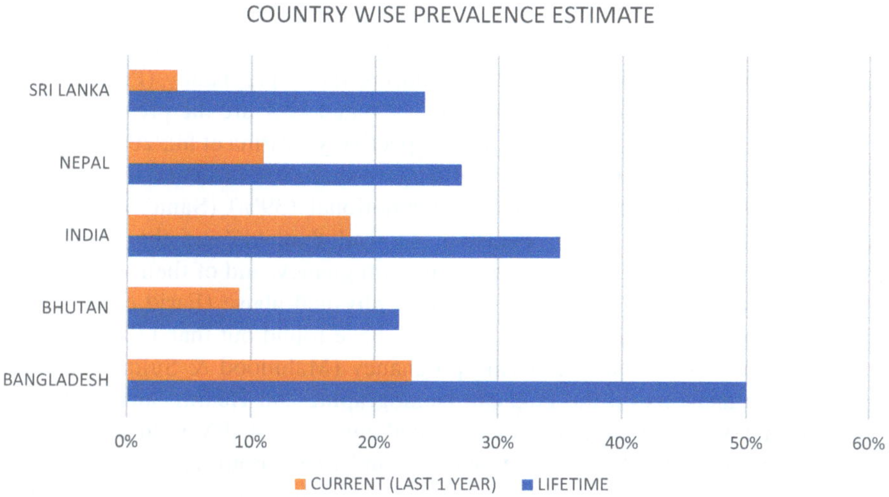

Fig. 12.1 Country-wise prevalence estimate of domestic violence in South Asian countries as per the WHO (Violence against Women Prevalence Estimates, 2018 – WHO South-East Asia Region)

3 Prevalence of Domestic Violence in Pregnancy with Focus on South Asia

The prevalence of domestic violence or intimate partner violence varies across studies. According to the WHO in their multi-country study, the rate of IPV is higher in developing countries (27.7%) as compared to developed countries (13.3%). The country-wise prevalence estimate of domestic violence in a lifetime and in the past 12 months among ever-married/partnered women aged 15–49 in various South Asian countries have been depicted in Fig. 12.1.

The report on violence against women (VAW) Survey in 2015 conducted in Bangladesh showed that almost two thirds (72.6%) have experienced one or more such forms of violence by their husband at least once in their lifetime and about half (54.7%) experienced violence during last 12 months. Out of all forms of IPV, controlling behaviour was most common (55.4%) followed by physical violence (49.6%), emotional violence (28.7% of women), sexual violence (27.3%) and economic violence (11.4%) (Bangladesh Bureau of Statistics, 2016). Another study from Bangladesh pointed out that IPV is pervasive in Bangladesh with more than half of the studied population being victims of IPV during pregnancy and lactation (Tran et al., 2020). In India the prevalence of IPV during pregnancy has ranged from 13% to 28% across various regions (Varma et al., 2007). A study from India done by INCLEN across seven sites (Bhopal, Chennai, Delhi, Lucknow, Nagpur, Thiruvananthapuram and Vellore) with data from family containing at least one woman (15–49 years of age) who has at least one child found out that of the total women who were hit in their lifetime, 48% were hit, 52% were kicked and 50% were beaten during pregnancy (Ahuja et al., 2000). Studies from other parts of the country showed a varied prevalence from 0.5% to 38% (Ramalingappa et al., 2018; Samal & Poornesh, 2022). Another study from Nagpur reports a prevalence of 22% of physical violence during index pregnancy (Purwar et al., 1999). A study from Bangalore found that 14% and 15% are the prevalence rates of physical and psychological violence, respectively (Varma et al., 2007). A study from Pakistan reported a prevalence of 41% of domestic violence in pregnancy, with the most common being verbal or emotional (39%) (Sana et al., 2023). Another study from Karachi, Pakistan, showed that 44% of the interviewed women experienced abuse during the current pregnancy, and of them 43% experienced emotional abuse, and 12.6% reported physical abuse (Farid et al., 2008). The Pakistan Democratic and Health Survey have found out that 11% of women experience domestic violence during pregnancy (Mahmood & Sultan, 2006). A retrospective analysis on the Pakistan Demographic and Health Survey (PDHS) revealed that 39% of individuals experienced any form of IPV with 26.1% experiencing physical IPV, 31.6% emotional IPV and 19.8% both (Zakar et al., 2016). A study from Sri Lanka done among pregnant women showed that the prevalence of ever-physical abuse is 18.3%, and current physical abuse is 10.6% with abuse during the current pregnancy being 4.7% and current sexual abuse being 2.7% (Moonesinghe, 2002). The Nepal Demographic and Health Survey 2016 had a domestic violence module which found out that 26% of married women faced spousal violence with the most common type being physical (23%), followed by emotional violence (12%) (Nepal, 2017). The prevalence rate of all South Asian countries overall was found to be 23.4% (ranging from 1.7% to 66.4%) with physical the form of IPV being 13.6%, sexual 8.5% and emotional 20.2% (Nepal et al., 2022). Although the prevalence rates have varied, it is very well established that IPV during pregnancy is common and a menace. Table 12.2 depicts the prevalence of DV in pregnancy across different studies of South Asian countries.

Table 12.2 Prevalence of DV in pregnancy found in different South Asian studies

Prevalence of violence during pregnancy	Afghanistan	Bangladesh	Bhutan	India	Nepal	Pakistan	Sri Lanka
Study details	Rahman et al. (2021)	Islam et al. (2021)	Study on the situation of violence against women in Bhutan by the National Commission for Women and Children	NFHS-5 2019–2020 (NFHS, 2022 n.d.)	Bhatta and Assanangkornchai (2019)	Karmaliani et al. (2008)	Muzrif et al. (2018)
Study population	2015 Afghanistan Demographic and Health Survey, reproductive-aged women (15–49)	426 new mothers, aged 15–49 years, who were in the first 6 months postpartum	Women aged 15–49 years with one women from each household	Ever-married women aged 18–49	Pregnant and postpartum mothers aged 15–49 years attending antenatal care	Antenatal women in their 20–26th week of gestation	
Overall	46%	66.4%	32.9%6		26.2%	47% (prior to pregnancy) 38% (during pregnancy)	38.6% overall and 15.9% during pregnancy
Physical	52.7%	35.2%	20.5%	3% (highest in the age group of 18–49 years, rural population)	9.4%	16% prior to 14% during pregnancy (physical and sexual abuse)	
Sexual	6.5%	18.5%	10.5%		16%		
Emotional/ psychological/ verbal		65%	23.2%		15%	31% (prior pregnancy) 24% (during pregnancy)	

4 Risk Factors Associated with Domestic Violence in Pregnancy

The various risk factors which predispose a woman for domestic violence can be categorized as individual (victim), partner (perpetrator), household and community factors. They are quite similar to the risk factors during the time the woman is not pregnant. Risk factors specific to pregnancy are the pregnancy being unintended/unwanted and doubt of the spouse that the child being born by the woman does not belong to him. Presence of violence even before pregnancy is also a risk factor (James et al., 2013; Nath et al., 2021). The risk factor in the South Asian setting is also special that the region falls under a low and middle socio-economic status. This vulnerability exposes women in this area to specific other risk factors. In a study from Bangladesh the various correlates found for domestic violence in pregnancy are analysed. It has been postulated that psycho-sociocultural characteristics have more influence than socio-economic status for IPV in developing countries. It was seen in that study that IPV can happen in all segments of the society due to its patriarchal norms. In such social context of developing countries, women are supposed to be perfect housewives and, thus the controlling behaviour of the husband becomes justified. Clinging to traditional gender roles, decision-making autonomy of women, demand of dowry and expectation of a male offspring are other unique factors of this region. The reduced energy and mobility with decreased physical capacity during pregnancy may hamper the role of a homemaker and may thus also contribute to IPV. Economic dependence on the male partner also increases the controlling behaviour of the husband (Islam et al., 2021). In-laws and their controlling behaviour also had an impact as the sociocultural set-up of this part of the world still follows a joint family set up as evident by a study in Nepal which showed that the DV in pregnancy was associated with high controlling behaviour of the mother-in-law (Bhatta & Assanangkornchai, 2019).

Various risk factors associated are enumerated (* marked for factors specific to South Asia):

1. *Individual/Victim Risk factors:-*
    a. Abuse before pregnancy
    b. Low socio-economic status
    c. Age of marriage less than 18 years *
    d. Lower educational level
    e. Pregnancy unwanted/unintended
    f. History of lifetime exposure to violence
    g. Marital/relationship discord
    h. Alcohol abuse/dependence
    i. Young age
    j. History of psychiatric disorders
    k. Clinging to traditional gender role*
    l. Reported dowry demand at marriage*
    m. Low decision-making autonomy during pregnancy*

2. *Partner/perpetrator Risk Factors:*
   a. Use of alcohol by the intimate partner
   b. Pregnancy unwanted/unintended
   c. Lower educational status*
   d. Employment status: unemployed or lowly employed*
3. *Household:*
   a. Low socio-economic status*
   b. Food insecurity*
   c. Less support from other family members/extended family members
   d. Educational discrepancy between spouses *
   e. High controlling behaviour of in-laws *
4. *Community:*
   a. Limited social support
   b. Consanguinity
   c. Preference for a son*
   d. Social inequality*
   e. Lack of access to services*

Whether pregnancy acts as a risk factor for IPV has been researched, and there are mixed results. It has been seen in some studies that the intensification may be associated with various changes of pregnancy-physical, emotional, social and economic with increased economic pressure and less physical relationships with partner. It has also been seen that the perpetrator also has a lot of new dynamics which can be stressful: economic stress of supporting a newborn, rage over unplanned pregnancy, jealousy that the attention of spouse have shifted towards the baby, less frequent sexual relationships and suspicion of fidelity of the baby (Brownridge et al., 2011; Islam et al., 2021). Some researchers have suggested that IPV in pregnancy is a continuum of already existing patterns, while some say that the pregnancy may act as a protective factor (Islam et al., 2021). A study from Pakistan has found out that the prevalence of all forms of DV decreased during pregnancy. It was seen that three-fourths of the women had the same severity of DV both prior to and during pregnancy, whereas for 17% it decreased in severity and for 8% it increased in severity (Karmaliani et al., 2008).

5 Effects of Domestic Violence During Pregnancy

There are various health consequences of domestic violence on pregnancy with both fatal and non-fatal outcomes. Figure 12.2 depicts the various possible impact on health.

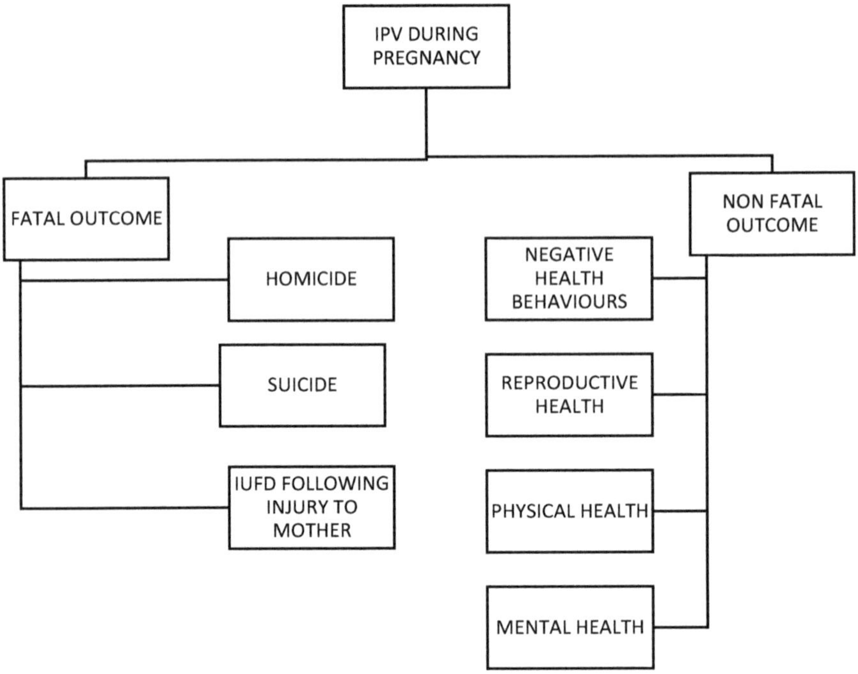

Fig. 12.2 Various health impacts of IPV during pregnancy

There can be various impacts of the IPV during pregnancy. The most extreme consequence of IPV can be homicide during pregnancy. There can also be severe depressive symptoms leading to a suicide attempt and finally to a completed suicide. Impulsive self-harm can also turn fatal sometimes. Injury to the abdomen of the pregnant lady can have adverse consequences for the foetus and may even can cause intra uterine foetal death (IUFD).

Non-fatal outcomes may include a detrimental effect to reproductive health which includes low birth weight, preterm labour or delivery, insufficient weight gain, unsafe abortions and sexually transmitted infections (STIs). Antepartum haemorrhage can also happen with both physical and sexual violence. IPV during pregnancy is also associated with a number of negative health behaviours like smoking, alcohol and drug abuse by the victim and delays in availing prenatal care. Smoking and other substance abuse also in turn predispose the individual to psychiatric disorders. Physical outcomes can include cuts, burns, broken teeth and bones, headaches and other non-fatal injuries. It has been seen that physical violence during pregnancy targeted the abdomen primarily. The partner also attacked other body parts like buttocks, breast, genitalia, head and neck and other extremities. Direct blows into the abdomen can cause both non-fatal and fatal injuries to the foetus. Mental health impact includes higher levels of depression, anxiety, stress, suicide attempts, lack of attachment with the child and post-traumatic stress disorder (PTSD). These are discussed in detail in the next sections. There is also an impact on the child as longitudinal studies have shown that maternal antenatal stress can predict behavioural and emotional problem in the child even after years. There is effect of maternal mood on the foetal brain development which is also discussed later in detail (Belay et al., 2019).

5.1 *Effects of Domestic Violence During Pregnancy: Impact on Mental Health*

It is imperative that living in fear of violent attacks and also experiencing it indeed create stress to the woman. Thus both the actual violence and the fear of violence are indeed stressful, and as stress is well associated with mental disorders, intimate partner violence can predispose, precipitate or perpetuate mental disorders. A meta-analysis on the impact of IPV on women showed that the mean prevalence of depression is 47.6% (ranging from 15% to 83%) in women exposed to IPV as compared to 10.2% in the general population of women. There is also a temporal association with the violence; thus, depression was associated with temporal proximity to the event and also remitted following the stoppage of violence. Also, the severity and duration of violence and depression were directly proportional. The prevalence of suicidality was also high among victims of IPV with a weighted mean of 17.9% (ranging from 4.6% to 77%). The prevalence of post-traumatic stress disorder was 63.8% (ranging from 31% to 84.4%), and the prevalence of alcohol abuse or dependence was 18.5% (ranging from 6.6% to 44%) (Golding, 1999). Pregnancy and the peripartum period on itself are a risk factor for mental health morbidity. Depression, anxiety disorders and somatoform disorders are common in the perinatal period, and untreated mental health morbidity also has adverse effects on the pregnancy outcome like birth weight of the baby, preterm delivery or fatal outcome of the neonate. It also increases the risk of post-partum depression and thus affects the attachment between the mother and child, overall caregiving and infant growth and development. For a country like India which falls under low- and lower-middle-income countries (LLMIC), the prevalence of mental disorders in pregnancy and post-partum is much higher than high-income countries, thus making Indian women more vulnerable in the pregnancy period (Halim et al., 2018). A meta- analysis of 92 studies estimating IPV during pregnancy among 23 LMIC showed its prevalence around 19.8% with a range of 12% in Bangladesh to 57% in Uganda. The prevalence in developing countries was 27.7% as compared to 13.3% for developed countries (Halim et al., 2018).

5.2 *Pathways Connecting Intimate Partner Violence in Pregnancy and Mental Health Disorders*

Intimate partner violence during pregnancy can contribute to mental health disorders through various pathways. Figure 12.3 gives an overview of how various factors can play a role as predisposing, precipitating or perpetuating factors. The link between IPV and mental disorders can be conceptually discussed through these pathways (Halim et al., 2018). A detailed discussion follows.

1. IPV is a significant stressful condition by itself and thus can directly play a causal role for perinatal mental disorder. Pregnant women may develop "physiological and psychological consequences of repeated chronic exposure to heightened neuroendocrine responses" as a response to the stress. The response of our body to stressful situations is mitigated through various neuroendocrine and epigenetic pathways (sympathetic nervous system hyperactivity, secretion of corticotrophin, malfunction in dopaminergic and serotonergic system and augmentation of allopregnanolone), these pathways are even heightened during pregnancy, thus acting as a precipitating factor in the causality of mental disorder (Osório et al., 2017).
2. Indirect psychological pathways may also play a role. Being exposed to frequent IPV can erode the self-esteem of the victim and thus hinder in the self-efficacy of the individual. This leads to an impaired coping ability when exposed to the stressful situation or adapting maladaptive coping strategies, all of which can precipitate mental disorders. It has been seen that exposure to IPV leads to avoidant coping and may even lead to PTSD (Dutton, 2009).
3. Behavioural pathways are also possible explanations for the increased mental health morbidity. Women with exposure to IPV initiate antenatal check-ups late or may even not go for antenatal check-ups. There can also be controlling behaviour of the spouse leading to decreased antenatal care of the woman.
4. Social, contextual factors also play a role. Being treated by a clinician with sparse knowledge of IPV or staying in a community where IPV is taken as a normal phenomenon and mental illness is taken as a stigma, which also can worsen the situation of IPV in pregnancy.
5. Endogenous factors like the presence of a mental disorder prior to conception or during pregnancy are also more susceptible to IPV during pregnancy. Genetic and hormonal susceptibility, presence of chronic disorder, medical illness, complications in pregnancy and rapid hormonal changes can also precipitate stress on the spouse and increase IPV in turn.
6. IPV and mental disorders can stay as concomitant factors without much impact on each other.

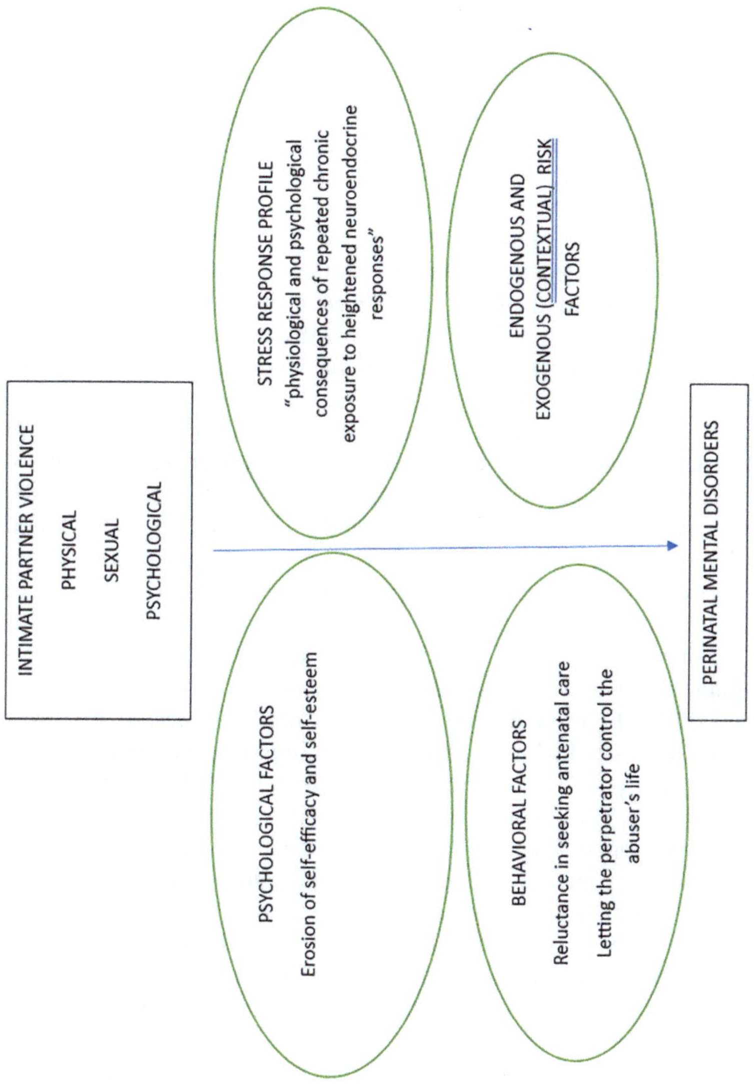

Fig. 12.3 Pathways connecting intimate partner violence in pregnancy and mental disorders

5.3 Mental Health Impacts on the Pregnant Woman

(A) Depression

Antepartum and post-partum depression both have been found to have increased if the pregnant woman is subjected to intimate partner violence. A scoping review on the impact of intimate partner violence in maternal health conducted in low- and middle-income countries showed that the chances of post-partum depression increased with the occurrence of intimate partner violence (Da Thi Tran et al., 2022). The two prospective studies conducted in Vietnam and Turkey both established an association of post-partum depression with IPV (Çankaya, 2020; Tho Nhi et al., 2019). Another cross-sectional study from Iran also showed that IPV during pregnancy is associated with post-partum depression (Afshari et al., 2020). Antepartum depression also was significantly associated with IPV during pregnancy in two studies (Belay et al., 2019; Manongi et al., 2020). Suicidal ideation and self-harm have also been reported in association with psychological IPV done at pregnancy (Teshome et al., 2021). Studies also report that IPV during pregnancy leads to financial instability which in turn can also cause depression (Ashaba et al., 2017). There has been consistent evidence from LMIC on the impact of IPV on pregnant women, but more prospective studies need to be done. Follow-up until 8 or 12 weeks post-partum has shown an association between IPV during pregnancy and post-partum depression, but scarcity of further follow-up studies could not throw light to the length and severity of such depressive episodes. There is also evidence that IPV during pregnancy is also associated with antepartum depression (Da Thi Tran et al., 2022). It has been seen that the direction of association between depression and IPV is bidirectional leading to increase in each other (Devries et al., 2011). A community study in India found out that IPV is a strong predictor of both antepartum and post-partum depression (Patel et al., 1999). Depressive symptoms were also associated with somatization pointing to a common emotional pathway. Somatic symptoms are expression of depressed affect in a more socially acceptable way. The cultural aspect of domestic violence being a private matter prevents the woman from seeking help a number of times, leading to internalization of stress giving rise to somatic symptoms (Varma et al., 2007). Depressive symptoms also lowered self-esteem which is also a major risk factor again for IPV in pregnancy. In a study from Bangladesh, it was seen that emotional IPV was associated with low decision-making autonomy which in turn perpetuated unhelpful behaviours leading to worsened mental health impact (Islam et al., 2021). Another study from Bangladesh also pointed out that women who were exposed to IPV were more likely to be depressed (Tran et al., 2020).

(B) Post-traumatic Stress Disorder

This entity is considered to be the most suitable diagnostic category for diagnosing the experiences resulting from IPV. Depressive symptoms are also present in PTSD and thus may overlap. The characteristic feature of PTSD is the presence of a trauma, and the violence here acts as the trauma. A nested ecological model can be used to explain the link of pathway between IPV and PTSD. The pattern of "coercive control" of IPV acts as mediator of the trauma. Greater severity and intensity of the violence are associated with greater PTSD. Presence of sexual violence and higher number of types of violence as associated with higher PTSD symptoms. Victims having history of childhood trauma, family history of psychiatric disorder and a pre-existing psychiatric illness in the victim increase the predisposition towards PTSD. Women belonging from low socio-economic status are also more vulnerable for PTSD. Being currently married has varied results, being both protective and perpetuating. History of childhood sexual trauma increased the risk for PTSD propensity. It specifically increased the hyperarousal symptoms. Witnessing maternal violence in childhood also works as a risk factor for development of PTSD. Coping self-efficacy is an individual's subjective appraisal that one can cope when faced with demands of stressful situation. This leads to negative self-behaviours in PTSD, thus complicating the situation even more. Emotional dysregulation present in PTSD may also regulate self-efficacy and hamper the situation. This poor self-efficacy also extends to physical health concerns, and as a result the victim's help-seeking behaviour for the physical angle also goes down, complicating it further. The presence of social support helps in mitigating these symptoms overall and thus acts as a protective factor. Revictimization also poses a challenge by not only influencing the course of PTSD but also that the PTSD can also predispose for further violence, specifically psychological violence. The functioning in PTSD victims is not only affected in the health front but also on other levels. It is related to decline in daily functioning, difficulty in parenting role and various other social obligations (Dutton, 2009).

(C) Suicidality

Domestic violence is a highly stressful event which can precipitate a suicide attempt. Suicide is a major global public health concern with more attempts done by women. In a study it was found that IPV is one of the consistent risk factors for attempted suicide in women after adjusting for mental disorders. Having a mother who had experienced intimate partner violence also serves as a risk factor (Devries et al., 2011). This is even more common in a low- and middle-income setting. Consumption of alcohol by spouse was associated with harsh physical violence, and use of alcohol in spouse also increases suicidal behaviour in married women. A study from Pakistan reported that 16% of women attempted suicide due to physical and verbal abuse during pregnancy (Karmaliani et al., 2008). A population-based cohort study from Goa showed that spousal violence acts as an independent risk factor for attempted suicide in women. Domestic violence can act as a stressor and precipitate a suicide attempt in a woman already having a family history of suicide attempt or high impulsivity. They also observed that attempted suicide was highest in sexual violence followed by physical and verbal abuse (Chowdhary & Patel, 2008). In a study from Kerala, a comparison was done between cases (women with suicide attempt), and domestic violence was found in 36.4% cases as compared to

8.5% in controls. Risk factors found in this study were younger age below 30 years, higher occupational status of spouse, poor social support, family history of psychiatric disorder, substance use disorder, past history of suicide attempt, high impulsivity and increased stressful life events. There was also a significant dose-response relationship between domestic violence and attempted suicide indicating that the odds of attempting suicide increased with the severity of violence. There is a proposed stress-diathesis model for suicidal behaviour. The risk for suicidal behaviour depends on state domains like stressful life event, depressive or psychotic episodes and a threshold domain or trait predisposition. The presence of a combination of risk factors over various domains increases the likelihood of a suicide attempt. Thus domestic violence is hailed as a significant stressor for attempting suicide (Indu et al., 2020). Other studies have also found that IPV is an independent risk factor for suicidality even after controlling depressive symptomology (Alhusen et al., 2015a).

(D) Miscellaneous

Injury caused due to physical violence can also have a mental health impact. The injury may harm the foetus leading to stress in the mother. There may also be severe injury to the foetus like placental abruption. All these have an impact on the mental health of the mother. Head injuries may lead to long-term damage and sequelae.

5.4 *Effect on Foetus, Newborn, Child and Adolescent*

1. Foetus and Newborn

There have been studies which show the impact of IPV during pregnancy on the foetal and newborn health. IPV has a direct impact on obstetric outcome; thus there may be low birth weight or premature babies being delivered. Physical IPV has been significantly associated with preterm birth and low birth weight (Agarwal et al., 2023), due to the impact of the blunt physical trauma to the mother. This low birth weight is detrimental to the long-term outcome of the infant. Emotional or sexual violence was associated with decreased breast feeding by the mother in the first year of life, leading to inadequate nutrition and frequent infections. Psychological IPV has also been linked to intrauterine growth restriction. Sexual violence during pregnancy also increases the odds of neonatal mortality (Da Thi Tran et al., 2022). Poor maternal nutrition and inadequate antenatal care also contribute to neonatal morbidity. Use of substance (tobacco, alcohol, etc.) by the pregnant woman also increases the chances of foetal alcohol syndrome and other teratogenic manifestations (Aeri & Farhoud, 2024). Psychological stress may aggravate ongoing physical disorders like hypertension or diabetes of the mother, which has an impact on the obstetric outcome and can thus impact the neonatal health. Exposure to heightened stress also induces the hypothalamic pituitary adrenal axis, including corticotrophin-releasing hormone, which can initiate premature labour and also compromise the uteroplacental circulation (Alhusen et al., 2015b). Another study from Brazil also showed that being small for gestational age is associated with domestic violence. In this study maternal negative behaviours like smoking, drinking and inadequate prenatal care were controlled, but still the impact was present showing that IPV during pregnancy itself is a risk factor for adverse neonatal outcomes (Ferraro et al., 2017). A study from Bangladesh found an inverse relationship with IPV and breastfeeding practices indicating that as IPV increased, the women would less likely be breastfeeding the child, which would be in turn detrimental for the newborn (Tran et al., 2020).

2. Children and Adolescents

Physical consequences to the children as a result of having low birth weight or born prematurely still continue until childhood and adolescence. Prenatal stress in the mother alters both maternal and foetal cortisol levels which in turn has an effect on foetal neurons, thus playing an important role in the child's emotional and social development. In a meta-analysis to find out the impact of IPV during pregnancy on the child after birth, it was seen that the child had behavioural problems and also externalizing and internalizing symptoms. The risk of behavioural symptoms increases by 82%, but it should also be interpreted cautiously. The possible confounding effect of violence continuing even after pregnancy was controlled as it may cause family dysfunction or even cause violence directly to the child, but still a higher rate was reported. The behavioural problems were measured by Child Behaviour Checklist (CBCL) and Rutter's scale, and a relative effect of 1.82 was found. Internalizing problems had an odds ratio (OR) of 2.10, and externalizing problems had an OR of 1.90. By performing subgroup analysis, it was found that the maximum effect was on the age group of <1–4 years age group. The possible explanation is that cerebral plasticity happens its highest in this age group, with neural circuits being more vulnerable. The constant state of fear and stress has an impact on the serotonergic system of the child's brain and thus reduces the hippocampal volume (Aeri & Farhoud, 2024). Traumatic events are also processed in a different way at this stage, and thus exposure to the trauma at the prenatal stage makes these children even more vulnerable. The social impact of disruption of parent-child relationship, exposure to ongoing violence and unstable home environment all play a role in the behavioural impact of the child. Data is sparse from developing countries and countries of eastern part of the world (Agarwal et al., 2023).

6 Impact of COVID-19 on IPV During Pregnancy

Studies conducted in various LMIC like Iran, Ethiopia, Jordan and South Africa showed that IPV was high during the COVID-19 phase. The study from Iran reported that one-third of women experienced IPV in pregnancy with the victims having lower quality of life in terms of mental health (Naghizadeh et al., 2021). The study from Ethiopia showed that 7.1% of women experienced IPV during pregnancy (Teshome et al., 2021). Another community-based study from Jordan showed that the level of IPV decreased during the pandemic from 65.1% to 50.2% for psychological violence, 30.7% to 13% for physical violence and 15.3% to 11.2% for sexual violence (Abujilban et al., 2022). A systematic review and meta-analysis on violence against women during pregnancy at the time of COVID-19 found out that the prevalence estimate is 23% (59% verbal-behavioral violence, 30% emotional violence, 14% sexual violence and 11% physical violence). Another meta-analysis conducted in non-COVID phases gave variable results as compared to these studies, with some reporting increased prevalence while others reporting decreased prevalence. As COVID and quarantine made people homebound, there are chances that domestic violence could have increased due to the higher time spent by the male partner at home. On the other hand, higher social support and networking can result in decreased violence as reported by other studies. Lack of social support in the form of social distancing played the role; otherwise, also closing off of counselling centres was also detrimental to victims of violence. Thus, the impact of COVID-19 had been mixed on domestic violence in pregnancy. The most common form of violence was verbal and controlling behaviour which could be due to the persistent stress related to the difficult economic and social situation during and after the pandemic. It has been seen that multiparous women had been facing more violence as compared to primiparous women. Evidence in high-income countries show that the COVID-19 pandemic worsened the mental health of the whole population and also increased the incidence of violence against women. Social distancing prevented women from taking help both for the IPV and the antenatal check-ups. Predictive factors for increased IPV were the mental health of the couple, drug and alcohol use history in spouse, low education level of the couple, multiparity, age over 35 years and presence of marital conflicts (Aghababaei et al., 2024).

7 Interventions

The antenatal period can be a suitable opportunity to mitigate intimate partner violence. It creates a chance for the woman to access healthcare and not only for a single point in time but for the entire duration of pregnancy. This ensures not only intervention but also possible follow-up. One of evidence-based managements is "empowerment counselling," which provides information to the woman about the types of abuse and the violence cycle and conducts an assessment to find out risks to the woman and provide options for safety which the child may consider. It develops a safety plan with the woman. Mental health screening thus should be an important part of a comprehensive perinatal health assessment. Despite that, it is imperative that healthcare providers are in a strategic position to intervene by identifying and referring as per necessary. It has been seen that there are various barriers. The presence of knowledge gaps, fear of offending patients and lack of intervention to address are some of the factors which act as impediments in providing intervention.

Thus mitigating this knowledge gap would ensure timely identification and mitigation of the factors.

Interventions that have been studied include perinatal home visit programmes, individual counselling and multifaceted counselling. Home visit programmes can be part of specific IPV screening or combined with existing home visit programmes already run by health workers. Programmes in line with Domestic Violence Enhanced Home Visitation Programme (DOVE) can be planned where six home visits are scheduled during pregnancy and the post-partum period. This method has a drawback in the form that the perpetrator is present in the home only, and thus this intervention can only work if the perpetrator does not live with them or privacy can be ensured from the perpetrator during the home visit (Mercier et al., 2024).

Screening during routine antenatal visits followed by referral is the most effective way of identifying women at risk. The goal of intervention is generally to prevent further abuse. It can be achieved by designing interventions to improve women's empowerment, enhance their independence and control or teach them safety measures for safeguarding themselves. The victims should be made aware of the legal provisions too. They should also be made aware of the provision of national helpline numbers to access help as when needed. Communication with others about the abusive relationship and taking help from the family network are other steps of intervention. The intervention may be done in a clinic consultation and can also be done through online methods. A systematic review done to find the effectiveness of interventions done for domestic violence among pregnant women showed that screening with interventions like counselling, home visits and psychotherapy had been effective. Use of cognitive behaviour therapy and other psychological therapies boosted self-esteem and was thus effective to reduce depressive symptoms. Focusing on social support, empathetic listening was also helpful (Sapkota et al., 2019). Identification of negative health behaviour like smoking and alcohol abuse should also be addressed adequately if present. Psychological counselling sessions for the victim based on cognitive behavioural therapy, interpersonal therapy, motivational interviewing and problem-solving can also be done (Jahanfar et al., 2014; Van Parys et al., 2014). Thus, universal screening followed by provision of adequate assistance and support is needed. Figure 12.4 summarizes a framework to address the issue of domestic violence during pregnancy in the context of South Asian countries.

Interventions done in South Asian settings are discussed in Table 12.3.

8 Preventing Violence Against Women

The main pillar of intervention also lies in the fact that domestic violence or intimate partner violence is actually preventable. Mitigation of the risk factors and promotion of protective factors play a paramount role. The WHO has come forward with strategies to prevent violence against women. It is known by the acronym "RESPECT": R, relationship skills strengthened (improve skills in interpersonal communication, conflict management and shared decision making); E,

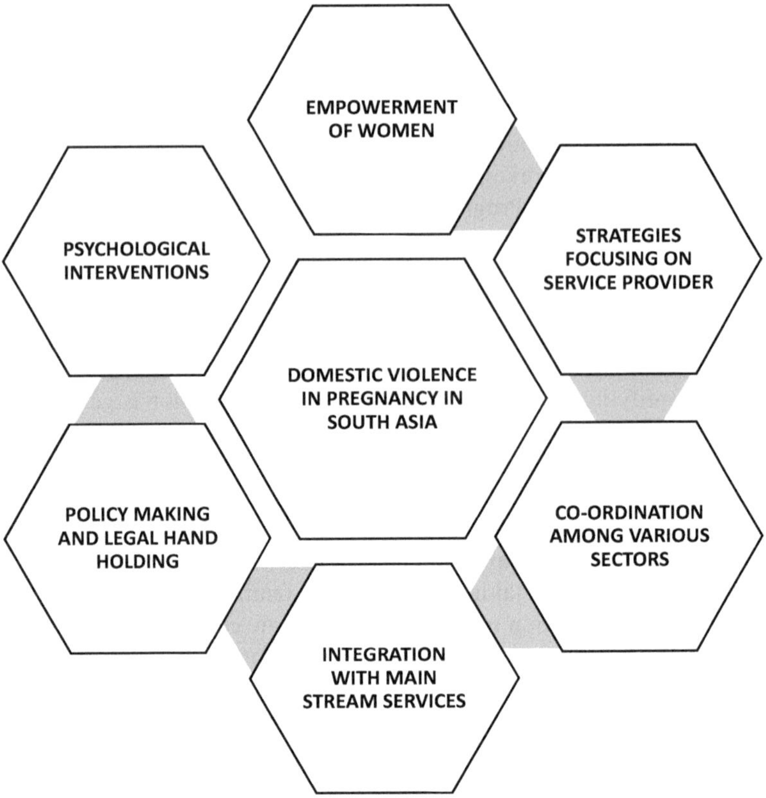

Fig. 12.4 Framework to address domestic violence during pregnancy in South Asian countries

empowerment of women (economic and social empowerment of women which includes inheritance and asset ownership, creation of safe spaces, building skills in self-efficacy, assertiveness, negotiation and self-confidence); S, services ensured (services encompassing social, legal, health and police should be provisioned); P, poverty reduced (alleviate poverty by cash transfers, savings, microfinance loans, labour force interventions); E, environment made safe (create safe schools, public spaces, work environments, etc.); C, child and adolescent abuse prevention (prevention of violence against children, nurturing family relationships, implementing parenting programmes); and T, transformed attitudes, beliefs and norms (strategies challenging harmful gender attitudes, stereotypes that uphold male privilege and female subordination like public campaigns, group education, to community mobilization efforts). Various programmes are run at the government and NGO levels to prevent IPV. The Multi-Sectoral Programme on Violence against Women is implemented by the Government of Bangladesh and led by the Ministry of Women and Children Affairs. Helplines are available at the country level and staffed by trained personnel to provide help to victims of abuse. Various legal frameworks exist in every country to support women from domestic violence. It is needed that women

Table 12.3 Interventions done in the South Asian setting

Author with year	Title of the study	Type of article	Sample	Intervention
India Suneeta Krishnan et al., 2012 (Krishnan et al., 2012)	Minimizing risks and monitoring safety of an antenatal care intervention to mitigate domestic violence among young Indian women: The Dil Mil trial	Randomized clinical trial	18–30-year-old married women with history of domestic violence with their mothers-in-law	Educational programme-based on participatory learning, role playing and discussion methods used, done separately and jointly to enhance the social support, knowledge and skills of participants Educated to interact in a respectful manner to ensure effective communication Knowledge about signs of seeking support
Nepal (Rishal et al., 2020)	Improving Safety Among Pregnant Women Reporting Domestic Violence in Nepal: A Pilot Study	Pretest post-test design	Antenatal women	All participating women were taught 15 safety measures by use of a locally developed flipchart Followed up in post-partum period and assessed on the use of safety behaviours
India Anita Raj et al., 2016 (Raj et al., 2016)	Cluster Randomized Controlled Trial Evaluation of a Gender Equity and Family Planning Intervention for Married Men and Couples in Rural India	Randomized clinical trial	Couples (1081 couples) recruited from 50 geographic clusters (25 clusters randomized to CHARM; 3 sessions of gender equity and family planning sessions and a control condition) Rural Maharashtra, India	The effect of CHARM intervention on men in relation to the use of contraceptives, unwanted pregnancies and attitude towards IPV Education about knowledge of family planning, mutual interaction and communication with a no violence policy

(continued)

Table 12.3 (continued)

Author with year	Title of the study	Type of article	Sample	Intervention
Nepal (Sapkota et al., 2020)	"We don't see because we don't ask": Qualitative exploration of service users' and health professionals' views regarding a psychosocial intervention targeting pregnant women experiencing domestic and family violence	Qualitative study	Antepartum women (24–34 weeks of gestation) and having history of domestic violence were recruited Seven healthcare providers were also interviewed	The study found out themes for improving intervention services like incorporating the intervention in routine healthcare services and having committed staff and sufficient resources

Table 12.4 Legal provisions on domestic violence

Country	Legal provisions
Afghanistan	Elimination of Violence against Women Law (2009)
Bangladesh	• Convention on the Elimination of All Forms of Discrimination against Women (1979) • The Dowry Prohibition Act (1980) • Suppression of Violence against Women and Children Act, 2000 (the Nari O Shishu Nirjatan Daman Ain, 2000 (NSA)) • Domestic Violence (Prevention and Protection) Act (2010) • Domestic Violence (Prevention and Protection) Rules (2013)
Bhutan	Domestic Violence Prevention Act of Bhutan 2013 (endorsed by The National Assembly, at the ninth Parliament Session, June–July 2012)
India	Domestic violence is considered a criminal offence under Indian Penal Code 498 A. Civil protection rights were enabled to victims of domestic violence under Protection of Women from Domestic Violence Act 2005 (PWDVA), which was operationalized in 2006
Nepal	2008 Domestic Violence (Offence and Punishment) Act2012/13–2016/17 National Strategy and Action Plan for Gender Empowerment to End Gender Based Violence
Pakistan	Domestic Violence (Prevention and Protection) Act passed in 2012 Domestic Violence Prevention and Protection Act (Sindh (2013) and Baluchistan (2014)) Prevention of Anti-Women Practices (Criminal Law Amendment) Act 2011
Sri Lanka	Prevention of Domestic Violence Act No. 34 of 2005 (PDVA) Articles 11 and 27 of the Constitution of Sri Lanka

are made aware of the legal provisions for help. Countries like Pakistan do not consider marital rape as illegal, thus perpetuating sexual abuse. It has been seen that there are other impediments too for help seeking, as there are fears that the abuse may increase, and there would be concern for confidentiality, embarrassment and fear of involving police. Pregnancy in particular is an even more difficult phase to take any action because of economic dependence and also to provide the child with a father (Karmaliani et al., 2008). The various legal helps available in South Asian countries are tabulated in Table 12.4.

9 Conclusion

Domestic violence in pregnancy is common in South Asia with a high prevalence reported from all the countries. The sociocultural make-up of this part of the world makes women vulnerable to violence of all types: physical, sexual, emotional or controlling behaviour. Financial dependence, low educational status, early age of marriage, low socio-economic status, demand for a male offspring and practice of dowry are some of the factors which make women in this region more exposed to DV. All types of violence are common with the most prominent being physical and psychological. Pregnancy is a period of special physiology in women, and exposure to DV then leads to neurobiological changes leading to mental health impacts like post-partum or antepartum depression or PTSD. Impact on the foetus is also present with high neonatal morbidity and late effects in childhood and adolescence (externalizing behaviours). Various interventions have been tried, but there is still a lot way left more to go. Antepartum visits by women can serve as a good opportunity for intervention both to prevent and mitigate DV in pregnancy. Research focused on south Asian countries are also scarce and need to be done to get a better picture of the situation for its effective prevention and control.

References

Abujilban, S., Mrayan, L., Hamaideh, S., Obeisat, S., & Damra, J. (2022). Intimate partner violence against pregnant jordanian women at the time of COVID-19 pandemic's quarantine. *Journal of Interpersonal Violence, 37*(5–6), NP2442–NP2464. https://doi.org/10.1177/0886260520984259

Aeri, R., & Farhoud, F. (2024). Intimate partner violence during pregnancy: impact on women and children: A review. *Journal of Social Behavior and Community Health, 8*(1), 1299–1305. https://doi.org/10.18502/jsbch.v8i1.15676

Afshari, P., Tadayon, M., Abedi, P., & Yazdizadeh, S. (2020). Prevalence and related factors of postpartum depression among reproductive aged women in Ahvaz, Iran. *Health Care for Women International, 41*(3), 255–265. https://doi.org/10.1080/07399332.2019.1578779

Agarwal, S., Prasad, R., Mantri, S., Chandrakar, R., Gupta, S., Babhulkar, V., Srivastav, S., Jaiswal, A., Wanjari, M. B., Babhulkar, V. P., IV, & Wanjari, M. (2023). A comprehensive review of intimate partner violence during pregnancy and its adverse effects on maternal and fetal health. *Cureus, 15*(5). https://doi.org/10.7759/cureus.39262

Aghababaei, S., Masoumi, Z., Tahmasebi, R., Jenabi, E., Toosi, Z., & Ghelichkhani, S. (2024). Violence against women during pregnancy and its dimensions in COVID-19 pandemic: A systematic review and meta-analysis. *Industrial Psychiatry Journal, 33*(Suppl 1), S8–S18. https://doi.org/10.4103/ipj.ipj_167_23

Ahuja, R. C., Bangdiwala, S., Bhambal, S. S., Jain, D., Jeyaseelan, L., Kumar, S., Lakshman, M., Mitra, M. K., Nair, M. K., Pillai, R., & Pandey, R. M. (2000). *Domestic violence in India – A summary report of a multi-site household survey*. International Center for Research on Women.

Alhusen, J. L., Frohman, N., & Purcell, G. (2015a). Intimate partner violence and suicidal ideation in pregnant women. *Archives of Women's Mental Health, 18*(4), 573–578. https://doi.org/10.1007/s00737-015-0515-2

Alhusen, J. L., Ray, E., Sharps, P., & Bullock, L. (2015b). Intimate partner violence during pregnancy: Maternal and neonatal outcomes. *Journal of Women's Health, 24*(1), 100–106. https://doi.org/10.1089/jwh.2014.4872

Ashaba, S., Kaida, A., Coleman, J. N., Burns, B. F., Dunkley, E., O'Neil, K., Kastner, J., Sanyu, N., Akatukwasa, C., & Bangsberg, D. R. (2017). Psychosocial challenges facing women living with HIV during the perinatal period in rural Uganda. *PLoS One, 12*(5), e0176256. https://doi.org/10.1371/journal.pone.0176256

Bangladesh Bureau of Statistics. (2016). *Bangladesh Violence against Women (VAW) Survey 2015.* Bangladesh Bureau of Statistics (BBS).

Belay, S., Astatkie, A., Emmelin, M., & Hinderaker, S. G. (2019). Intimate partner violence and maternal depression during pregnancy: A community-based cross-sectional study in Ethiopia. *PLoS One, 14*(7), e0220003. https://doi.org/10.1371/journal.pone.0220003

Bhatta, N., & Assanangkornchai, S. (2019). Patterns of domestic violence against women during pregnancy and the postpartum period in Kathmandu, Nepal. *Asia-Pacific Psychiatry, 11*(1), e12342. https://doi.org/10.1111/appy.12342

Brownridge, D. A., Taillieu, T. L., Tyler, K. A., Tiwari, A., Chan, K. L., & Santos, S. C. (2011). Pregnancy and intimate partner violence: Risk factors, severity, and health effects. *Violence Against Women, 17*(7), 858–881. https://doi.org/10.1177/1077801211412547

Çankaya, S. (2020). The effect of psychosocial risk factors on postpartum depression in antenatal period: A prospective study. *Archives of Psychiatric Nursing, 34*(3), 176–183. https://doi.org/10.1016/j.apnu.2020.04.007

Chowdhary, N., & Patel, V. (2008). The effect of spousal violence on women's health: Findings from the Stree Arogya Shodh in Goa, India. *Journal of Postgraduate Medicine, 54*(4), 306–312. https://doi.org/10.4103/0022-3859.43514

Da Thi Tran, T., Murray, L., & Van Vo, T. (2022). Intimate partner violence during pregnancy and maternal and child health outcomes: A scoping review of the literature from low-and-middle income countries from 2016-2021. *BMC Pregnancy and Childbirth, 22*(1), 315. https://doi.org/10.1186/s12884-022-04604-3

Devries, K., Watts, C., Yoshihama, M., Kiss, L., Schraiber, L. B., Deyessa, N., Heise, L., Durand, J., Mbwambo, J., & Jansen, H. (2011). Violence against women is strongly associated with suicide attempts: Evidence from the WHO multi-country study on women's health and domestic violence against women. *Social Science and Medicine, 73*(1), 79–86. https://doi.org/10.1016/j.socscimed.2011.05.006

Dutton, M. A. (2009). Pathways linking intimate partner violence and posttraumatic disorder. *Trauma, Violence, and Abuse, 10*(3), 211–224. https://doi.org/10.1177/1524838009334451

Farid, M., Saleem, S., Karim, M. S., & Hatcher, J. (2008). Spousal abuse during pregnancy in Karachi, Pakistan. *International Journal of Gynecology and Obstetrics, 101*(2), 141–145. https://doi.org/10.1016/j.ijgo.2007.11.015

Ferraro, A. A., Rohde, L. A., Polanczyk, G. V., Argeu, A., Miguel, E. C., Grisi, S. J. F. E., & Fleitlich-Bilyk, B. (2017). The specific and combined role of domestic violence and mental health disorders during pregnancy on new-born health. *BMC Pregnancy and Childbirth, 17*(1), 257. https://doi.org/10.1186/s12884-017-1438-x

Golding, J. M. (1999). Intimate partner violence as a risk factor for mental disorders: A meta-analysis. *Journal of Family Violence, 14*(2), 99–132. https://doi.org/10.1023/A:1022079418229

Halim, N., Beard, J., Mesic, A., Patel, A., Henderson, D., & Hibberd, P. (2018). Intimate partner violence during pregnancy and perinatal mental disorders in low and lower middle income countries: A systematic review of literature, 1990–2017. *Clinical Psychology Review, 66*, 117–135. https://doi.org/10.1016/j.cpr.2017.11.0044

India Code: Protection of Women from Domestic Violence Act, 2005. Retrieved April 1, 2025, from https://www.indiacode.nic.in/handle/123456789/2021

Indu, P. V., Remadevi, S., Vidhukumar, K., Shah Navas, P. M., Anilkumar, T. V., & Subha, N. (2020). Domestic violence as a risk factor for attempted suicide in married women. *Journal of Interpersonal Violence, 35*(23–24), 5753–5771. https://doi.org/10.1177/0886260517721896

Islam, M. J., Mazerolle, P., Broidy, L., & Baird, K. (2021). Exploring the prevalence and correlates associated with intimate partner violence during pregnancy in Bangladesh. *Journal of Interpersonal Violence, 36*(1–2), 663–690. https://doi.org/10.1177/0886260517730029

Jahanfar, S., Howard, L. M., & Medley, N. (2014). Interventions for preventing or reducing domestic violence against pregnant women. *Cochrane Database of Systematic Reviews, 11*. https://www.cochranelibrary.com/cdsr/doi/10.1002/14651858.CD009414.pub3/abstract

James, L., Brody, D., & Hamilton, Z. (2013). Risk factors for domestic violence during pregnancy: A meta-analytic review. *Violence and Victims, 28*(3), 359–380. https://doi.org/10.1891/0886-6708.vv-d-12-00034

Karmaliani, R., Irfan, F., Bann, C. M., Mcclure, E. M., Moss, N., Pasha, O., & Goldenberg, R. L. (2008). Domestic violence prior to and during pregnancy among Pakistani women. *Acta Obstetricia et Gynecologica Scandinavica, 87*(11), 1194–1201. https://doi.org/10.1080/00016340802460263

Krishnan, S., Subbiah, K., Chandra, P., & Srinivasan, K. (2012). Minimizing risks and monitoring safety of an antenatal care intervention to mitigate domestic violence among young Indian women: The Dil Mil trial. *BMC Public Health, 12*(1), 943. https://doi.org/10.1186/1471-2458-12-943

Mahmood, A., & Sultan, M. (2006). National Institute of Population Studies (NIPS) (Pakistan), and Macro International Inc. *Pakistan Demographic and Health Survey, 7*(2), 123–145.

Manongi, R., Rogathi, J., Sigalla, G., Mushi, D., Rasch, V., Gammeltoft, T., & Meyrowitsch, D. W. (2020). The association between intimate partner violence and signs of depression during pregnancy in Kilimanjaro Region, Northern Tanzania. *Journal of Interpersonal Violence, 35*(23–24), 5797–5811. https://doi.org/10.1177/0886260517724256

Mercier, O., Fu, S. Y., Filler, R., Leclerc, A., Sampsel, K., Fournier, K., Walker, M., Wen, S. W., & Muldoon, K. (2024). Interventions for intimate partner violence during the perinatal period: A scoping review. *Campbell Systematic Reviews, 20*(3), e1423. https://doi.org/10.1002/cl2.1423

Moonesinghe, L. N. (2002). *The prevalence and correlates of physical abuse within marriage in a cohort of pregnant women in the Badulla district* [PhD Thesis]. http://librepository.pgim.cmb.ac.lk/bitstream/handle/1/1003/D-981-AB.pdf?sequence=2

Muzrif, M. M., Perera, D., Wijewardena, K., Schei, B., & Swahnberg, K. (2018). Domestic violence: A cross-sectional study among pregnant women in different regions of Sri Lanka. *BMJ Open, 8*(2), e017745. https://doi.org/10.1136/bmjopen-2017-017745

Naghizadeh, S., Mirghafourvand, M., & Mohammadirad, R. (2021). Domestic violence and its relationship with quality of life in pregnant women during the outbreak of COVID-19 disease. *BMC Pregnancy and Childbirth, 21*(1), 88. https://doi.org/10.1186/s12884-021-03579-x

Nath, A., Venkatesh, S., Vindhya, J., Balan, S., & Metgud, C. S. (2021). Prevalence of intimate partner violence among pregnant women attending a public sector hospital in Bengaluru, southern India. *National Medical Journal of India, 34*(3) https://www.nmji.in/content/141/2021/34/3/pdf/NMJI-34-132.pdf

Nepal, U. (2017). *Population situation analysis of Nepal*. UNFPA Nepal. https://eeca.unfpa.org/sites/default/files/pub-pdf/Nepal%20Population%20Situation%20Analysis.pdf

Nepal, S., Atreya, A., Shrestha, D. B., Budhathoki, P., Lamichhane, S., Nepal, S., Marahatta, A., & Dhital, R. (2022). Intimate partner violence during pregnancy in South Asia: Systematic review and meta-analysis. *Journal of Nepal Health Research Council, 20*(3), 562–569. https://doi.org/10.33314/jnhrc.v20i3.3983

NFHS. (2022 n.d.). Retrieved April 1, 2025, from https://www.nfhsiips.in/nfhsuser/nfhs5.php

Osório, C., Probert, T., Jones, E., Young, A. H., & Robbins, I. (2017). Adapting to stress: Understanding the neurobiology of resilience. *Behavioral Medicine, 43*(4), 307–322. https://doi.org/10.1080/08964289.2016.1170661

Patel, V., Araya, R., De Lima, M., Ludermir, A., & Todd, C. (1999). Women, poverty and common mental disorders in four restructuring societies. *Social Science and Medicine, 49*(11), 1461–1471.

Purwar, M. B., Jeyaseelan, L., Varhadpande, U., Motghare, V., & Pimplakute, S. (1999). Survey of physical abuse during pregnancy GMCH, Nagpur, India. *Journal of Obstetrics and Gynaecology Research, 25*(3), 165–171. https://doi.org/10.1111/j.1447-0756.1999.tb01142.x

Rahman, M., Saha, P., Anwar, N., & Hossain, A. (2021). He hurts her womb: Physical-sexual violence and pregnancy complications among women in Afghanistan. *Health Promotion Perspectives, 11*(4), 485.

Raj, A., Ghule, M., Ritter, J., Battala, M., Gajanan, V., Nair, S., Dasgupta, A., Silverman, J. G., Balaiah, D., & Saggurti, N. (2016). Cluster randomized controlled trial evaluation of a gender equity and family planning intervention for married men and couples in rural India. *PLoS One, 11*(5), e0153190. https://doi.org/10.1371/journal.pone.0153190

Ramalingappa, P., Akhila, M. V., Anjali, R., & Sowmya, K. P. (2018). Domestic violence in pregnancy and its adverse maternal and perinatal outcome: A prospective cohort study. *International Journal of Clinical Obstetrics and Gynaecology, 2*(3), 16–20. https://doi.org/10.33545/gynae.2018.v2.i3a.71

Rishal, P., Devi Pun, K., Schei, B., Bhandari, B., Kumar Joshi, S., Swahnberg, K., Infanti, J. J., Lukasse, M., & Group, A. S. (2020). Improving safety among pregnant women reporting domestic violence in Nepal—A pilot study. *International Journal of Environmental Research and Public Health, 17*(7), 2268. https://doi.org/10.3390/ijerph17072268

Samal, S., & Poornesh, S. (2022). Prevalence of domestic violence among pregnant women: A cross-sectional Study from a Tertiary Care Centre, Puducherry, India. *Journal of Clinical and Diagnostic Research, 16*(4). https://doi.org/10.7860/JCDR/2022/50428.16213

Sana, S. H., Makhdoom, S., Husain, S., Hira, A., Bano, K., & Yasmin, H. (2023). Frequency of domestic violence in pregnancy and its adverse maternal outcomes among Pakistani women. *African Health Sciences, 23*(4), 406–414. https://doi.org/10.4314/ahs.v23i4.44

Sapkota, D., Baird, K., Saito, A., & Anderson, D. (2019). Interventions for reducing and/or controlling domestic violence among pregnant women in low- and middle-income countries: A systematic review. *Systematic Reviews, 8*(1), 79. https://doi.org/10.1186/s13643-019-0998-4

Sapkota, D., Baird, K., Saito, A., Rijal, P., Pokharel, R., & Anderson, D. (2020). 'We don't see because we don't ask': Qualitative exploration of service users' and health professionals' views regarding a psychosocial intervention targeting pregnant women experiencing domestic and family violence. *PLoS One, 15*(3), e0230069. https://doi.org/10.1371/journal.pone.0230069

Shrestha, S. K., Thapa, S., Vicendese, D., & Erbas, B. (2022). Women's attitude towards intimate partner violence and utilization of contraceptive methods and maternal health care services: An analysis of nationally representative cross-sectional surveys from four South Asian countries. *BMC Women's Health, 22*(1), 215. https://doi.org/10.1186/s12905-022-01780-4

Teshome, A., Gudu, W., Bekele, D., Asfaw, M., Enyew, R., & Compton, S. D. (2021). Intimate partner violence among prenatal care attendees amidst the COVID-19 crisis: The incidence in Ethiopia. *International Journal of Gynecology and Obstetrics, 153*(1), 45–50. https://doi.org/10.1002/ijgo.13566

Tho Nhi, T., Hanh, N. T. T., Hinh, N. D., Toan, N. V., Gammeltoft, T., Rasch, V., & Meyrowitsch, D. W. (2019). Intimate Partner Violence among Pregnant Women and Postpartum Depression in Vietnam: A longitudinal study. *BioMed Research International, 2019*, 1–9. https://doi.org/10.1155/2019/4717485

Tran, L. M., Nguyen, P. H., Naved, R. T., & Menon, P. (2020). Intimate partner violence is associated with poorer maternal mental health and breastfeeding practices in Bangladesh. *Health Policy and Planning, 35*(Supplement_1), i19–i29. https://doi.org/10.1093/heapol/czaa106

United Nations. (2023). *What is domestic abuse?* . Retrieved April 1, 2025, from https://www.un.org/en/coronavirus/what-is-domestic-abuse

Van Parys, A.-S., Verhamme, A., Temmerman, M., & Verstraelen, H. (2014). Intimate partner violence and pregnancy: A systematic review of interventions. *PLoS One, 9*(1), e85084. https://doi.org/10.1371/journal.pone.0085084

Varma, D., Chandra, P. S., Thomas, T., & Carey, M. P. (2007). Intimate partner violence and sexual coercion among pregnant women in India: Relationship with depression and post-traumatic stress disorder. *Journal of Affective Disorders, 102*(1–3), 227–235. https://doi.org/10.1016/j.jad.2006.09.026

Zakar, R., Nasrullah, M., Zakar, M. Z., & Ali, H. (2016). The association of intimate partner violence with unintended pregnancy and pregnancy loss in Pakistan. *International Journal of Gynecology and Obstetrics, 133*(1), 26–31. https://doi.org/10.1016/j.ijgo.2015.09.009

Chapter 13
Reproductive Mental Health of Marginalised Women in South Asia

Ankita Chattopadhyay, Sudha Srinivasa Ragavan, Sayani Bisoi, and Sayan Saha

1 Introduction

The realm of reproductive mental health, a critical yet often neglected dimension of well-being, assumes a particularly complex and urgent character within the context of marginalised women in South Asia. Literature defines marginalised women as a diverse group facing multiple layers of systemic exclusion and discrimination due to intersecting sociocultural, economic, and political factors. In the context of South Asia, it includes, but is not limited to, women from lower castes, Rohingya women in Myanmar and Bangladesh, rural and tribal women, refugee and displaced women, women subjected to harmful traditional practices, transgender women, sex workers or women being victims of human trafficking, etc. Even in the modern era, instances of women in South Asia being denied their socio-economic and legal rights continue to happen. They exist within a system dominated by patriarchal norms, religious directives, tribal customs, economic disparities, gender-based violence, and discriminatory laws, inadequate healthcare access, and stigma surrounding mental illness (Niaz & Hassan, 2006). These factors contribute to a high burden of reproductive mental health issues, including depression, anxiety, and trauma related to pregnancy, childbirth, and infertility among marginalised women in South Asia.

A. Chattopadhyay (✉) · S. S. Ragavan
Department of Psychiatry, Jawaharlal Institute of Postgraduate Medical Education and Research (JIPMER), Puducherry, India

S. Bisoi
Department of Psychiatry, All India Institute of Medical Sciences (AIIMS), Kalyani, Kalyani, West Bengal, India

S. Saha
Department of Psychiatry, National Institute of Mental Health and Neurosciences (NIMHANS), Bengaluru, Karnataka, India

P. Kukreti et al. (eds.), *Women's Reproductive Mental Health in South Asia*, South Asian Perspectives in Mental Health and Psychology,
https://doi.org/10.1007/978-981-96-9219-4_13

2 Epidemiology of Reproductive Mental Health Disorders Among Marginalised Women of South Asia

2.1 Perinatal Period

This period of psychological vulnerability may not only contribute to relapses of pre-existing mental health conditions but can precipitate the start of new onset psychiatric conditions such as postnatal depression and, more rarely, puerperal psychosis.

Perinatal mental health (PMH) is a global public health concern that transcends cultural boundaries and has varied social, cultural, biological, and psychological underpinnings (Insan et al., 2022). According to the World Health Organisation (WHO), South Asia has some of the highest rates of maternal mortality and morbidity globally, with marginalised women being disproportionately affected (WHO, 2020). Perinatal depression is one of the most common reproductive mental health disorders in South Asia. Studies on marginalised women in South Asian countries like India, Pakistan, and Nepal have shown varying prevalence across studies and regions, ranging from around 15% to 35% which is higher than the global average. Financial stress, ethnic minority, lack of social support, domestic violence, and cultural dogma make them particularly vulnerable to stress, isolation, and discrimination during this period. Lack of accessible infrastructure further worsens the situation by increasing the number of undiagnosed and untreated cases. Maternal depression in turn affects development as studies of mothers from rural areas of Bangladesh showed that maternal depression and perceived infant irritability were associated with poor development of infant cognitive skills (Black et al., 2007). Studies have identified economic constraints, malnutrition, immigration, unemployment of husbands, poor living conditions, and pressure to bear male children as risk factors. Post-partum rituals in regions of South Asia are believed to support new mothers and babies but lack substantial research (Klainin & Arthur, 2009). Marginalised women in South Asia face multiple stressors including fear of childbirth and cultural beliefs and socio-economic uncertainties surrounding, food insecurity, and poverty which make them more vulnerable to develop anxiety during pregnancy or post childbirth. Although studies on post-partum psychosis or post-partum blues are lacking, their vulnerabilities do increase the probability of developing these disorders in marginalised women.

2.2 Perinatal Mental Health of Women Victims of Sex Trafficking

Every year 1–two million women, men, and children are trafficked worldwide, and around 225,000 of them are reported to be from South Asia (Huda, 2006). Majority of them (58%) are girls or women.

Victims of sex trafficking experience anxiety, depression, isolation, disorientation, aggression, suicidal ideation, attention deficit, psychotic disorders, behavioural disturbances, and post-traumatic stress disorder (PTSD) (Suwetty et al., 2019). Women who are victims of sex trafficking report constant social exclusion, anxiety, and lack of support from society. With at least one in four women with sex trafficking reportedly ending up in pregnancy, the burden of perinatal mental health of women victims of sex trafficking is manifold. Maternity mental care in these cases needs to be guided by trauma-informed care and respectful maternity care.

2.3 *Perinatal Mental Health of Migrant and Refugee Women*

In a review of studies reporting perinatal depression among migrant women, pooled prevalence was 31% [95% confidence interval (CI) 23%–40%] for any depressive disorder and 17% (95% CI 12–23%) for major depressive disorder (Fellmeth et al., 2017). Perinatal outcomes were predominantly worse among migrant women, particularly mental health, maternal mortality, preterm birth, and congenital anomalies. Access and use of care were obstructed by structural, organisational, social, personal, and cultural barriers. Migrant women's experiences of care included negative communication, discrimination, poor relationships with health professionals, cultural clashes, and negative experiences of clinical intervention (Heslehurst et al., 2018).

2.4 *Perinatal Mental Health in Tribal Women*

Depression and anxiety are highly prevalent among the tribal population of India, which is home to the second largest tribal population in the world, with 705 indigenous groups. According to the latest National Family Health Survey (NFHS-5, 2019–2021), the under-5 mortality rate among Scheduled Tribes is 50.3 per 1000 live births, which is significantly higher than the average of 41.9 across the country. These high rates of under-5 mortality rates leading to exploration of associated factors bring to the front the burden of perinatal mental health issues of tribal women (Singh & Kumar, 2025). Since the figure of under-5 deaths among scheduled tribes has been considerably high for long, the contribution of maternal illness like depression and anxiety can contribute to the child's survival issues as mentioned by the authors.

In a study on postnatal women of two tribal communities of Odisha, India, to study the prevalence of postnatal depression, high scores of >15 on Edinburgh Postnatal Depression Scale (EPDS) indicative of possible depression were reported in 54.2% women. Variables like caste, gender of the child (male), and *General Health Questionnaire-12* (GHQ-12) scores as proxy of familial stress were found significant for high EPDS score in logistic regression model. The authors here point out that despite the availability of a robust healthcare delivery system, socio-familial factors such as family perceptions and spousal role in terms of nonacceptance or casual approach to contraceptive use, with a skewed gender bias observed for the female child, compound poor mental health in postnatal tribal women in India and act as barriers for success of these services (Kar et al., 2024).

The concept of ethnic minorities and the policies that are used for handling perinatal mental health problems in such population were discussed by 24 healthcare professionals (including mental health staff, midwifery, primary care, social care professionals) in a study by Bains and colleagues. Lack of awareness and understanding of perinatal mental illness and service structure was noted interestingly in both patients of ethnic minorities and healthcare professionals treating them (Bains et al., 2023).

3 Psychological Effects Related to Unintended Pregnancies and Contraception Among Marginalised Women in South Asia

The marginalised women are at heightened risk of unintended pregnancies, closely spaced childbirths, complications from unsafe pregnancies, and increased maternal mortality rates. These women are also more vulnerable to sexual violence, exploitation, and abuse, thus enhancing their risk of having sexually transmitted diseases (STDs) mandating the need of contraception use in them. Use of contraception has a profound psychological impact on marginalised women of South Asia due to societal stigma, cultural taboos, and gender norms. Contraception use is envisioned as defying traditional roles in patriarchal societies of South Asia as women with a reported expectation to bear multiple children, particularly sons. Thus using contraception results in family disputes, shame, guilt, fear of judgement, and ostracisation. Often they have to use contraception secretly leading to constant fear and anxiety. Studies on Rohingya women in refugee camps have shown that they face verbal and physical violence and even marriage dissolution for using contraception against the will of husbands or in-laws, further deteriorating their mental health. Additionally, fear of side effects, permanent infertility, birth defects, and anomalies owing to lack of knowledge and misperceptions limit the use of contraceptives among these women. Use of hormonal contraceptives associated with irregular and improper usage among these populations leads to increased side effects including weight gain, body aches, and irregular and prolonged bleeding, hampering their mental health. Thus the fear of social and health repercussions imposes a continuous psychological burden on these women (Islam & Habib, 2024). While some women face challenges in accessing contraception, forced or coerced sterilisation or incentivised sterilisation is also practiced in regions of South Asia among targeted women including ethnic and racial minorities and poor and lower caste women mostly without proper consent. Thus, by violating human rights, it compromises with individual autonomy and enhances systemic discrimination (Hardee et al., 2014; Wilson, 2018). There are even reports of deaths following forced sterilisation, thus bringing into light the poor unhygienic quality of operative and post-operative care provided to the marginalised women during forced sterilisation. These malpractices can lead to depression, fear, and emotional distress in these women. Along the years, increased usage of contraception among these women has been instrumental in alleviating their anxiety related to childbirth and conferring them with a sense of reproductive autonomy and social empowerment. The situation is similar for medical termination of pregnancy (MTP). It is deeply intertwined with societal stigma, misperceptions, cultural beliefs, accessibility, and lack of proper care. Although it has been legalised in some countries like India and Nepal, it is still considered illegal and sin among the majority of these communities in some places in South Asia. Additionally, studies have shown that marginalised women face challenges in accessing abortion services from public-funded institutions including long delays, repeated visits, and denial, further accentuating their socio-economic hardships (Sunil, 2022). Rather risky self-managed abortions still seem to be a common practice among marginalised women. Thus, the decision of MTP is faced with fear of judgement, guilt, and shame. Often financial constraints force them to adopt unsafe means leading to anxiety, panic attacks, and fear of complications and infertility. Increased risk of sexual assault makes them more vulnerable to forced or unsafe abortions with increased probability of developing depression or post-traumatic stress disorder. Limited reproductive autonomy among these women often leads to forced abortion, thus leaving them with a sense of helplessness and despair.

4 Menarche and Mental Health Issues Among Marginalised Women in South Asia

The journey starts from menstruation. It is faced with numerous challenges owing to its attached stigma including restrictions on bathing, mobility, religious activities, untouchability, and using unhygienic practices during this time. Studies revealed inadequate knowledge and misinformation regarding menstruation thus inviting it as a shock coupled with shame, embarrassment, fear, and guilt (McCammon et al., 2020; Mahon & Fernandes, 2010). Physical illness related to unhygienic practices can also lead to profound psychological stress among these population.

The mental health issues surrounding menarche start with the lack of awareness on menstruation among girls, especially those in marginalised communities. There have been various reports of girls being unaware of menstruation up to and until menarche, and this number is as high as 48.67% in marginalised communities (Kumari et al., 2021). The menstrual health management challenges of different marginalised communities are fundamentally "period poverty" leading to lack of adequate period care products, lack of water sanitation and hygiene (WASH) facilities or safe sanitation facilities, taboos regarding menstruation, negative views on menstruation, and lack of medical assistance in girls who need medical care for problems related to menarche and menstruation. The myths around menstruation, the concept of being impure during menstruation, isolation, not gaining access to clean water due to taboo, restriction of movement, etc., are found to have a negative impact on the mental health of girls (Maiti & Samantaray, 2020) (Sharma & Thakur, 2019). These problems have aggravated effect when combined with period poverty, restrictions to attend school, school dropout, and lack of education. The stigma surrounding menstruation can lead to various psychological problems like frustration, anxiety, depression, etc. Early menarche could be an important factor affecting the mental health of girls. It has particularly been noted that girls are more likely to drop out of school after menarche if they belong to those castes with restrictive gender norms in India. The gender-specific social norms and concerns for safety of the girls are amplified after menarche (Khanna, 2019).

Challenges and barriers are more in transgender and gender-diverse (TGD) menstruators, that is, the individuals assigned female at birth, who retain the capacity to menstruate and have a gender identity that differs from their sex at birth. The considerations around the reproductive health and reproductive mental health of transgender individuals are described by Arshed et al. as follows: social stigma around menstruation in transgenders, access to period care products, lack of inclusive sanitary facilities, the consensus and policy on gender affirmation, menstrual suppression, hysterectomy and fertility preservation, inclusive pregnancy care, etc. (Arshed et al., 2024).

5 Menopause and Mental Health Issues of Marginalised Women in South Asia

Awareness about menopause and its varied presentations is low among women of deprived background and in marginalised societies. Qualitative analysis reports many women being aware of changes in their body but unaware of the cause and services available for the same. Timing of menopause also varies across population. In India, the mean menopausal age varies from 43.7 years among the Ahom of Assam to 54.6 years among the Hindu Harijans of Punjab with the country average being 46.7 years. And in the tribal women, it varies from 43 years among Kamar women of Chhattisgarh, 46.63 years among Iruliga women of Karnataka, to 51.33 years among Nagas of Nagaland (Dakshayani et al., 2007). Ethnic minority women usually hesitate to seek professional medical help and try to help themselves through various natural and complementary interventions, like taking natural supplements, herbal products, traditional medicine, etc., with the incorporation of lifestyle changes and getting support from family. But that will be insufficient in some cases when menopause is associated with various psychiatric symptoms like anxiety, depression, insomnia, sexual dysfunction, vasomotor symptoms, and cognitive decline along with physical risk of higher incidence of cardiovascular disease such as metabolic syndrome, insulin resistance and diabetes, central obesity, hypertension, and mental morbidity as well (Prasad, 2023). Pooled prevalence of depression in perimenopausal and postmenopausal women was 42.47% in India (Yadav et al., 2021). Literature on specific concerns of different minority groups and marginalised women around menopause transition and the mental health outcomes is scarce in South Asian countries. It is to be noted that mental health issues around aging and menopause are less researched even in the general population in these countries.

6 Suicide and Suicidality Risk of Marginalised Women in South Asia

Though the exact statistics of the distribution of suicide deaths across the reproductive period of the women are not available, the overall high rates of suicidality in this age group anyways point to the vulnerability to suicide. Women's vulnerability to suicide in the region is deeply influenced by sociocultural factors, including early marriage and dowry (bride price) pressures, expectations to bear children and associated societal demands, and gender-based violence, including domestic abuse (Vijayakumar, 2015).

The risk factors vary across countries, highlighting the compounding effects of gender inequalities. For example, in Nepal, the female suicide rate is 20 per 100,000, making it the third leading cause of death among women. In this scenario, the heightened vulnerability has been found to be linked to factors like limited personal agency and decision-making power, low levels of education, early marriage and restrictive patriarchal norms, and limited freedom of movement, self-expression, and life choices (Marahatta et al., 2017).

6.1 Sexual Minorities

Majority of research exploring sexual minority status (persons who self-identify as lesbian, gay, bisexual, transgender, queer/questioning, and intersex, i.e. LGBTQI+) and suicidal risk has been mostly done in high-income countries. The extent of social, economic, and legal barriers faced by this group makes it challenging for them to overcome those barriers in South Asia which majorly consists of low- and middle-income countries. Such sustained discrimination can trigger suicidality but needs to be explored specifically (Vijayakumar et al., 2021). Study in gender minorities in Nepal has highlighted that perceived discrimination acts as an independent risk factor for suicidal ideation in this population (Thapaliya et al., 2018).

6.2 Tribal

In the Idu Mishmi tribe of Arunachal Pradesh, suicide attempt rate was 14.22%, which was higher than the urban population in general, and females were at higher risk. Depression, anxiety syndrome, alcohol abuse, and eating disorder like binge eating and bulimia nervosa were recorded as risk factors for suicide in this tribe (Singh et al., 2013).

6.3 Refugee

A substantial proportion of refugees and forcibly displaced populations have been settling in low- and middle-income countries (LMICs) in South Asia, but assessing and addressing suicide and mental health concerns in these low-resource settings present several challenges, including limited availability of mental health professionals, leading to gaps in care compounded by low rates of help-seeking behaviour in this group pf women due to stigma, cultural beliefs, or lack of awareness.

According to social integration theory, the sense of isolation, weakened social ties, and displacement-related tensions are deeply distressing and can contribute to higher suicide rates among refugee populations (Vijayakumar et al., 2021). However, research on suicide risk and prevention in refugee populations remains limited compared to other high-risk groups.

In a study, suicide attempts were found in 6.1% of the Sri Lankan refugees staying in South India, majority being women (Vijayakumar, 2017). There were more number of suicidal attempts among women than men in a Bhutanese refugee population in a settlement in Eastern Nepal, the presence of gender-based violence (GBV) among the refugees being a significant risk factor for both suicidal attempts and completion (Thapaliya et al., 2018). Overall women of ethnic minority are at increased risk of suicidality due to vulnerability factors like social roles, cultural identity, and low educational level with maintaining factors like acculturation stress and lack of social support or help-seeking or appropriate services along with precipitating factors like interpersonal issues, marital conflict, and domestic violence (Khan & Waheed, 2009).

6.4 Female Sex Workers (FSW)

Female sex workers (FSWs) are among the most vulnerable population groups anywhere in the world. Among the reported deaths, maternity-related complications and suicide contribute to more than half of the deaths. A meta-analysis of FSWs in LMICs including South Asian countries estimated a pooled prevalence of suicidal ideation of 22.8% (past year) and 25% (lifetime). The range of suicide attempt rates was wide (2.6–44.2%). However, specific data on suicide as a cause of death among FSWs remains limited. The authors tried using the community knowledge approach to determine cause-specific deaths and get new insights into suicide-related mortality among FSWs in LMICs. Around 14% of reported FSW deaths were attributed to suicide, with nearly two-thirds of these suicides being maternal suicides. Another critical finding of this study was that the majority of maternal suicides occurred during the prenatal period, highlighting a critical need for targeted mental health interventions during pregnancy (Macias-Konstantopoulos et al., 2024).

A study of suicidal behaviour prevalence and its associated factors among female sex workers in Goa, India, revealed that in the past 3 months suicidal ideation was present in 34.9%, suicide planning in 25.6%, and suicide attempts in 18.7% of women. About 41% of attempters were less than 20 years old. Both structural factors like gender inequality and the context of sex work and individual factors like poor mental health were independently associated with the suicidal behaviours (Shahmanesh et al., 2009).

7 Substance Use of Marginalised Women in South Asia

Challenges, barriers to help seeking, and the differential needs of women with substance use highlight that socio-economic status and poverty are very important reasons behind poor help seeking among women with substance use disorders. Women being an overall marginalised population, poverty in women adds to this and hence needs more public health interventions for balancing the inequalities in delivery of de-addiction services to this population (Motyka et al., 2022).

7.1 Sexual Minorities

Substance use in gender minorities is a complex interplay of stressors, social isolation, stigma, peer pressure, psychological vulnerability, and minority stress. Newer problems of chemsex and growing issue of sexually transmitted infections (STIs) and novel drugs add to the burden of disease. Various studies have concluded that bisexuals and sexual minorities have higher prevalence of substance use disorders. There is a report of about 33.9% using alcohol frequently and 11.5% using illicit substances, among 4607 trans women in India. The authors also emphasise on the need for identifying the syndemic of substance use, HIV, and sexual violence for devising better public health strategies for the same (Chakrapani et al., 2022).

7.2 *Tribal*

The extent of substance use, especially alcohol and tobacco among tribal women, is a problem that requires more research and mitigation strategies as studies show prevalence as high as 38% among communities in Northeast India, where alcohol use is ceremonial. In tribal population of Rajasthan, the prevalence of opium use was more in women, and socio-economic factors such as occupation, education, and marital status were associated with opium use. Prevalence of alcohol use has been reported to be higher in females, probably due to increased access to home-made rice brew generally prepared by tribal women in Arunachal Pradesh. A household survey from Changlang district of Arunachal Pradesh revealed that there was a strong association between opium use and age, occupation, marital status, religion, and ethnicity among both sexes of STs, particularly among Singhpho and Khamti (Chaturvedi et al., 2016).

7.3 *Refugee and Displaced Population*

As mentioned in the World Drug Report 2023, the refugee and displaced population face a higher risk of substance use and substance use disorders compared to the general population. This heightened vulnerability is driven by several factors, like increased exposure to risk factors of family disruption and separation, chronic stress due to displacement, uncertainty, trauma, and limited access to mental health support and coping resources. Also, with the absence of protective factors such as family monitoring, stable and safe living environments, and social and community support networks, the combination of these factors amplifies the risk of substance use. But studies focusing on substance use in the female migrant population in South Asia are specifically lacking.

7.4 *Female Sex Workers (FSWs)*

Substance use as a means to alleviate stress or due to other reasons is seen in this vulnerable group of FSWs. In a study of alcohol-using female sex workers, majority (74%) were using tobacco, 14% were using opioids, and 12% were on cannabis and cocaine. Comorbid depression was present in 71% of women, while 42% had comorbid anxiety disorder. They had physical comorbidity also in measure of 22% suffering from sexually transmitted diseases and 2% suffering from HIV (Pandiyan et al., 2012).

8 Current Status of Services, Policies, and Resources Among Marginalised Women of South Asia

In South Asia, reproductive mental health policies are often integrated within broader reproductive health and mental health frameworks, with varying degrees of emphasis across different countries. While specific policies exclusively targeting reproductive mental health may be limited, several initiatives and programmes address aspects of this intersection. India has several programmes catering to the welfare of females in the reproductive age groups, such as the National Mental Health Programme (NMHP) and the Reproductive and Child Health (RCH) Programme, which aim to address mental health and reproductive health, respectively. In all the policies, strategies, programmes, and laws, the primary focus lies on physical health during the perinatal period to reduce adverse maternal and newborn and child outcomes and barely considers mental health. Counselling programmes recommended under the maternity program are specific to unintended, unwanted, or mistimed pregnancy, contraception, and family planning rather than to maternal mental health needs. Recent efforts include promoting the linkages with psychiatry departments of tertiary institutes or medical colleges for staff training and professional support as a part of community-based treatment and care programmes. Efforts have been made to integrate successful national health policies into reproductive healthcare, focusing on perinatal mental health and the psychological well-being of women. State-based initiatives like Amma Manasu (Mother's Mind) in Kerala and Thayi Card in Karnataka for integrating mental health into routine maternity care provide local examples of feasibility to address this critical gap in public health. The government's National Health Mission has also started discussing ways of integrating perinatal mental health into existing mother and child programmes. Experts have proposed several policy options to enhance maternal mental health services within the existing programmes, such as strengthening and including a "maternal" component in the National Mental Health Programme (NMHP) or integrating mental health into Reproductive, Maternal, Newborn, Child, and Adolescent Health (RMNCH+A) (Priyadarshini et al., 2023). However, challenges persist in seamless integration and implementation, especially in catering to marginalised women. Overall, South Asian countries have different population policies aiming to reduce maternal mortality. But issues in implementation of services to the otherwise difficult to reach women of marginalised community in the background of differential policies to manage maternal health, like restrictive abortion laws, pose unique challenges to women's reproductive health in this group, potentially impacting their mental health due to stress and consequences of unintended pregnancies. There is a need for a comprehensive approach to develop policies to address perinatal mental health needs, considering the high disease burden and several sociocultural barriers amplified in marginalised women.

In South Asia, specialised perinatal mental health services are notably scarce even though LMICs have high birth rates and post-partum psychiatric disorders requiring specialised services during this period. India has initiated some efforts, such as establishing perinatal psychiatry services with dedicated inpatient or outpatient perinatal psychiatry service in tertiary care centres. The concept of mother-baby unit (MBU) offering inpatient psychiatric care, allowing joint admission of mothers and their infants up to 2 years old with provision of liaison services with obstetricians, neurologists, and paediatricians, is helpful in addressing the mental health needs of pregnant and post-partum women, emphasising mother-infant bonding and providing psychotherapy and education on mental health conditions (Chandra et al., 2015). While some tertiary care hospitals may offer such perinatal mental health services, the integration of mental healthcare into routine maternal health services remains largely limited leading to poor utilisation by the marginalised women.

In Bangladesh and Pakistan, research highlights a significant gap in addressing psychological and sociocultural challenges faced by couples during the perinatal period, emphasising the need for culturally sensitive mental health interventions (Insan et al., 2022; Shafiq, 2024). However, this structured perinatal mental health service remains underdeveloped, and mental healthcare is often integrated into general maternal health services without a specialised focus on the couple. Across the regions, limited resources, societal stigma, shortage of trained professionals, and limited resources allocated for these marginalised populations remain barriers to accessing reproductive mental health care. The South Asian Marcé Association (SAMA), founded in 2023, is an organisation of trained professionals who aim to address these challenges by promoting interdisciplinary interventions tailored to South Asia's socio-economic and cultural contexts..

9 Available Research and Gaps

9.1 Psychological Impact of Reproductive Issues

Although the prevalence of mental illness in those suffering from infertility is less documented, it is similar to those associated with other serious medical conditions. Lower socio-economic status (SES) can significantly impact mental health in individuals facing infertility. Global studies suggest that individuals with lower SES often experience higher levels of stress, anxiety, and depression due to limited access to healthcare, financial constraints, and societal pressures (Bagade et al., 2023). However, there are limited studies from Southern Asia evaluating the related social determinants. In the South Asian context, the ability to conceive is frequently equated with a woman's worth and a family's honour, leading to immense stigma and emotional distress for those facing fertility challenges. Women, in particular, may experience blame, isolation, or even rejection, adding to the already present sociocultural difficulties due to marginalisation (Niaz & Hassan, 2006).

9.2 Perinatal Mental Health

Perinatal psychiatry in South Asian countries has garnered increasing attention, leading to a range of studies that explore the prevalence, risk factors, and interventions associated with perinatal mental health disorders. A systematic review of the prevalence of common perinatal mental disorders in women in LMICs resulted in a weighted mean prevalence of 15.6% antenatally and 19.8% postnatally, with an essential risk factor being socio-economic disadvantage (Fisher et al., 2012). Thirty-eight studies involving 20,043 women yielded perinatal depression of 22% in India (Upadhyay et al., 2017). Prevalence of common antenatal mental disorders was found to be up to 21.87%, associated with several sociocultural determinants derived from metanalysis of 27 studies involving 7780 women (Kalra et al., 2021). In Bangladesh the prevalence of perinatal depression lies between 10% and 39%. Several region-specific clinical and psychosocial characteristics associated with perinatal psychiatric illness have been identified. A study found depression rates ranging from 9.8% to 36.7% and anxiety up to 55.7% in pregnant women and emphasised the necessity of integrating mental health services into routine prenatal care to address these challenges effectively (Choedon et al., 2023; Arafat & Rajkumar, 2024).

There is a dearth of research data covering the geographically and culturally marginalised groups. Other than prevalence studies, several studies were carried out to develop effective treatment strategies for perinatal mental illness. In South Asia, the development of perinatal psychiatry scales tailored to the region's unique socio-cultural context is limited. Researchers have primarily focused on adapting and validating existing tools to ensure their relevance and effectiveness for South Asian populations. Although several attempts were made to develop and validate culture-specific approaches related to mental health assessments, most of the studies have validated the Edinburgh Postnatal Depression Scale (EPDS) in identifying perinatal depression, especially in the Indian setting (Fellmeth et al., 2021a, 2021b). The NIMHANS Maternal Behaviour Scale (NIMBUS) and Developmental Assessment Scale for Indian Infants are other assessment tools in perinatal psychiatry developed in India and applicable in LMIC or South Asian contexts. Other than pharmacotherapeutic strategies, psychotherapeutic strategies were modified to enhance their feasibility and accessibility, especially for marginalised sections. One study has ascertained the feasibility of a mobile-based interactive voice response system (IVRS) for preventing and managing perinatal depression in a rural district of Bihar, India (Seshu et al., 2021). A module for brief psychological intervention for postpartum depression (BIND-P) has been developed to effectively screen and widen the coverage of healthcare services among the isolated population (Ransing et al., 2021). Initially tested in four regions of India, this model is now being adopted in other countries, including Nepal, Thailand, and Tunisia, reflecting its potential for broader applicability. The Maternal and Perinatal Health Research Collaboration India (MaatHRI) is a collaboration between the National Perinatal Epidemiology Unit (NPEU), the University of Oxford, and 15 hospitals across 5 states in India to address the evidence gaps of perinatal psychiatry in India, facilitate diagnosis, and be better positioned to offer appropriate support and treatment to women with special emphasis on the rural and marginalised population groups (Fellmeth et al., 2021a, 2021b). The SMARThealth Pregnancy and Mental Health (PRAMH) study is a situational analysis to understand mental health problems during pregnancy and in the first year following birth with an intention to develop an implementation framework for future interventions especially in rural India which has already been implemented in several HIC countries (Votruba et al., 2023).

The mental health issues of single mothers are influenced by various factors like lack of support, traumatic past life, and ongoing physical morbidity along with unemployment and poverty. It is widely accepted that single mothers are mostly marginalised with systematic exclusion from mainstream health policies too, but specific evidence from South Asian countries is particularly lacking in this regard. There is also less research from South Asian countries in the area of problems faced by parents in same-sex marriages, adoption in same-sex marriages, and their mental health implications. With increasing numbers of single mothers all over the world and specifically in South Asia, there is a pressing need for bootstrapping mental health services designed for them.

10 Challenges and the Way Forward

Despite the aforementioned initiatives, research on reproductive mental health in South Asia has identified several critical gaps that need to be addressed to improve outcomes for women (Fellmeth et al., 2021a, 2021b).

1. Limited validation of screening tools since mental health screening instruments used in South Asia are adapted from other cultures without proper validation for local contexts
2. Underrepresentation of diverse populations since research often overlooks rural, low-income, and marginalised communities, despite these groups being at higher risk for perinatal mental health issues due to factors such as socio-economic deprivation, intimate partner violence, and traditional confinement practices after childbirth
3. Insufficient focus on certain disorders
   While depression during the perinatal period has been extensively studied, other mental illnesses like anxiety disorders, substance use disorder, and post-traumatic stress disorder (PTSD) remain under-researched. Given the high prevalence of somatoform disorders as a common expression of emotional distress among women in South Asia, it has not been sufficiently studied among pregnant or postpartum marginalised women.
4. Lack of longitudinal studies
   Most existing studies are cross-sectional, providing limited insight into the progression and long-term effects of perinatal mental health disorders.

5. Stigma and awareness
   The stigma surrounding mental health remains a substantial barrier, preventing many women, especially those from marginalised background, from seeking help. Strategies to assess and address stigma specific to perinatal mental health need further research and understanding.

   Perinatal mental health services need to be a stepped approach with predetermined multiple approachable care pathways taking into account the varying sociocultural disparities between the regions and the barriers and facilitators to accessing mental health services for maternal mental health problems. Capacity building of healthcare providers is essential to sensitise and train in perinatal mental health, especially to screen out at-risk patients from marginalised background. In both the public and private sectors, primary care nurses, midwives, and doctors require separate training to provide suitable and evidence-based interventions in order to establish appropriate care pathways for women screening positive for mental health issues. There is a pressing need for the development and integration of dedicated perinatal mental health services within the existing healthcare infrastructure to better support mothers and families in the region. Separate mother and baby psychiatric units in district and teaching hospitals, which are low resource and designed to meet cultural needs, require further development (Ganjekar et al., 2019). Integration of maternal mental health in maternity and mental health policies to address unmet perinatal mental health needs of women needs to be a top priority in South Asian countries. Deciphering and addressing the challenges in providing specialised mental health care in geographically, economically, and socioculturally marginalised populations seem like a distant goal at present. However, such targets need to be achieved in order to ensure effective implementation of all the reforms in policies and advancement in treatment strategies.

11 Conclusion

Reproductive mental health in marginalised women in South Asia is an area with immediate need for rigorous research and policy implementations with effects that will reach far and wide. To be able to have inclusive care and tailor-made accessible mental healthcare for these women, there needs to be collaborative efforts from various segments of the society including the state and active public participation. Mental health problems around menarche, childbirth, and menopause in women of marginalised sections of the society need to be addressed with an approach sensitive to their needs and vulnerabilities, paying attention to the various unique problems that they face in these phases of life.

References

Arafat, S. M. Y., & Rajkumar, R. P. (2024). Mental disorders during pregnancy and postpartum in Bangladesh: A narrative review. *Health Science Reports, 7*(9), e70027. https://doi.org/10.1002/hsr2.70027

Arshed, A., Madanes, S., Pottinger, S., Ackerman, M. G., & Deutch, A. B. (2024). Menstrual management in transgender and gender diverse individuals: Psychiatric and psychosocial considerations. *Frontiers in Psychiatry, 15*, 1422333. https://doi.org/10.3389/fpsyt.2024.1422333

Bagade, T., Mersha, A. G., & Majeed, T. (2023). The social determinants of mental health disorders among women with infertility: A systematic review. *BMC Women's Health, 23*(1), 668. https://doi.org/10.1186/s12905-023-02828-9

Bains, K., Bicknell, S., Jovanović, N., et al. (2023). Healthcare professionals' views on the accessibility and acceptability of perinatal mental health services for South Asian and Black women: A qualitative study. *BMC Medicine, 21*, 370. https://doi.org/10.1186/s12916-023-02978-5

Black, M. M., Baqui, A. H., Zaman, K., McNary, S. W., Le, K., Arifeen, S. E., Hamadani, J. D., Parveen, M., Yunus, M. D., & Black, R. E. (2007). Depressive symptoms among rural Bangladeshi mothers: Implications for infant development. *Journal of Child Psychology and Psychiatry, and Allied Disciplines, 48*(8), 764–772.

Chakrapani, V., Lakshmi, P. V. M., Newman, P. A., Kaur, J., Tsai, A. C., Vijin, P. P., et al. (2022). Syndemic violence victimization, alcohol and drug use, and HIV transmission risk behavior among HIV-negative transgender women in India: A cross-sectional, population-based study. *PLOS Glob Public Health, 2*(10), e0000437. https://doi.org/10.1371/journal.pgph.0000437

Chandra, P. S., Desai, G., Reddy, D., Thippeswamy, H., & Saraf, G. (2015). The establishment of a mother-baby inpatient psychiatry unit in India: Adaptation of a Western model to meet local cultural and resource needs. *Indian Journal of Psychiatry, 57*(3), 290–294. https://doi.org/10.4103/0019-5545.166621

Chaturvedi, H. K., Bajpai, R. C., & Pandey, A. (2016). Predictors of substance use in the tribal population of Northeast India: Retrospective analysis of a cross-sectional survey. *Journal of Addiction Research and Therapy, 7*, 295. https://doi.org/10.4172/2155-6105.1000295

Choedon, T., Sethi, V., Killeen, S. L., Ganjekar, S., Satyanarayana, V., Ghosh, S., et al. (2023). Integrating nutrition and mental health screening, risk identification and management in prenatal health programs in India. *International Journal of Gynecology & Obstetrics, 162*(3), 792–801. https://doi.org/10.1002/ijgo.14728

Dakshayani, B., Chandran, M. S., & Gangadhar, M. R. (2007). Menarche and menopause among the Iruliga tribal women. *The Anthropologist., 9*(3), 255–256.

Fellmeth, G., Fazel, M., & Plugge, E. (2017). Migration and perinatal mental health in women from low- and middle-income countries: A systematic review and meta-analysis. *BJOG: An International Journal of Obstetrics and Gynaecology, 124*(5), 742–752. https://doi.org/10.1111/1471-0528.14184

Fellmeth, G., Harrison, S., Opondo, C., Nair, M., Kurinczuk, J. J., & Alderdice, F. (2021a). Validated screening tools to identify common mental disorders in perinatal and postpartum women in India: A systematic review and meta-analysis. *BMC Psychiatry, 21*(1), 200. https://doi.org/10.1186/s12888-021-03190-6

Fellmeth, G., Kishore, M. T., Verma, A., Desai, G., Bharti, O., Kanwar, P., et al. (2021b). Perinatal mental health in India: Protocol for a validation and cohort study. *Journal of Public Health (Oxford, England), 43*(Suppl 2), ii35–ii42.

Fisher, J., Mello, M. C., Patel, V., Rahman, A., Tran, T., Holton, S., & Holmes, W. (2012). Prevalence and determinants of common perinatal mental disorders in women in low-and lower-middle-income countries: A systematic review. *Bulletin of the World Health Organization, 90*, 139–149. https://doi.org/10.2471/BLT.11.091850

Ganjekar, S., Thekkethayyil, A. V., & Chandra, P. S. (2019). Perinatal mental health around the world: Priorities for research and service development in India. *BJPsych International, 17*(1), 2–5.

Hardee, K., Harris, S., Rodriguez, M., Kumar, J., Bakamjian, L., Newman, K., & Brown, W. (2014). Achieving the goal of the London Summit on Family Planning by adhering to voluntary, rights-based family planning: What can we learn from past experiences with coercion? *International Perspectives on Sexual and Reproductive Health, 40*(4), 206–214. https://doi.org/10.1363/4020614

Heslehurst, N., Brown, H., Pemu, A., Coleman, H., & Rankin, J. (2018). Perinatal health outcomes and care among asylum seekers and refugees: A systematic review of systematic reviews. *BMC Medicine, 16*, 89. https://doi.org/10.1186/s12916-018-1064-0

Huda, S. (2006). Sex trafficking in South Asia. *International Journal of Gynecology & Obstetrics, 94*, 374–381. https://doi.org/10.1016/j.ijgo.2006.04.027

Insan, N., Weke, A., Rankin, J., & Forrest, S. (2022). Perceptions and attitudes around perinatal mental health in Bangladesh, India and Pakistan: A systematic review of qualitative data. *BMC Pregnancy and Childbirth, 22*(1), 293. https://doi.org/10.1186/s12884-022-04642-x

Islam, M., & Habib, S. E. (2024). "I don't want my marriage to end": A qualitative investigation of the sociocultural factors influencing contraceptive use among married Rohingya women residing in refugee camps in Bangladesh. *Reproductive Health, 21*(1), 32. https://doi.org/10.1186/s12978-024-01763-8

Kalra, H., Tran, T. D., Romero, L., Chandra, P., & Fisher, J. (2021). Prevalence and determinants of antenatal common mental disorders among women in India: A systematic review and meta-analysis. *Archives of Women's Mental Health, 24*(1), 29–53.

Kar, S., Samantaray, P. C., Patnaik, L., Mishra, A., & Lakshmi, P. (2024). Family and facility care variables attributing to postnatal depression among women in two tribal-dominated districts of Odisha: Log model analysis to suggest intervention. *Journal of Family Medicine and Primary Care, 13*(3), 958–963. https://doi.org/10.4103/jfmpc.jfmpc_1367_23

Khan, F., & Waheed, W. (2009). Suicide and self-harm in South Asian immigrants. *Psychiatry, 8*(7), 261–264.

Khanna, M. (2019). The precocious period: The impact of early menarche on schooling in India. *SSRN Electronic Journal*. https://doi.org/10.2139/ssrn.3419041

Klainin, P., & Arthur, D. G. (2009). Postpartum depression in Asian cultures: A literature review. *International Journal of Nursing Studies, 46*(10), 1355–1373. https://doi.org/10.1016/j.ijnurstu.2009.02.012

Kumari, S., Sood, S., Davis, S., & Chaudhury, S. (2021). Knowledge and practices related to menstruation among tribal adolescent girls. *Industrial Psychiatry Journal, 30*(Suppl 1), S160–S165. https://doi.org/10.4103/0972-6748.328808

Macias-Konstantopoulos, W. L., Willis, B., Weerasinghe, S., Perttu, E., & Bennett, I. M. (2024). Suicide during pregnancy as a major contributor to maternal suicide among female sex workers in eight low-and middle-income countries: A community knowledge approach investigation. *Cambridge Prisms: Global Mental Health, 11*, e107.

Mahon, T., & Fernandes, M. (2010). Menstrual hygiene in South Asia: A neglected issue for WASH (water, sanitation and hygiene) programmes. *Gender and Development, 18*(1), 99–113. https://doi.org/10.1080/13552071003600083

Maiti, A., & Samantaray, S. (2020). Menstrual hygiene practices among tribal adolescent girls in Odisha, India. *Journal of Preventive and Curative Medicine*. https://www.jptcp.com/index.php/jptcp/article/view/4014

Marahatta, K., Samuel, R., Sharma, P., Dixit, L., & Shrestha, B. R. (2017). Suicide burden and prevention in Nepal: The need for a national strategy. *WHO South-East Asia Journal of Public Health, 6*(1), 45–49.

McCammon, E., Bansal, S., Hebert, L. E., Yan, S., Menendez, A., & Gilliam, M. (2020). Exploring young women's menstruation-related challenges in Uttar Pradesh, India, using the socio-ecological framework. *Sexual and Reproductive Health Matters, 28*(1), 1749342. https://doi.org/10.1080/26410397.2020.1749342

Motyka, M. A., Al-Imam, A., Haligowska, A., & Michalak, M. (2022). Helping women suffering from drug addiction: Needs, barriers, and challenges. *International Journal of Environmental Research and Public Health, 19*(21), 14039. https://doi.org/10.3390/ijerph192114039

Niaz, U., & Hassan, S. (2006). Culture and mental health of women in South-East Asia. *World Psychiatry, 5*(2), 118.

Pandiyan, K., Chandrasekhar, H., & Madhusudhan, S. (2012). Psychological morbidity among female commercial sex workers with alcohol and drug abuse. *Indian Journal of Psychiatry, 54*(4), 349–351.

Prasad, S. (2023). Menopause in ethnic minority women. *Post Reproductive Health, 29*(4), 236–239. https://doi.org/10.1177/20533691231186562

Priyadarshini, U., Rao, A. P., & Dash, S. (2023). Recommendations for maternal mental health policy in India. *Journal of Public Health Policy, 44*(1), 90–101.

Ransing, R., Kukreti, P., Raghuveer, P., Mahadevaiah, M., Puri, M., Pemde, H., et al. (2021). Development of a brief psychological intervention for perinatal depression (BIND-P). *Asia-Pacific Psychiatry, 13*(1), e12436.

Seshu, U., Khan, H. A., Bhardwaj, M., Sangeetha, C., Aarthi, G., John, S., et al. (2021). A qualitative study on the use of mobile-based intervention for perinatal depression among perinatal mothers in rural Bihar, India. *International Journal of Social Psychiatry, 67*(5), 467–471.

Shafiq, S. (2024). An exploration of psychological and socio-cultural facets in perinatal distress of Pakistani couples: A triangulated qualitative study. *BMC Pregnancy and Childbirth, 24*(1), 596.

Shahmanesh, M., Wayal, S., Cowan, F., Mabey, D., Copas, A., & Patel, V. (2009). Suicidal behavior among female sex workers in Goa, India: The silent epidemic. *American Journal of Public Health, 99*(7), 1239–1246.

Sharma, N., & Thakur, K. (2019). Attitudes towards menstruation among Purig tribe adolescents in Jammu and Kashmir, India. *Asian Journal of Health Science*. https://www.i-scholar.in/index.php/Ajhs/article/view/63316

Singh, T., & Kumar, D. (2025). Children under 5-year mortality and the risk of maternal mental illness among India's scheduled tribe. *Indian Journal of Psychiatry, 67*(3), 350–353. https://doi.org/10.4103/indianjpsychiatry.indianjpsychiatry_1136_2

Singh, P. K., Singh, R. K., Biswas, A., & Rao, V. R. (2013). High rate of suicide attempt and associated psychological traits in an isolated tribal population of North-East India. *Journal of Affective Disorders, 151*(2), 673–678.

Sunil, B. (2022). Running an obstacle-course: A qualitative study of women's experiences with abortion-seeking in Tamil Nadu, India. *Sexual and Reproductive Health Matters, 29*(2), 1966218. https://doi.org/10.1080/26410397.2021.1966218

Suwetty, A. M., Astari, A. M., & Wihastuti, T. A. (2019). Mental health of human trafficking; A systematic review. *Research Journal of Life Science, 6*(2), 130–140. https://doi.org/10.21776/ub.rjls.2019.006.02.7

Thapaliya, S., Sharma, P., & Upadhyaya, K. (2018). Suicide and self harm in Nepal: A scoping review. *Asian Journal of Psychiatry, 32*, 20–26.

Upadhyay, R. P., Chowdhury, R., Salehi, A., Sarkar, K., Singh, S. K., Sinha, B., Pawar, A., Rajalakshmi, A. K., & Kumar, A. (2017). Postpartum depression in India: A systematic review and meta-analysis. *Bulletin of the World Health Organization, 95*(10), 706–717. https://doi.org/10.2471/BLT.17.192237

Vijayakumar, L. (2015). Suicide in women. *Indian Journal of Psychiatry, 57*(Suppl 2), S233–S238.

Vijayakumar, L. (2017). Challenges and opportunities in suicide prevention in South-East Asia. *WHO South-East Asia Journal of Public Health, 6*(1), 30–33.

Vijayakumar, L., Ray, S., Fernandes, T. N., & Pathare, S. (2021). A descriptive mapping review of suicide in vulnerable populations in low and middle countries. *Asia-Pacific Psychiatry, 13*(3), e12472.

Votruba, N., Praveen, D., Mellers, L., Rajan, E., Thout, S. R., Arora, V., Malik, Y., Kashyap, A., Majumdar, S., Hirst, J., & Maulik, P. K. (2023). SMARThealth PRegnancy And Mental Health study: protocol for a situational analysis of perinatal mental health in women living in rural India. *Frontiers in global women's health*, 4, 1143880. https://doi.org/10.3389/fgwh.2023.1143880

Wilson, K. (2018). For reproductive justice in an era of Gates and Modi: The violence of India's population policies. *Feminist Review, 119*(1), 89–105. https://doi.org/10.1057/s41305-018-0112-0

World Health Organization. (2020). *Maternal mortality in South Asia: Trends and challenges*. WHO Regional Office for South-East Asia.

Yadav, V., Jain, A., Dabar, D., Goel, A. D., Sood, A., Joshi, A., Agarwal, S. S., Nandeshwar, S. (2021). A meta-analysis on the prevalence of depression in perimenopausal and postmenopausal women in India. *Asian Journal of Psychiatry, 57*, 102581. https://doi.org/10.1016/j.ajp.2021.102581

Chapter 14
Mental Health Challenges Among Single Mothers in South Asia

Rashmi Shukla, Ankita Saroj, Nalin Shukla, and Su Mon Hein

1 Introduction

Motherhood is often portrayed as a journey of love, sacrifice, and fulfilment. However, for single mothers in South Asia, this journey is fraught with unique challenges that significantly impact their mental well-being. In societies with predominantly patriarchal family structures, single mothers often encounter social stigma, economic hardship, and emotional isolation. Unlike in many Western countries, where single parenthood is more accepted and institutionally supported, South Asian societies tend to place an immense burden on women who raise children alone (Dube, 1997).

Mental health remains a stigmatized subject in the region, making it even harder for single mothers to seek help. Many struggle with anxiety, depression, and chronic stress, yet their struggles are often overlooked. Instead of receiving support, they frequently encounter blame, exclusion, and judgment. These challenges, compounded by a lack of institutional support and deeply ingrained cultural norms, create an environment that significantly impacts their psychological well-being (Nahar et al., 2020).

R. Shukla (✉)
Department of Psychiatry, King George's Medical University, Lucknow, Uttar Pradesh, India

A. Saroj
King George's Medical University, Lucknow, Uttar Pradesh, India

N. Shukla
Hind Institute of Medical Sciences, Atarita, Sitapur, Uttar Pradesh, India

S. M. Hein
North East London NHS Foundation Trust, Dagenham, UK

P. Kukreti et al. (eds.), *Women's Reproductive Mental Health in South Asia*, South Asian Perspectives in Mental Health and Psychology,
https://doi.org/10.1007/978-981-96-9219-4_14

Concepts of single motherhood in South Asia are shaped by historical and political contexts that reinforce traditional family structures. Heteronormative ideals position two-parent families as the norm, marginalizing other family models and rendering them socially undesirable. One of the biggest challenges single mothers face is societal attitudes toward them. Single motherhood can result from various circumstances divorce, the death of a spouse, being unmarried, or by choice. A 2019 UN Women study found that there are 4.5 crore single mothers in India (Nigam, 2019a, b). Single mothers frequently receive unsolicited advice from family, neighbors, and even strangers, making it stressful to manage everything alone while still falling short of societal expectations (Dube, 1997). This chapter explores the key factors contributing to the mental health struggles of single mothers in South Asia, highlighting the urgent need for societal and policy-level interventions.

2 Key Factors Contributing to Mental Health Challenges Among Single Mothers

2.1 Stigma and Cultural Expectations

South Asian societies traditionally emphasize the role of women as devoted wives and mothers within a marital unit. When a woman becomes a single mother whether through divorce, separation, or widowhood, she often faces harsh societal judgment. Many communities view single mothers as having "failed" in their marital roles, leading to social exclusion (Nigam, 2024a, b).

Divorced women, in particular, experience heightened scrutiny as marriage is viewed as a lifelong commitment. Widowed mothers, on the other hand, may be expected to live a life of restraint and sacrifice. In some conservative communities, they are discouraged from remarrying or seeking companionship, further isolating them emotionally (Dharani & Balamurugan, 2024). These cultural norms intensify feelings of loneliness, guilt, and shame, contributing to depression and low self-esteem (Nigam, 2024a, b).

2.2 Economic Hardships and Financial Struggles

Financial insecurity is one of the most pressing challenges faced by single mothers in South Asia. Many women rely on their spouses or extended families for economic stability. Following divorce or abandonment, legal systems often fail to enforce alimony or child support, forcing single mothers into low-paying jobs with exploitative conditions (Nigam, 2019a, b). Widowed mothers may depend on other family members for financial survival but face discrimination in inheritance rights.

Economic insecurity leads to chronic stress, anxiety, and vulnerability to mental health issues (Munir et al., 2024).

2.3 *Lack of Emotional and Social Support*

In many South Asian cultures, divorce and single motherhood are heavily stigmatized, often leading to social exclusion. Single mothers may be denied participation in community events, religious gatherings, or even housing opportunities. The absence of social support networks significantly increases their risk of anxiety, chronic stress, and postpartum depression. Many single mothers suppress their emotions for the sake of their children, resulting in emotional exhaustion and burnout (Dharani & Balamurugan, 2024; Nigam, 2024a, b).

2.4 *Parental Pressure and Childcare Burden*

Raising a child alone in a society where parenting is traditionally a shared responsibility is overwhelming. Single mothers often face judgment regarding their ability to raise children without a male figure, leading to self-doubt and heightened anxiety. Balancing work, childcare, and household responsibilities can lead to mental fatigue, self-neglect, and emotional breakdowns, exacerbated by financial constraints and societal expectations (Dharani & Balamurugan, 2024; Nigam, 2019a, b).

2.5 *Legal and Institutional Barriers*

Many South Asian countries' legal systems do not provide sufficient protection or support for single mothers. Custody battles, inheritance disputes, and bureaucratic hurdles make life an uphill battle. For instance, unmarried or divorced mothers may face challenges in obtaining legal guardianship documents, enrolling their children in schools, or accessing healthcare services without a male guardian's consent. The lack of state-sponsored welfare programs further exacerbates financial and emotional distress (Nigam, 2024a, b).

3 Mental Health Issues in Single Mothers

Single mothers in South Asia face disproportionately high rates of mental health disorders (Agnafors et al., 2019). Studies indicate that single mothers have nearly twice the rate of moderate to severe mental health disabilities compared to partnered mothers (Crosier et al., 2007). When considering factors like sociodemographics, household income, financial hardship, and social support, 94% of the link between single motherhood and poor mental health is explained. Financial hardship and social support are the strongest predictors of this association (Crosier et al., 2007).

Bangladesh, India, and Pakistan, which are lower- to middle-income countries (LMICs) in South Asia, share cultural and social similarities despite their differences. These commonalities contribute to similar challenges and social inequalities faced by women in these countries, making them often studied together to better understand health issues in the region (Ahmed & Lemkau, 2000).

3.1 *Depression, Anxiety, and Substance Use*

In recent years, mental health has become a crucial policy issue, with a significant rise in depression among women (Wittchen et al., 2011). Single mothers experience depression at nearly three times the rate of partnered mothers (Targosz et al., 2003). The etiological model of depression in single mother illustrates interaction of childhood and earlier adult experiences through protective and risk factors (Fig. 14.1). The study "Single Mothers, Poverty, and Depression" by George W. Brown and Patricia M. Moran explores the connections between marital status, poverty, and depression among inner-city women (Brown & Moran, 1997).

Furthermore, pregnancy brings significant psychological changes, making women more vulnerable to depression and anxiety. Systematic reviews indicate that perinatal depression is highly prevalent in LMICs, affecting about one in four women during pregnancy and one in five women after childbirth (Gelaye et al., 2016). The prevalence is higher in Bangladesh, India, and Pakistan compared to high-income countries, due to poor understanding and a lack of mental health

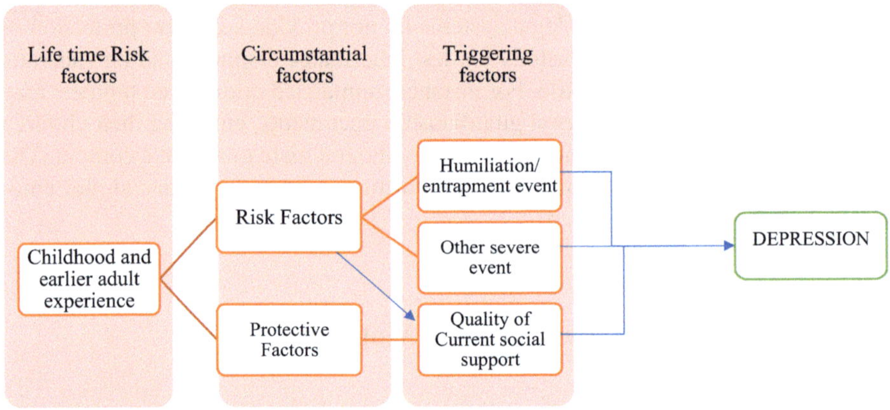

Fig. 14.1 Interaction of various factors in the genesis of depressive symptoms in a single mother (Brown & Moran, 1997)

integration in antenatal care. Additionally, antenatal depression and anxiety are linked to adverse outcomes, including postnatal depression, low birth weight, and impaired fetal development (Gelaye et al., 2016).

The systematic review and meta-analysis identified significant predictors of antenatal depression in Bangladesh, India, and Pakistan, including partner violence, male gender preference, poor relationships with spouse, parents, and unplanned pregnancies. These significant stressors could potentially cause single parenthood. These findings are crucial for developing targeted interventions to prevent and screen for antenatal depression and anxiety in South Asia (Insan et al., 2022).

In addition to mental health issues, substance use among women in South Asia is a growing public health issue. Single mothers, particularly those facing financial hardship and social isolation, may turn to alcohol, opioids, cannabis, solvents, or sedatives as coping mechanisms. The underlying causes include poverty, peer pressure, domestic violence, and restricted access to mental health services (Shozi, 2020).

3.2 Social Isolation, Stress, Caregiving Burden, and Burnout

Single mothers navigate a complex emotional journey, balancing the joys of parenting with the challenges of financial stress and loneliness. Stress factors include low parenting self-efficacy, having at least one child with a disability, low perceived social support, entering a new partnership, and the developmental stage of the youngest child (Sartor et al., 2023). Many single mothers manage household expenses and childcare costs alone, often facing unemployment or part-time work with insufficient income.

The absence of a co-parent can heighten feelings of loneliness and emotional exhaustion. Without shared accountabilities, single mothers take on the full responsibility of childcare, making it difficult to maintain a social life, meet new people, or find time for self-care. Despite progress toward gender equality, societal attitudes often hold single mothers to different standards, resulting in unfair judgment and criticism.

Rani's (2006) research on poor and working-class single mothers in India revealed that those without formal education are often relegated to unskilled jobs. Additionally, patriarchal state policies fail to offer childcare support, reinforcing the stigma against single motherhood (Rani, 2006). Working mothers must arrange childcare, leading to constant anxiety about their children's well-being. Many single mothers experience sleeplessness, restlessness, anxiety, sadness, feelings of unworthiness, aggression, and even suicidal thoughts. Financial difficulties, lack of social support, and increased caregiving demands contribute significantly to their stress (Dor, 2021; Mishra et al., 2021).

3.3 Emotional Trauma from Divorce, Abandonment, or Widowhood

The relationship between divorce and post-traumatic stress disorder (PTSD) is complex. While not every divorce results in PTSD, the significant emotional and psychological turmoil of ending a marriage can lead to trauma. Cross-sectional studies consistently link marital status to life satisfaction, with married individuals reporting higher levels of well-being than those who are divorced. A longitudinal study in Germany found that people adapt to marriage relatively quickly (within about 2 years) but take much longer to adjust to the death of a spouse (around 8 years) (Haring-Hidore et al., 1985; Lucas, 2005).

The death of a partner in later life is generally experienced as the most stressful normative life event. Multiple reviews have found adverse health outcomes for individuals experiencing spousal loss, particularly an increased risk of mortality—a phenomenon known as the widowhood effect (Holm & Severinsson, 2012).

Halter suggested that psychological distress following the loss of a spouse is characterized by two main processes: affective and expressive responses, which include profound sadness, grief, and depression, and evaluative and introspective processes, which involve how the bereaved individual adapts to new circumstances, including self-efficacy, mastery, and self-esteem (Halter, 2014). Kleber's study found that widowed women experience more health problems compared to their married counterparts further highlighting the need for targeted mental health interventions (Kleber, 2019).

4 Impact of Single Parenthood on Children

Single parents often struggle with balancing dual responsibilities while facing social stigma and limited support. This lack of resources and time can make it challenging for them to provide adequate emotional and academic support to their children. Higher stress levels among single mothers are often attributed to childhood behavioral problems, chronic illnesses, or disabilities of their children (Table 14.1). For instance, 35% of single parents report problems with their children, compared to 25% of parents in two-parent families (Hatzmann et al., 2014). Consequently, children raised in such households may experience academic challenges, reduced social interactions, and increased risk of emotional or behavioral issues (Fig. 14.2).

However, research suggests that resilience-building strategies, strong parental bonding, and community support can mitigate these challenges, leading to positive long-term outcomes. Globally, about 6.8% of children live in single-parent households, with India reporting a rate of 5% (Kramer et al., 2019; Chavda & Nisarga, 2023). A Swedish study found that children from single-parent households have higher likelihood of developing mental health conditions such as anxiety, depression, and substance use disorders. Economic difficulties, negative parenting

Table 14.1 The impacts of single parenting on children across various age groups (Chavda & Nisarga, 2023)

Age group	Impact
Neonatal outcomes (0 < 28 days)	Higher risk of low birth weight, preterm birth, and neonatal intensive care admission due to socioeconomic factors and maternal health behaviors
Infants and toddlers (0–3 years)	Distress through irritability, poor sleep, separation anxiety, and developmental regression
Young children (2–6 years)	Feel fearful and abandoned during parental separation but adapt quickly
Children (7–12 years)	Better at expressing emotions and accepting parental separation but may face social and emotional problems
Adolescents (12–17 years)	Struggle the most with parental divorce, showing difficulties in emotional expression and higher risks of abandoning home

behaviors, and exposure to stressful life events were identified as major contributing factors (Goodrum et al., 2012; Weitoft et al., 2003).

Additionally, low socioeconomic status (SES) is associated with both early and single motherhood. Researchers have noted that structural inequalities persist across generations, increasing the risk of mental health challenges for both mothers and their children (Bradley & Corwyn, 2002). A study conducted in Pakistan found that women experiencing antepartum depression were nearly twice as likely to give birth to low birth weight infants compared to nondepressed mothers, further emphasizing the impact of maternal mental health on child outcomes (Rahman et al., 2007).

5 Role of Mental Health Professionals (MHPs) in Supporting Single Mothers

MHPs play a crucial role in providing both individual and group therapy, offering a safe place where mothers can express their emotions, develop coping strategies, and rebuild confidence. These sessions empower them to navigate their challenges without fear of judgment (Yee Theng et al., 2022). Beyond therapy, MHPs can advocate for policy changes to improve single mothers' access to mental healthcare and financial support. By pushing for affordable services and government-funded mental health programs, they help ensure that struggling mothers receive necessary care (Yee Theng et al., 2022).

Additionally, MHPs facilitate peer support groups where single mothers can connect with others facing similar challenges. These groups foster a sense of belonging, allowing women to share experiences, offer guidance, and provide emotional support (Thara & Padmavati, 2013). In many South Asian communities, mental health support remains stigmatized. Mental health professionals play a vital role in changing these perceptions through awareness campaigns, workshops, and media outreach (Singla et al., 2014; Thara & Padmavati, 2013).

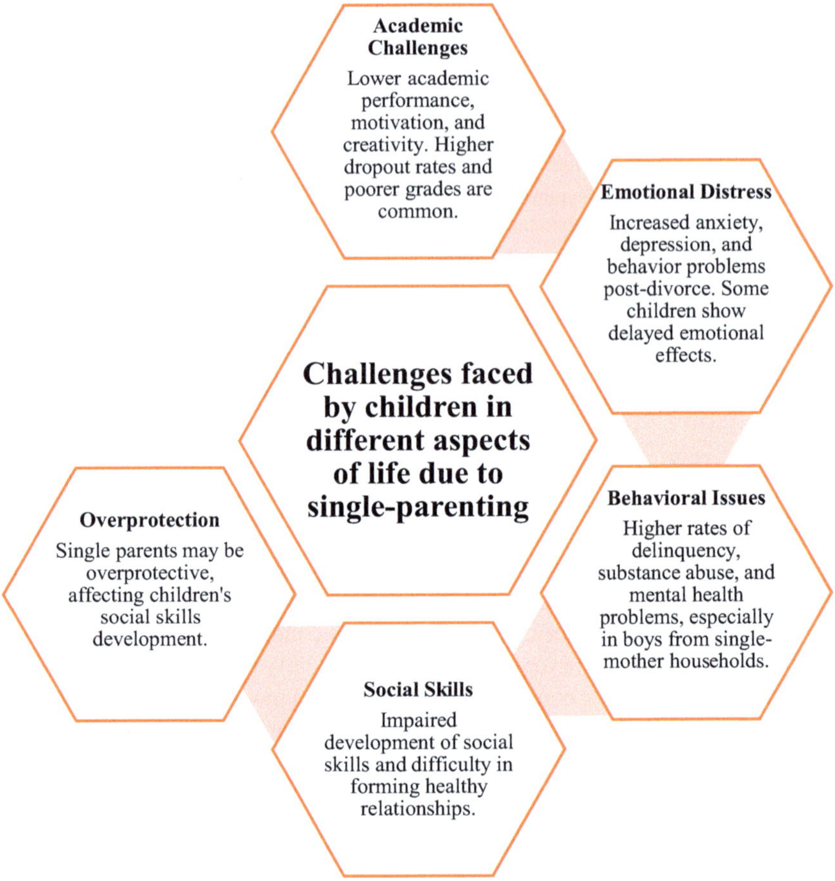

Fig. 14.2 Challenges faced by children in different aspects of life due to single parenting (Chavda & Nisarga, 2023)

6 Government Schemes and Benefits for Single Mothers

The government has implemented a variety of schemes focused on monetary aid, healthcare, and social welfare which can be utilized for the single mothers as well. One such initiative is the *Pradhan Mantri Matru Vandana Yojana (PMMVY)* which offers partial financial support to pregnant and lactating mothers to compensate for income loss during maternity, encouraging them to seek better healthcare. The program also accommodates cases of miscarriage, stillbirth, and infant mortality, recognizing the economic impact on affected women (Behera, 2023).

For economic empowerment, the *Stand-Up India Scheme* offers bank loans between ₹10 lakhs and ₹1 crore to promote entrepreneurship, requiring every bank branch to extend at least one loan to a women entrepreneur (Rani, 2017). Meanwhile The *National Food Security Act 2013 (NFSA)* ensures food security for vulnerable population particularly women and children. Under the Integrated Child Development Services (ICDS), pregnant and lactating mothers receive free meals and maternity benefits, while children are provided nutritious meals at schools and Anganwadi centers (Tanksale & Jha, 2015).

Several states have also introduced targeted welfare programs. *Maharashtra's Mukhyamantri Majhi Ladki Bahin Yojana* provides financial aid to women aged 21–65, helping them achieve economic self-sufficiency. Through a monthly stipend, the scheme aims to ease immediate financial burdens, allowing women to prioritize their health, education, and overall quality of life (Ambedkar_Ovhal & Shinde, 2025).

Likewise in Bangladesh, the government has introduced a maternal health voucher scheme which provides vouchers for antenatal care, delivery, and postnatal services targeting poor pregnant women (Ahmed & Khan, 2011). For fostering inclusive growth, the government of Nepal has social protection programs which provide in-kind or cash transfers through a system or providing employment in public sector at guaranteed salary to vulnerable population including single mothers (Adhikari et al., 2024). To alleviate poverty, Sri Lanka introduced the *Samurdhi Program*, offering financial and nutritional support to underprivileged groups, including single mothers (Ilma & Shantha, 2024). The social safety net program in Pakistan, known as *Benazir Income Support Program*, is also an example of a government-led initiative to curb extreme and chronic poverty (Ijaz, 2021).

However, despite existence of these schemes, many single mothers struggle to access them due to bureaucratic hurdles, cumbersome documentation processes, lack of awareness, and delays in approvals. Insufficient outreach efforts further limit the effectiveness of these programs, leaving many eligible women unaware of the support available to them. To truly empower single mothers, it is essential to streamline application process, enhance public awareness, and improve accessibility to these resources.

7 Conclusion and Recommendations

Supporting single mothers necessitates a multifaceted approach that combines financial aid, social support, affordable, accessible mental health services, and legal reforms. Several high-income countries have implemented successful strategies that can serve as models for adaptation in South Asian regions. For example, Canada and Sweden train healthcare providers to identify and address postpartum depression (World Health Organization, 2008), while Denmark and the United Kingdom offer financial assistance through direct cash transfers and subsidized childcare (Aerts et al., 2022). Germany and Australia emphasize vocational training to enhance economic independence, whereas Japan and the United States foster community support networks (Bosch & Charest, 2008). The Netherlands and Norway focus on legal reforms and anti-stigma campaigns, strategies that could be adapted to improve the socioeconomic well-being of single mothers in South Asian countries (Leproni & Azara, 2025).

In LMICs, one of the main challenges for such adaptations is lack of awareness and low recognition of mental disorders by primary care health workers, partly due to a shortage of clinicians with specialized training in assessing and managing these conditions. This also highlights the need for holistic interventions that consider the interplay of stressors in single mothers in cultural contexts.

Key recommendations include establishing protocols for the early identification, treatment, and prevention of perinatal mental health issues. Policies should emphasize on early intervention for alcohol-related issues, while vocational training programs can empower single mothers by enhancing their financial independence. Expanding access to social support services, community resources, and mental health services is crucial in reducing negative impacts and promoting well-being. Additionally, premarital counselling and health education can help prevent family breakdowns after divorce or separation. A collaboration approach between government and nongovernment organizations is vital to improving the quality of life for single mothers. Further research in also needed to assess their hardships and mental health challenges, ensuring that policies and interventions are evidence based and effective.

References

Adhikari, M., Kishore, A., Koirala, P., Rashid, S., & Chand, I. (2024). *Social safety nets in Nepal: A review*. The Cereal Systems Initiative for South Asia (CSISA) & Transforming Agrifood Systems in South Asia (TAFSSA). Kathmandu. https://hdl.handle.net/10883/34956

Aerts, E., Marx, I., & Parolin, Z. (2022). Income support policies for single parents in Europe and the United States: What works best? *The Annals of the American Academy of Political and Social Science, 702*(1), 55–76. https://doi.org/10.1177/00027162221120448

Agnafors, S., Bladh, M., Svedin, C. G., & Sydsjö, G. (2019). Mental health in young mothers, single mothers and their children. *BMC Psychiatry, 19*(1), 112. https://doi.org/10.1186/s12888-019-2082-y

Ahmed, S., & Khan, M. M. (2011). Is demand-side financing equity enhancing? Lessons from a maternal health voucher scheme in Bangladesh. *Social Science and Medicine, 72*(10), 1704–1710. https://doi.org/10.1016/j.socscimed.2011.03.031

Ahmed, S. M., & Lemkau, J. P. (2000). Cultural issues in the primary care of South Asians. *Journal of Immigrant Health, 2*(2), 89–96. https://doi.org/10.1023/A:1009585918590

Ambedkar_Ovhal, V. V., & Shinde, R. (2025). Impact of mukhyamantri mazi ladki bahin yojana on women in Maharashtra: An analytical study. *International Journal of Management (IJM), 16*(1).

Behera, S. (2023). *Pradhan Mantri Matru Vandana Yojana (PMMVY): A*. https://www.academia.edu/download/105633386/pradhan_mantri_yojna_review_Dr._Sasmita_Behera.pdf.

Bosch, G., & Charest, J. (2008). Vocational training and the labour market in liberal and coordinated economies. *Industrial Relations Journal, 39*(5), 428–447. https://doi.org/10.1111/j.1468-2338.2008.00497.x

Bradley, R. H., & Corwyn, R. F. (2002). Socioeconomic Status and Child Development. *Annual Review of Psychology, 53*, 371–399. https://doi.org/10.1146/annurev.psych.53.100901.135233

Brown, G. W., & Moran, P. M. (1997). Single mothers, poverty and depression. *Psychological Medicine, 27*(1), 21–33. https://doi.org/10.1017/S0033291796004060

Chavda, K., & Nisarga, V. (2023). Single parenting: Impact on child's development. *Journal of Indian Association for Child and Adolescent Mental Health, 19*(1), 14–20. https://doi.org/10.1177/09731342231179017

Crosier, T., Butterworth, P., & Rodgers, B. (2007). Mental health problems among single and partnered mothers. *Social Psychiatry and Psychiatric Epidemiology, 42*(1), 6–13. https://doi.org/10.1007/s00127-006-0125-4

Dharani, M. K., & Balamurugan, J. (2024). The psychosocial impact on single mothers' well-being—A literature review. *Journal of Education and Health Promotion, 13*(1), 148. https://doi.org/10.4103/jehp.jehp_1045_23

Dor, A. (2021). Single motherhood by choice: Difficulties and advantages. *Journal of Educational and Developmental Psychology, 11*(1), 1–18.

Dube, L. (1997). *Women and kinship: Comparative perspectives on gender in South and South-East Asia.* http://collections.unu.edu/view/UNU:2377.

Gelaye, B., Rondon, M. B., Araya, R., & Williams, M. A. (2016). Epidemiology of maternal depression, risk factors, and child outcomes in low-income and middle-income countries. *The Lancet Psychiatry, 3*(10), 973–982. https://doi.org/10.1016/S2215-0366(16)30284-X

Goodrum, N. M., Jones, D. J., Kincaid, C. Y., Cuellar, J., & Parent, J. M. (2012). Youth externalizing problems in African American single-mother families: A culturally relevant model. *Couple and Family Psychology: Research and Practice, 1*(4), 294–305. https://doi.org/10.1037/a0029421

Halter, M. J. (2014). *Varcarolis' foundations of psychiatric mental health nursing.* Elsevier Health Sciences.

Haring-Hidore, M., Stock, W. A., Okun, M. A., & Witter, R. A. (1985). Marital status and subjective well-being: A research synthesis. *Journal of Marriage and Family, 47*(4), 947–953. https://doi.org/10.2307/352338

Hatzmann, J., Peek, N., Heymans, H., Maurice-Stam, H., & Grootenhuis, M. (2014). Consequences of caring for a child with a chronic disease: Employment and leisure time of parents. *Journal of Child Health Care: For Professionals Working with Children in the Hospital and Community, 18*(4), 346–357. https://doi.org/10.1177/1367493513496668

Holm, A. L., & Severinsson, E. (2012). Systematic review of the emotional state and self-management of widows. *Nursing & Health Sciences, 14*(1), 109–120. https://doi.org/10.1111/j.1442-2018.2011.00656.x

Ijaz, U. (2021). Impact of benazir income support program (BISP) on consumption, health and education. *Economic Consultant, 4(36)*, Article 4.

Ilma, A. A. F., & Shantha, M. S. (2024). *The role of microcredit on women empowerment in Sri Lanka: Evidence from Samurdhi Program Beneficiaries in Weligama Divisional Secretariat Division.* http://repo.lib.sab.ac.lk:8080/xmlui/handle/susl/4456

Insan, N., Weke, A., Forrest, S., & Rankin, J. (2022). Social determinants of antenatal depression and anxiety among women in South Asia: A systematic review & meta-analysis. *PLoS One, 17*(2), e0263760. https://doi.org/10.1371/journal.pone.0263760

Kleber, R. J. (2019). Trauma and public mental health: A focused review. *Frontiers in Psychiatry, 10.* https://doi.org/10.3389/fpsyt.2019.00451

Kramer, S., Hackett, C., Schiller, A., & Nolan, H. (2019). *Religion and living arrangements around the world.* Religion and Living Arrangements Around the World.

Leproni, R., & Azara, L. (2025). "Women must not be left behind": The UNESCO path towards women's empowerment. In *Scars of war: Migration, security and sustainable future* (pp. 21–46). Emerald Publishing Limited. https://doi.org/10.1108/S0895-993520250000030004

Lucas, R. E. (2005). Time does not heal all wounds: A longitudinal study of reaction and adaptation to divorce. *Psychological Science, 16*(12), 945–950. https://doi.org/10.1111/j.1467-9280.2005.01642.x

Mishra, P. S., Thamminaina, A., & Mishra, N. (2021). Single mothers: Strategies of family management and support systems in relation to health. *Journal of International Women's Studies, 22*(5), 393–406.

Munir, M., Yuda, T. K., Kusumah, E. P., & Suwandi, M. A. (2024). An exploratory study on women single parents' experiences in coping with socioeconomic insecurity. *International Journal of Sociology and Social Policy, 44*(7/8), 643–656.

Nahar, J. S., Algin, S., Sajib, M. W. H., Ahmed, S., & Arafat, S. M. Y. (2020). Depressive and anxiety disorders among single mothers in Dhaka. *The International Journal of Social Psychiatry, 66*(5), 485–488. https://doi.org/10.1177/0020764020920671

Nigam, S. (2019a). Gender specific laws on violence in India. *Nigam Shalu, Gender specific laws on violence in India, In Training manual for legal empowerment of women and girls with physical disabilities in India, Editor Renu Addlakha, Center for Women's Development Studies, New Delhi.* https://papers.ssrn.com/sol3/Delivery.cfm?abstractid=3498382

Nigam, S. (2019b). *Women and domestic violence law in India: A quest for justice.* Routledge India. Retrieved March 16, 2025, from https://www.taylorfrancis.com/books/mono/10.4324/9780429343575/women-domestic-violence-law-india-shalu-nigam

Nigam, A. D. S. (2024a). *Single mothers, patriarchy and citizenship in India: Rethinking lone motherhood through the lens of socio-legal and policy framework.* Shalu Nigam.

Nigam, S. (2024b). Guardianship Law in India: Examining the principle of 'best interests' of minors and the rights of single mothers as sole guardians. *Indian Journal of Gender Studies, 31*(3), 308–327. https://doi.org/10.1177/09715215241262137

Rahman, A., Bunn, J., Lovel, H., & Creed, F. (2007). Association between antenatal depression and low birthweight in a developing country. *Acta Psychiatrica Scandinavica, 115*(6), 481–486. https://doi.org/10.1111/j.1600-0447.2006.00950.x

Rani, N. I. (2006). Child care by poor single mothers: Study of mother-headed families in India. *Journal of Comparative Family Studies, 37*(1), 75–91. https://doi.org/10.3138/jcfs.37.1.75

Rani, M. A. (2017). Startup India: Opportunities & challenges "Start up India stand up India". *ACADEMICIA: An International Multidisciplinary Research Journal, 7*(1), 104–113.

Sartor, T., Lange, S., & Tröster, H. (2023). Cumulative stress of single mothers—An exploration of potential risk factors. *The Family Journal, 31*(1), 88–94. https://doi.org/10.1177/10664807221104134

Shozi, P. N. (2020). *The influence of single mothers alcohol misuse on the well being of their families: Reflections of social service providers* [PhD Thesis, Stellenbosch: Stellenbosch University]. https://scholar.sun.ac.za/handle/10019.1/107856

Singla, D., Lazarus, A., Atif, N., Sikander, S., Bhatia, U., Ahmad, I., Nisar, A., Khan, S., Fuhr, D., Patel, V., & Rahman, A. (2014). "Someone like us": Delivering maternal mental health through peers in two South Asian contexts. *Journal of Affective Disorders, 168*, 452–458. https://doi.org/10.1016/j.jad.2014.07.017

Tanksale, A., & Jha, J. K. (2015). Implementing national food security act in India: Issues and challenges. *British Food Journal, 117*(4), 1315–1335.

Targosz, S., Bebbington, P., Lewis, G., Brugha, T., Jenkins, R., Farrell, M., & Meltzer, H. (2003). Lone mothers, social exclusion and depression. *Psychological Medicine, 33*(4), 715–722. https://doi.org/10.1017/S0033291703007347

Thara, R., & Padmavati, R. (2013). Community mental health care in South Asia. *World Psychiatry, 12*(2), 176–177. https://doi.org/10.1002/wps.20042

Weitoft, G. R., Hjern, A., Haglund, B., & Rosén, M. (2003). Mortality, severe morbidity, and injury in children living with single parents in Sweden: A population-based study. *The Lancet, 361*(9354), 289–295. https://doi.org/10.1016/S0140-6736(03)12324-0

Wittchen, H. U., Jacobi, F., Rehm, J., Gustavsson, A., Svensson, M., Jönsson, B., Olesen, J., Allgulander, C., Alonso, J., Faravelli, C., Fratiglioni, L., Jennum, P., Lieb, R., Maercker, A., van Os, J., Preisig, M., Salvador-Carulla, L., Simon, R., & Steinhausen, H.-C. (2011). The size and burden of mental disorders and other disorders of the brain in Europe 2010. *European Neuropsychopharmacology, 21*(9), 655–679. https://doi.org/10.1016/j.euroneuro.2011.07.018

World Health Organization, W. O. of N., Academies, & Physicians, A. A. of G. P. (2008). *Integrating mental health into primary care: A global perspective*. World Health Organization.
Yee Theng, L., Abdul Rahman, R., & Ismail, S. B. (2022). Determinants of depression among malay single mothers living in community in Perak, Malaysia. *The Malaysian Journal of Medical Sciences: MJMS, 29*(2), 80–93. https://doi.org/10.21315/mjms2022.29.2.8

Chapter 15
Sexuality in Perinatal Period

Chandrima Naskar and Harshita Biswas

1 Introduction

The perinatal period is a unique milestone in life accompanied by new emotions, challenges, and developments. The commonly accepted definition of perinatal period (PNP) or the peripartum period describes it to be extending from the time of conception till 1 year post-childbirth. However, the International Classification of Diseases (ICD 10) has a shortened definition of the PNP extending from the 22nd week of gestation till 7 days after birth. The Diagnostic and Statistical Manual of Mental Disorders (DSM 5) defines the PNP from conception to 4 weeks after the childbirth, while ICD 11 extends it till 6 weeks after the childbirth. The definition becomes further difficult when the pregnancy ends in a spontaneous or medical termination. While this period is heterogeneous with its dynamic and novel challenges, sexuality during the perinatal period is not commonly discussed, formally assessed, or extensively researched.

Sexuality encompasses a wide range of physiological, behavioral, psychological, and social elements that go beyond the singular action of sexual intercourse between partners.

So that brings to us several questions:

(i) What happens to natural sexuality during the perinatal period?
(ii) What are the factors that play a role?

C. Naskar (✉)
Old Age Psychiatry, Kingsway Hospital, Derbyshire Healthcare Foundation Trust, NHS, UK

H. Biswas
Tata Main Hospital, Jamshedpur, Jharkhand, India
e-mail: harshita.biswas@tatasteel.com

P. Kukreti et al. (eds.), *Women's Reproductive Mental Health in South Asia*, South Asian Perspectives in Mental Health and Psychology,
https://doi.org/10.1007/978-981-96-9219-4_15

(iii) What happens in in vitro fertilization (IVF), medical termination of pregnancy (MTP), intrauterine fetal death (IUFD), older mother, and other complicated pregnancies?
(iv) When to assess, why to assess, and how to assess?
(v) When to intervene and how to intervene?

2 Normal Sexuality in Perinatal Period

Normal sexuality in the perinatal period varies greatly between individuals and couples. Some women have increased sexual desire as a result of enhanced blood circulation and hormonal changes, while others experience decreased libido due to multiple reasons (Pauleta et al., 2010). Sexual function may take some time to restore after delivery (Leeman & Rogers, 2012). Fluctuations in sexual desire and activity are of typical occurrence, and medical consultation, together with effective communication between partners, can help to overcome this. The consensus states that females experience a significant decrease in "sexual interest, desire, frequency of sexual intercourse, sexual enjoyment, coital activity, orgasm, and satisfaction." In many cases, the reduction persists long after childbirth for variable individual durations (Yıldız, 2015). However, a few authors who have used specially designed questionnaires to assess the sexual satisfaction and desire during pregnancy and peripartum period have noted that in about 40–50% of women, the desire and satisfaction remain unchanged even if there is a decline in the frequency of sexual activity. Also, it is important to note that, at a cognitive level, about a quarter of the women report having a fear of causing harm or distress to the fetus if they take part in sexual act (Pauleta et al., 2010). This belief or fear might end up coloring their intent or interest of sexual activities. Research in these domains focusing specifically on couples originating and/or staying in the South Asian countries is scarce. From our clinical experience, we can comment that sexuality is most commonly avoided as a topic of discussion by both the partners as well as the medical professionals during the peripartum period. Sometimes this avoidance is intentional, due to embarrassment, shame, and belief that it is impure to think of sexuality or considering it to be abnormal or unacceptable. At other times, it is missed out unintentionally since the limited resource for medical help is more concerned on providing the basic care to sustain the mother's physical health.

2.1 *Sexuality During Pregnancy*

Both psychological and physiological aspects affect sexual functioning during pregnancy. Hormonal differences, such as increased progesterone and estrogen levels, can lead to heightened sensitivity in some women, while others experience decreased libido due to fatigue, nausea, or physical discomfort (Brtnicka et al., 2009).

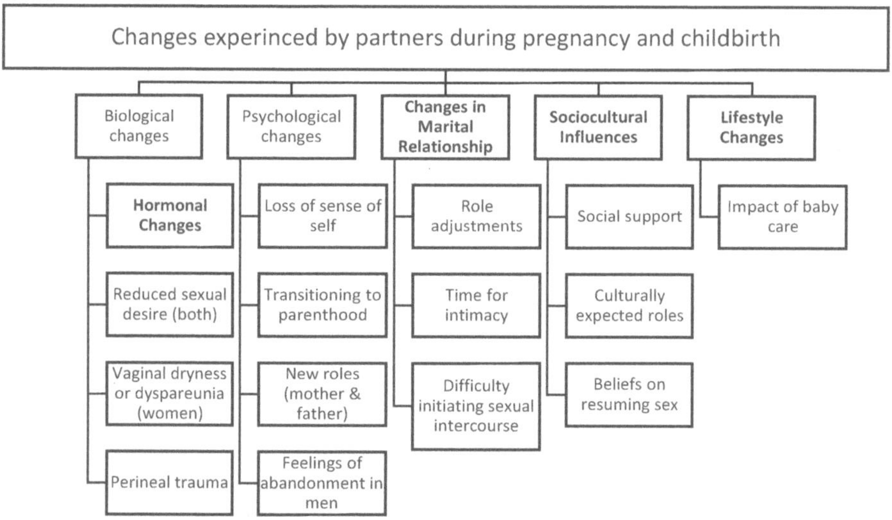

Fig. 15.1 Changes experienced by partners during the peripartum period

Figure 15.1 attempts to briefly summarize the alterations that occur in various biopsychosocial domains of the couple in the peripartum period. A meta-analysis by Von Sydow (1999) established that sexual frequency decreases during pregnancy, most significantly in the third trimester, because of concerns about fetal safety and discomfort. The decline is slight in the first trimester, fluctuating in the second trimester, and marked in the third trimester (Yıldız, 2015). Emotional well-being also plays a role in sexual functioning. Anxiety and depressive symptoms, which are typical in pregnancy, have been linked with a decrease in sexual desire and satisfaction (Faisal-Cury et al., 2013). Also, cultural norms influence sexual behavior during pregnancy. Traditional beliefs in South Asian cultures generally discourage sexual behavior because it might hurt the baby or displease religious norms (Withers et al., 2018). Such perspectives may lead to reduced sexual frequency and communication gaps between partners.

2.2 *Sexuality in the Postpartum Period*

The postpartum period introduces new challenges, including hormonal shifts, physical recovery, sleep deprivation, and psychological stress. Studies have shown that a large number of women suffer from perinatal sexual dysfunction, which is characterized by low libido, vaginal dryness, painful intercourse, and body image issues (Leeman & Rogers, 2012; McBride & Kwee, 2017). In a longitudinal study conducted by Wallwiener et al. (2017), they determined that almost 60% of the women suffered from some sexual dysfunction in the first 6 months after childbirth, improving gradually over the years. Psychosocial issues also impact postpartum sexuality.

The occurrence of depressive or anxiety symptoms negatively affects sexual desire and functioning (Faisal-Cury et al., 2013). In addition, the quality of the relationship between a couple and communication is essential. Fitzpatrick et al. (2021) emphasize that emotional support among partners and an understanding between partners can ease the transition to postpartum intimacy. Also, the method of childbirth has been found to impact sexual functioning in the postpartum period. Assisted vaginal deliveries and caesarean deliveries have been found to have worse sexual functioning postpartum, when compared to normal vaginal deliveries in some assessment, while others have found no statistically significant difference between the two groups (Fanshawe et al., 2023). Overall, low partnership quality, breastfeeding, higher maternal education, caesarean delivery, and postpartum mood symptoms have been the main factors negatively affecting sexual functioning in the postpartum period (Wallwiener et al., 2017).

2.3 *Factors Affecting Sexuality in Perinatal Period*

As discussed in the above paragraphs, many factors play an intertwined role in determining the peripartum sexual experiences. In the following part, we try to discuss the most significant factors, which can be addressed in a clinical scenario.

(i) **Preexisting interpersonal relationship between partners:** A longitudinal study by Yıldız (2015) attempted to find out the relationship between the preexisting sexual relationship between couples and the changes in sexuality during pregnancy and the postpartum period. It was found that the preexisting sexual pattern was carried into the first two trimesters, even when the frequency of sexual contact altered during this period. Also, it was found that couples who had preexisting sexual dysfunction continued to experience higher prevalence of sexual dysfunction in the pregnancy and postpartum periods. However, what was interesting was that new-onset sexual dysfunction during pregnancy did not continue to effect postpartum sexuality. The overall conclusion was that healthy prepregnancy sexuality can help in preserving sexual function during pregnancy and immediate postpartum sexuality (Yıldız, 2015).

(ii) **High-risk or complicated pregnancy:** It is common for treating doctors to suggest the pregnant couple that they can continue sexual activity as usual and as per their own sense of comfort throughout most of the pregnancy. However, the difficulty arises when the pregnancy is complicated due to some medical or other reasons (a valuable pregnancy, past bad obstetric history, shortened cervix, multiple fetuses, etc.). In these scenarios, sexual intercourse needs to be discouraged or even completely forbidden. In these situations, instead of just advising "pelvic rest" or vaguely suggesting "abstain from all sexual activities," it is important to have a conversation with the couple regarding their concerns and queries. Unaddressed concerns can lead to practices that might harm the couple's relationship, emotional state, anxiety and worries, and even the pregnancy outcome at times (Simetinger & Gianotten, 2023). An Indian study tried to assess the impact of hysterectomy during childbirth for postpartum hemorrhage on the sexual experience and quality of life of the mothers. It was found that though the sexual experience was unaffected, the overall quality of life was reduced than the control group (Jha et al., 2025).

(iii) **Religion, morality, and social factors:** While focusing on the South Asian countries, religion and social and cultural traditions play an important role. A few studies spanning over both the Hindu- and Muslim-predominant countries across South Asia have reported that social traditions describe feelings as well as discussion about sexuality as a taboo, more so in the peripartum period. The studies have also identified a sense of conflict within the new mothers where the individual's internal perception of sexuality is in dissonance with the social role of mother, which shuns sexuality and paints mothers as "pious and pure" (Cantarino et al., 2016; Grussu et al., 2021; Lamba et al., 2023). Also, a common practice in the South Asian families is that the mother and child are kept in the maternal house of the female for 4–6 months after the child's birth. These moral dissonances and the physical distance can further complicate the rebuilding of sexual functioning in postpartum period.

(iv) **Gender of the partner:** While some research is available regarding the women's experience of peripartum changes in sexuality, similar research primarily focusing on their male partners is remarkably lacking. The available research shows that hormonal changes also occur in the male partners during the pregnancy period, including alteration in cortisol, oxytocin, and testosterone levels (Clephane & Lorenz, 2021). However, it is also common that the male sexuality returns to prepregnancy levels almost immediately after the childbirth, not in keeping with their female partners. This difference, if not addressed and normalized, can lead to significant emotional and marital problems (MacAdam et al., 2011).

3 Psychological Effects of MTP, Unsuccessful Pregnancy, and Complicated Perinatal Period

Medical termination of pregnancy (MTP), loss of pregnancy, and complications at childbirth can bring about severe psychological distress in both partners. In societies of South Asia, these experiences are much more complicated, as cultural, religious, and social factors shape people's views on pregnancy loss.

3.1 Psychological Effects of MTP

Owing to the psychology involved, MTP, whether elective or medically necessary, may lead to lasting consequences. Studies report that abortion may carry the risk of post-traumatic stress disorder, depression, and some kind of difficulty with interpersonal relationships. In South Asia, where abortion is highly stigmatized and bound by religious and societal standards, the psychological burden can even be heavier. Women might suffer from alienation from society, or there can be rumors about wedding discord (Withers et al., 2018). Moreover, mental health problems are compounded by limited access to safe abortion services and legal prohibition in select Asian countries. Women resorting to unsafe abortions suffer the greater trauma, fear, and depression (Ganatra et al., 2017). Support services for psychology are often unavailable to address the distress following MTP.

3.2 Psychological Impact of Unsuccessful Pregnancy

Miscarriage, stillbirth, and recurrent pregnancy loss are linked to a significant prevalence of depression, anxiety, and post-traumatic stress disorder (PTSD) (Faisal-Cury et al., 2013). In South Asia, this psychological impact gets aggravated by cultural expectations of motherhood and internal family pressures on having children (Wallwiener et al., 2017). Women who go through unsuccessful pregnancies may face blame, experience domestic strain, and even deal with marital instability. Research shows that, in South Asia, societal norms toward pregnancy loss often discourage talk, causing many women to grieve alone (Fernández-Sola et al., 2018). Rituals connected to miscarriage and stillbirth differ from South Asian cultures, whereby some allow for a structured grieving process, while others entrench silence and stigma (Withers et al., 2018). Inaccessibility of opportunities for psychological counseling prevents women from seeking help.

3.3 Psychological Consequences of a Complicated Perinatal Period

Women who face complications during pregnancy or childbirth, such as preeclampsia, hemorrhage, or emergency C-sections, frequently report increased anxiety and depressive symptoms (Leeman & Rogers, 2012). In South Asia, where maternal mortality rates are still alarmingly high, these complications can be life-threatening and lead to significant psychological distress (Wood et al., 2022). Increased anxiety and depressive symptoms arise from worries about maternal health, worries about neonatal health, and inadequate medical support. This period is salient for maternal mental health. High prevalence is reported for postpartum depression in South Asia yet remains mostly undiagnosed, due to culturally competitive expectations of prioritizing family over women's health needs (Lévesque et al., 2021). The presence of extended family can have mixed effects; while it offers social support, it can also create additional pressure and limit the autonomy of the couple (Fitzpatrick et al., 2021).

Thus, it is inevitable that these scenarios in the peripartum period affect the couple's sexual encounters as much as, or even more than, that in normal pregnancy. The grief, self-blame, ideas of guilt, and worthlessness, in the presence or absence of any depressive or anxiety disorder, can affect either or both the partner's libido and sexual functions. The overall dysfunction can continue to exaggerate all the associated symptoms in the form of a vicious cycle as described in Fig. 15.2.

4 Perinatal Education of Parents: Is the Topic of Sexuality Covered?

Perinatal education is central to preparing parents, at multiple levels, for challenges related to childbirth and the postpartum period. Maternal and infant health comprises the bulk of the discussion, and parameters around sexual health remain a muted subject, especially in the Indian subcontinent. In spite of the physiological, emotional, and relationship-based changes a couple experiences during the perinatal period, cultural taboos and a lack of discussion about sexual health in primary healthcare settings often prevent any open conversation on this subject.

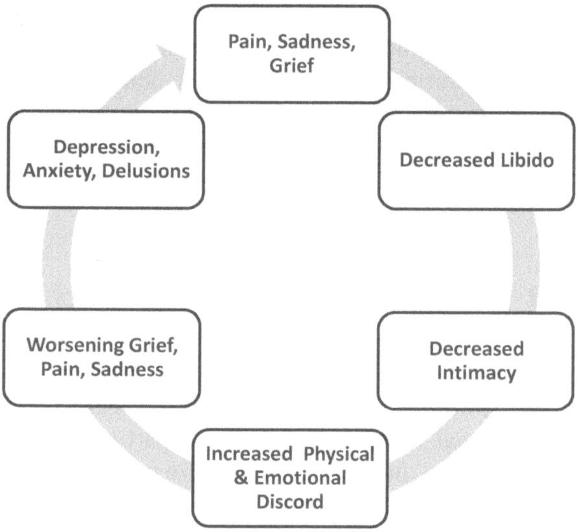

Fig. 15.2 The vicious cycle of sexual dysfunction and mood symptoms

4.1 Perinatal Education and the Omission of Sexuality

In South Asia, perinatal education programs predominantly focus on maternal nutrition, fetal development, labor and delivery, and newborn care. But discussions related to recovery postpartum, in which sexuality would be included, are largely absent due to sociocultural barriers (Withers et al., 2018). A study by von Sydow (1999) indicates that sexual function changes significantly during pregnancy and postpartum; women in very conservative hesitate to seek information or support.

Healthcare providers in South Asian countries often avoid discussing sexuality due to personal discomfort or fear of social backlash. Even when perinatal classes exist, they rarely address topics such as libido changes, vaginal dryness, dyspareunia, or the emotional impact of childbirth on intimate relationships (Brtnicka et al., 2009). In sharp contrast, the Western countries, including the USA, Canada, and portions of Europe, integrate sexual health into perinatal care, normalizing discussions about intimacy, contraception, and postnatal sexual dysfunction (Leeman & Rogers, 2012).

4.2 Service Utilization Patterns in South Asia

Service utilization for perinatal education in South Asia is limited due to multiple factors, including low healthcare accessibility, socioeconomic disparities, and gender norms that discourage women from seeking knowledge independently (Wood et al., 2022). Many pregnant women rely on informal sources, such as elders, traditional birth attendants, and social media, rather than structured healthcare programs (Fitzpatrick et al., 2021).

Given an inquiry on sexual health, South Asian women are more likely to consult, firstly, their female relatives or other unqualified practitioners than trained medical practitioners (Yıldız, 2015). A dearth of culturally sensitive educational materials further discourages engagement with formal perinatal education programs. In contrast, high-income countries have existing structured classes through hospitals, midwifery services, and online avenues that allow active discussion on postpartum intimacy (McBride & Kwee, 2017).

4.3 Comparative Global Perspectives

Globally, the integration of sexuality into perinatal education varies. Scandinavian countries, known for progressive sexual health policies, include discussions on perinatal sexual function as a standard part of maternal care (Bitzer & Alder, 2000). Australia and the UK also emphasize open communication between healthcare providers and expecting parents, incorporating psychoeducational resources into antenatal visits (Serrano Drozdowskyj et al., 2020). In contrast, Asian studies highlighted the cultural denial of discussion regarding sexuality and negative experiences, including discomfort, shyness, embarrassment, fear of intimidation, etc. (Ellin et al., 2024).

The absence of sexuality in perinatal education programs in Asia reflects broader sociocultural attitudes toward discussing sexual health. Addressing these gaps requires targeted policy interventions, culturally sensitive educational materials, and training programs for healthcare professionals to normalize discussions on sexuality during the perinatal period.

When the couple is not counseled during pregnancy regarding the alterations and the expectations related to sexuality, it can lead to false beliefs and untoward practices, which can affect the whole experience of peripartum period negatively. Unlike common belief and the usual shunning of the topic, sexuality is an important part of the peripartum period and a broader approach than only intercourse needs to be adopted, and the practices need to be adapted related to the physical changes and emotional needs (Fernández-Sola et al., 2018).

5 Country-Specific Challenges

5.1 Global and Social Perspectives in Addressing Perinatal Sexuality

In Western societies, open discussion of perinatal sexuality and medical interventions like pelvic floor therapy are more prevalent, and hence awareness and management of sexual dysfunction are increased (Fitzpatrick et al., 2021). In South Asian cultures, however, conventional postpartum confinement practices are more dominant, which may prolong periods of sexual abstinence but offer structured social support to new mother (Withers et al., 2018). Further, although trends worldwide suggest that sexual activity declines during pregnancy and the postpartum period, the reasons for such a decline differ: in Western societies, personal comfort and medical recommendations are highly influential, while in South Asia, sociocultural and religious norms influence more strongly (Al Bustan et al., 1995). Recognizing these differences is essential in creating culturally appropriate strategies for sexual health during the perinatal period.

5.2 The Interplay of Sociocultural Factors

Postpartum confinement customs and traditions in South Asia significantly influence sexuality. Many cultures promote a period of abstinence lasting at least 40 days for both religious and health reasons (Withers et al., 2018). While these practices can assist in the mother's recovery, they may also lead to prolonged periods of sexual inactivity and tension within the relationship. Al Bustan et al. (1995) learned that community norms and religious beliefs play a crucial role in shaping postpartum sexual behavior among Kuwaiti Muslim women. Additionally, family dynamics, such as the involvement of extended family, often impact a couple's intimacy and privacy during the perinatal period in countries like India and Pakistan (Withers et al., 2018).

Addressing the psychological implications in order to mitigate the psychological toll on maternal trauma, pregnancy loss, and perinatal complications is of paramount importance for the implementation of culturally competent mental health interventions. Raising awareness on perinatal mental health, embedding psychological support in maternal healthcare, and challenging cultural stigma around fetal loss and abortion are some ways through which distress can be alleviated (Serrano Drozdowskyj et al., 2020).

Restrictive societal norms in Asia often limit discussions on mental health, making it difficult for women to seek psychological help. Stigma and adherence to traditional beliefs dampen conversations about mental health problems, causing underreporting among these women when seeking available services. Asian nations often rely on family networks for support, which may not always be conducive to addressing mental health concerns. The values associated with maintaining family honor and societal reputation may hinder open conversations about mental health, which often leads in many instances to women remaining without assistance (Chen et al., 2012).

6 Perinatal Sexual Dysfunction

Having alteration in sexuality and sexual activity during the pregnancy and post-childbirth period is the usual norm. However, in a fraction of couples, the alteration can be associated with significant dysfunction and disruption of their usual marital relationship. There exists no diagnostic category, specifically adapted assessment tool, or clinical guideline for classifying perinatal sexual dysfunction. That makes it challenging for any clinician, be it an obstetrician, general physician, or a psychiatrist/mental health professional to objectively determine when to actively intervene. While clear diagnostic criteria remain for female sexual dysfunction and the subtype of FSD following pelvic surgeries, no such criteria have been developed yet for understanding pregnancy and childbirth-related sexual dysfunctions (Raina et al., 2007).

However, the principle for a clinical intervention can be drawn in the similar way to any other cause of sexual dysfunction. When the couple or either of the partner experiences significant distress, dissatisfaction, or mood and anxiety symptoms primarily related to their sexual intimacy or the lack of it, assessment and treatment must be initiated. Since the etiology to perinatal sexual dysfunction is biopsychosocial and is further colored by cultural and traditional beliefs and practices, the assessment and intervention should also be in the same line.

7 Interventions that Might Be Helpful

(i) *Preemptive education of the couples regarding what changes they might expect during the perinatal period in regard to sexuality and sexual functioning*: Studies have shown that hardly 20% of expecting partners receive any such knowledge and education in their prepregnancy or pregnancy period. But it is also evident that individuals who have received such information adapt better to the expected changes and develop individual patterns and methods to cope with the same (Fitzpatrick et al., 2021).

(ii) *Helping communication between partners*: Many a time, the stigma and shame associated with sexuality and sexual needs make it impossible for partners to discuss their concerns, ultimately compounding their distress and dysfunction. That is why easing them into conversation with each other and also the healthcare worker is beneficial.

(iii) *Training them in nonphysical aspects of sexuality and sensuality*: A few qualitative studies have found that couples who have successfully managed to traverse through the peripartum period without significant sexual discord tend to develop non-body-focused methods of enjoying each other's presence. The physical changes during and after pregnancy and the body-related concerns can be a major deterrent in sexuality, and thus this method can be helpful in such scenarios.

(iv) *Pelvic floor exercises*: While a handful of small-sampled research has been done to assess the efficacy of pelvic muscle contractions like Kegel's method to improve sexuality and sexual functioning in the peripartum period, there are not many randomized controlled trials (RCTs) in this area. Individual studies report usefulness of the pelvic floor exercises, but a systematic meta-analysis could only conclude a minimal positive effect of the same. However, since these exercises are overall safe and have been shown to maintain pelvic floor muscle tone and organization, it might be of no harm to teach pregnant women about these methods and their usefulness (Karaahmet et al., 2022).

(v) *Medical management*: When the psychosocial interventions might not be adequate, hormonal interventions, adequate pain management, and assessing and reducing inflammation might be needed for attaining enjoyable sexual functioning. At times, psychiatric conditions like depression, anxiety, and grief related to pregnancy loss tend to be the primary underlying factor for the alteration in sexuality (Faisal-Cury et al., 2013). In those scenarios, adequate treatment for the underlying disorder is essential.

8 Conclusions

Research is deficient for male partners' sexuality, sexual activity, noncoital sexual interests, and sexual thoughts. Most of the research tend to equate sexuality with intercourse frequency and satisfaction, thus overlooking the much larger aspect of the concept. Also the lack of tools to specifically assess the sexuality during this special life period leads to questionable reliability and validity of the studies that are available (von Sydow, 1999). However, despite the challenges and the lack of robust information, the overarching pattern in terms of perinatal sexuality can be summarized as follows: (i) childbirth and the presence of a newborn alter the sexuality and sexual functioning in both partners; (ii) the pregnancy and postpartum period does not necessarily lead to decreased sexual satisfaction, and thus any persistent negative pattern in sexual satisfaction should be addressed and intervened; (iii) with a transition to parenthood, most couples tend to modify their patterns of sexuality and find a new balance (Lévesque et al., 2021).

References

Al Bustan, M. A., El Tomi, N. F., Faiwalla, M. F., & Manav, V. (1995). Maternal sexuality during pregnancy and after childbirth in muslim Kuwaiti women. *Archives of Sexual Behavior, 24*(2), 207–215. https://doi.org/10.1007/BF01541581

Bitzer, J., & Alder, J. (2000). Sexuality during pregnancy and the postpartum period. *Journal of Sex Education and Therapy, 25*(1), 49–58. https://doi.org/10.1080/01614576.2000.11074329

Brtnicka, H., Weiss, P., & Zverina, J. (2009). Human sexuality during pregnancy and the postpartum period. *Bratislavské Lekárske Listy, 110*, 427–431.

Cantarino, S. G., Pinto, J. M. d. M., Fabião, J. A. d. S. A. d. O., García, A. M. C., Abellán, M. V., & Rodrigues, M. A. (2016). The importance of religiosity/Spirituality in the sexuality of pregnant and postpartum women. *PLoS One, 11*(6), e0156809. https://doi.org/10.1371/journal.pone.0156809

Chen, Y.-Y., Wu, K. C.-C., Yousuf, S., & Yip, P. S. F. (2012). Suicide in Asia: Opportunities and challenges. *Epidemiologic Reviews, 34*, 129–144. https://doi.org/10.1093/epirev/mxr025

Clephane, K., & Lorenz, T. K. (2021). Putative mental, physical, and social mechanisms of hormonal influences on postpartum sexuality. *Current Sexual Health Reports, 13*(4), 136–148. https://doi.org/10.1007/s11930-021-00321-8

Ellin, M. R. B., Hazariah, A. H. S. B., Arifin, S. R. M., Hasan, H. B., Othman, S. B., & Zain, N. M. B. (2024). Examining asian parents' perspectives and challenges in sexual and reproductive health education with implications for public health: A systematic review. *Indian Journal of Public Health, 68*(3), 407–417. https://doi.org/10.4103/ijph.ijph_1281_23

Faisal-Cury, A., Huang, H., Chan, Y.-F., & Menezes, P. R. (2013). The relationship between depressive/anxiety symptoms during pregnancy/postpartum and sexual life decline after delivery. *The Journal of Sexual Medicine, 10*(5), 1343–1349. https://doi.org/10.1111/jsm.12092

Fanshawe, A.-M., De Jonge, A., Ginter, N., Takács, L., Dahlen, H. G., Swertz, M. A., & Peters, L. L. (2023). The impact of mode of birth, and episiotomy, on postpartum sexual function in the medium- and longer-term: An integrative systematic review. *International Journal of Environmental Research and Public Health, 20*(7), Article 7. https://doi.org/10.3390/ijerph20075252

Fernández-Sola, C., Huancara-Kana, D., Granero-Molina, J., Carmona-Samper, E., López-Rodríguez, M. d. M., & Hernández-Padilla, J. M. (2018). Sexuality throughout all the stages of pregnancy: Experiences of expectant mothers. *Acta Paulista de Enfermagem, 31*, 305–312. https://doi.org/10.1590/1982-0194201800043

Fitzpatrick, E. T., Kolbuszewska, M. T., & Dawson, S. J. (2021). Perinatal sexual dysfunction: The importance of the interpersonal context. *Current Sexual Health Reports, 13*(3), 55–65. https://doi.org/10.1007/s11930-021-00313-8

Ganatra, B., Gerdts, C., Rossier, C., Johnson, B. R., Tunçalp, Ö., Assifi, A., Sedgh, G., Singh, S., Bankole, A., Popinchalk, A., Bearak, J., Kang, Z., & Alkema, L. (2017). Global, regional, and subregional classification of abortions by safety, 2010–14: Estimates from a Bayesian hierarchical model. *The Lancet, 390*(10110), 2372–2381. https://doi.org/10.1016/S0140-6736(17)31794-4

Grussu, P., Vicini, B., & Quatraro, R. M. (2021). Sexuality in the perinatal period: A systematic review of reviews and recommendations for practice. *Sexual and Reproductive Healthcare, 30*, 100668. https://doi.org/10.1016/j.srhc.2021.100668

Jha, N., Palepu, P. M., Pampapati, V., Mukherjee, M. P., Karthikeyan, K., Anuja, M., Deodhare, K. G., & Pannirselvan, K. (2025). Quality of life and sexual health of women with peripartum hysterectomy: A single-center experience from South India. *International Journal of Gynecology & Obstetrics*, 1–7. https://doi.org/10.1002/ijgo.70058

Karaahmet, A. Y., Gençturk, N., Boyacıoğlu, N. E., & lcin. (2022). Does perinatal period pelvic floor muscle exercises affect sexuality and pelvic muscle strength? A systematic review and meta-analysis of randomized controlled trials. *Revista da Associação Médica Brasileira, 68*, 1033–1041. https://doi.org/10.1590/1806-9282.20220133

Lamba, A., Mohajir, N., & Rahman, S. (2023). A review of the psychosocial factors that contribute to sexuality, female sexual dysfunction, and sexual pain among Muslim women. *Sexual Medicine Reviews, 11*(3), 156–173. https://doi.org/10.1093/sxmrev/qead019

Leeman, L. M., & Rogers, R. G. (2012). Sex after childbirth: Postpartum sexual function. *Obstetrics and Gynecology, 119*(3), 647–655. https://doi.org/10.1097/AOG.0b013e3182479611

Lévesque, S., Bisson, V., Fernet, M., & Charton, L. (2021). A study of the transition to parenthood: New parents' perspectives on their sexual intimacy during the perinatal period. *Sexual and Relationship Therapy, 36*(2–3), 238–255. https://doi.org/10.1080/14681994.2019.1675870

MacAdam, R., Huuva, E., & Berterö, C. (2011). Fathers' experiences after having a child: Sexuality becomes tailored according to circumstances. *Midwifery, 27*(5), e149–e155. https://doi.org/10.1016/j.midw.2009.12.007

McBride, H. L., & Kwee, J. L. (2017). Sex after baby: Women's sexual function in the postpartum period. *Current Sexual Health Reports, 9*(3), 142–149. https://doi.org/10.1007/s11930-017-0116-3

Pauleta, J. R., Pereira, N. M., & Graça, L. M. (2010). Sexuality during pregnancy. *The Journal of Sexual Medicine, 7*(1_Part_1), 136–142. https://doi.org/10.1111/j.1743-6109.2009.01538.x

Raina, R., Pahalajani, G., Khan, S., Gupta, S., Agarwal, A., & Zippe, C. D. (2007). Female sexual dysfunction: Classification, pathophysiology, and management. *Fertility and Sterility, 88*(5), 1273–1284. https://doi.org/10.1016/j.fertnstert.2007.09.012

Serrano Drozdowskyj, E., Gimeno Castro, E., Trigo López, E., Bárcenas Taland, I., & Chiclana Actis, C. (2020). Factors influencing couples' sexuality in the puerperium: A systematic review. *Sexual Medicine Reviews, 8*(1), 38–47. https://doi.org/10.1016/j.sxmr.2019.07.002

Simetinger, G., & Gianotten, W. L. (2023). Sexual aspects of high-risk and complicated pregnancy. In S. Geuens, A. Polona Mivšek, & Woet L. Gianotten (Eds.), Midwifery and sexuality (pp. 141–153). Springer International Publishing. https://doi.org/10.1007/978-3-031-18432-1_12.

von Sydow, K. (1999). Sexuality during pregnancy and after childbirth: A metacontent analysis of 59 studies. *Journal of Psychosomatic Research, 47*(1), 27–49. https://doi.org/10.1016/S0022-3999(98)00106-8

Wallwiener, S., Müller, M., Doster, A., Kuon, R. J., Plewniok, K., Feller, S., Wallwiener, M., Reck, C., Matthies, L. M., & Wallwiener, C. (2017). Sexual activity and sexual dysfunction of women in the perinatal period: A longitudinal study. *Archives of Gynecology and Obstetrics, 295*(4), 873–883. https://doi.org/10.1007/s00404-017-4305-0

Withers, M., Kharazmi, N., & Lim, E. (2018). Traditional beliefs and practices in pregnancy, childbirth and postpartum: A review of the evidence from Asian countries. *Midwifery, 56*, 158–170. https://doi.org/10.1016/j.midw.2017.10.019

Wood, S. N., Pigott, A., Thomas, H. L., Wood, C., & Zimmerman, L. A. (2022). A scoping review on women's sexual health in the postpartum period: Opportunities for research and practice within low-and middle-income countries. *Reproductive Health, 19*(1), 112. https://doi.org/10.1186/s12978-022-01399-6

Yıldız, H. (2015). The relation between prepregnancy sexuality and sexual function during pregnancy and the postpartum period: A prospective study. *Journal of Sex and Marital Therapy, 41*(1), 49–59. https://doi.org/10.1080/0092623X.2013.811452

Chapter 16
Forensic Issues in Perinatal Psychiatry in South Asia

Prerna Kukreti, Sanyam Tyagi, and Ravi Yadav

1 Introduction

Perinatal psychiatry is a specialized field that addresses mental health disorders during pregnancy and the first year following childbirth (O'Hara & Wisner, 2014). Psychiatric conditions, including postpartum depression, psychosis, and anxiety, are prevalent during this period and can significantly impact maternal well-being, at times leading to situations involving mother coming in conflict with law (Friedman et al., 2024). This chapter explores the forensic issues surrounding perinatal psychiatry, especially in the South Asian context, where the legal, cultural, and healthcare systems are frequently ill-equipped to address these complex conditions.

In South Asia, perinatal mental health disorders are often misunderstood because of prevailing stigma (Insan et al., 2022), leading to a lack of appropriate legal safeguards and psychiatric care for mothers. Infanticide, pseudocyesis, and child abandonment are some criminal offenses that can be seen among women in the perinatal period, but mothers in such cases are frequently tried like an ordinary criminal without considering the mental health conditions underlying these actions (Sapkota et al., 2024) leading to criminal evaluations, custody disputes, and incarceration rather than diversion to treatment. This chapter critically examines the legal systems in South Asian countries highlighting the gaps in current laws, forensic psychiatric evaluations, and available healthcare services.

P. Kukreti (✉)
Department of Psychiatry, Lady Hardinge Medical College,
New Delhi, Delhi, India

S. Tyagi · R. Yadav
Department of Psychiatry, Lady Hardinge Medical College and Associated Hospitals,
New Delhi, India

P. Kukreti et al. (eds.), *Women's Reproductive Mental Health in South Asia*,
South Asian Perspectives in Mental Health and Psychology,
https://doi.org/10.1007/978-981-96-9219-4_16

2 Forensic Psychiatry Issues in the Perinatal Period

Forensic psychiatry in the perinatal period involves applying psychiatric expertise to legal contexts, including maternal assessment for criminal responsibility, capacity assessments, and assessment of child welfare. Certain issues which can be of relevance in forensic psychiatry assessments with regard to perinatal psychiatry are as follows.

2.1 *Infanticide*

Infanticide refers to the killing of a child, often by the mother, within a short time after birth. In forensic psychiatry, infanticide is often linked to severe psychiatric conditions such as postpartum depression or psychosis.

But it is important to understand that in South Asian societies, infanticide is also deeply interwoven with sociocultural contexts, gender discrimination, and family honor codes. Notoriously, female infanticide, historically practiced due to patriarchal norms, preference for sons, and economic pressures associated with dowry, still remains a concerning issue, especially in rural areas of India (Saravanan, 2002), Pakistan, Bangladesh, and Nepal (Shoib et al., 2023). Additionally, societal stigma surrounding maternal mental illness, inadequate support for new mothers, familial isolation, and domestic violence may also significantly increase the risk of maternal infanticide (Srivastava, 2001).

Understanding the psychological basis of maternal infanticide involves differentiating between intentional, impulsive, and psychotic acts where intentional acts often reflect severe distress, hopelessness, or rationalizations based on cultural or personal beliefs, impulsive acts occur under acute stress or psychological crises, while psychotic infanticide results from delusions or hallucinations due to underlying psychiatric disorders (Anand, 2010). This distinction is the key in determining the concept of "mens rea" which may decide the fate of the mother. A recent case law (Savita Chaudhari v. State of Maharashtra, 2017) saw a mother being acquitted for infanticide due to postpartum depression, highlighting the importance of psychiatric testimony in such cases.

2.2 *Pseudocyesis and Delusional Pregnancy*

Pseudocyesis commonly referred to as "false pregnancy" is a condition in which a woman believes she is pregnant despite the absence of an actual fetus. This belief can be accompanied by bodily changes resembling pregnancy, such as abdominal enlargement and breast tenderness. Delusional pregnancy, by contrast, is primarily observed in individuals with psychotic disorders—most notably schizophrenia—where the conviction of being pregnant persists despite clear medical evidence to the contrary (Yadav et al., 2012).

Pseudocyesis is rare in most of the developed countries but continues to appear in clinical settings like of South Asia, where social and cultural pressures on women to conceive are high (Goyal et al., 2020). In South Asian nations, a strong emphasis on fertility and motherhood may exacerbate the emotional distress of childlessness which may potentially exacerbate such condition. It has also been known that women with limited social support, a history of infertility, or repeated pregnancy losses are more susceptible to developing this condition though psychiatric disorders such as depression, anxiety, and personality disorders have also been found as potential risk factors (Bera & Sarkar, 2015).

In forensic settings, both these conditions can result in coming into conflict with the law, especially when women act out on their delusions, such as attempting to conceal a nonexistent pregnancy or even attempting to kidnap a child (Seeman, 2014). Such cases present significant challenges for forensic evaluators, as they involve psychiatric disorders that may not be immediately apparent but significantly influence behavior.

2.3 *Baby Snatching and Forced Separation and Custody Loss*

In certain situations, women with mental illnesses may engage in baby snatching, often driven by delusions or intense desires to care for a child. This behavior is complicated by the legal and social system's inability to properly address mental health issues. For example, women may abduct children to fulfill their delusional belief that they are mothers, even if they do not have a biological child (D'Orbán, 1982).

Mothers with mental illness in such cases often risk losing custody under family laws. In India, the Guardians and Wards Act, 1890, assesses "fitness to care," for a mother often neglecting the need of providing support for child care as part of "reasonable accommodation" and right of a person with mental illness. Forced separation may occur if a mother is deemed unfit to take care of child on ground of mental illness. Such cases pose ethical dilemma of balancing "child's welfare" versus mother's right to care for her child if she is capable of doing so (Kenny, 2018).

2.4 *Fitness to Take Care of Child for Mothers with Mental Illness*

Mothers suffering from mental illnesses often face challenges in proving their ability to care for their children and, in cases mentioned above, may often be sent for evaluation of fitness to take care of their child. In South Asia, where stigma surrounding mental illness is prevalent, many mothers are also unjustly deemed unfit to care for their children. Western guidelines, like those from the *American Academy of Forensic Psychiatry (AAFP)*, emphasize structured assessments in such cases, but no such guidelines exist in any of the South Asian countries.

2.5 Denial and Concealment of Pregnancy

In some cases, women with mental illness deny their pregnancy, concealing it from both healthcare providers and family members. This can lead to criminal issues, particularly if the pregnancy results in the abandonment or harm of the child (Jenkins et al., 2011). Legal systems in South Asia often fail to recognize the psychiatric underpinnings of such behaviors and instead focus on the criminal aspects of the case. In Bangladesh, early marriage is common, but as per old hostel rules of university, married and pregnant female students were not allowed to stay in the dormitory hall of hostel, which was detrimental to the idea of supporting mothers during the perinatal period. Rather such rules were impediment to women empowerment and right to safe motherhood and posed as a risk factor for concealment of pregnancy. After protest, such rule was abolished in December 2021 (Arafat et al., 2022).

2.6 Mothers with Mental Illness in Prison and Mother-Baby Units

In many South Asian countries, women with mental illnesses who are incarcerated are separated from their children (United Nations Office on Drugs and Crime, 2008). Prisons lack appropriate infrastructure to support women with psychiatric conditions and their children, leading to both maternal and child suffering. The absence of mother-baby units (MBU) in these facilities further exacerbates the issue. International best practices suggest the establishment of mother-baby units to allow incarcerated mothers to remain with their infants (Dolan, 2018), promoting better mental health outcomes for both, but such care facilities are nonexistent in South Asian context for prisons.

2.7 Juvenile Justice and Separation of Children from Mothers

Under the Juvenile Justice Act (Government of India, 2015) in India, children may be removed from their mothers if the latter are deemed unfit to care for them due to mental illness or other factors. This raises ethical questions about whether the removal of the child is in the best interest of both parties. It also presents challenges in ensuring that these children are placed in safe and supportive environments while ensuring the mother's rights are not infringed upon.

2.8 Mental Health Care Act's Role

Among all South Asian Countries, The Mental Health Care Act (MHCA) 2017 (Government of India, 2017) of India is the only law which specifically talks about safeguarding separation of mother and child less than 3 years on grounds of mental illness. Under Section 21(4) of MHCA 2017, a child under 3 years cannot be separated from the mother in any mental health facility unless necessary for the child's safety, based on the psychiatrist's opinion. Such separation must be reviewed every 15 days, and it should be terminated as soon as conditions warranting separation cease to exist. The Act tries to finely balance right of motherhood and child welfare rights.

3 Evaluation of Perinatal Psychiatry Cases in Western Countries

In contrast to South Asia, many Western countries have well-established legal standards for the forensic evaluation of psychiatric conditions, including those that arise during the perinatal period. Western countries have comprehensive guidelines and expert systems for evaluating the mental state of mothers during the perinatal period and considering the impact of mental illness on criminal responsibility.

3.1 United States

In the United States, forensic psychiatric evaluations during the perinatal period are guided by established principles outlined by American Academy of Forensic Psychology (AAFP) and the *American Psychiatric Association (APA)* (Friedman et al., 2024). The key areas of evaluation include:

1. **Mental State at the Time of the Offense (MSO):** The forensic psychiatrist evaluates whether the mother's mental illness affected her behavior at the time of the alleged offense (Rogers & Shuman, 2000). This involves a detailed assessment of the psychiatric history, the presence of any perinatal disorders (such as postpartum depression or psychosis), and an understanding of the individual's mental state during the criminal act (Sher, 2015).

2. **Fitness to Stand Trial:** The psychiatrist assesses whether the individual is competent to stand trial, focusing on their ability to understand the nature of the proceedings and assist in their own defense (Sher, 2015).
3. **Postpartum Disorders:** In the United States, the AAFP recognizes the significance of postpartum psychosis and depression in the criminal justice system. The presence of these conditions can result in reduced criminal responsibility or a recommendation for mental health treatment instead of punitive measures (Friedman et al., 2024).

The landmark case of "Texas v. Andrea Yates" involved Andrea Yates who drowned her five children in 2001. Her delusions—including the belief that she was Satan and bore the "mark of the beast"—were evident signs of psychosis, yet the trial featured conflicting psychiatric testimonies and lacked a consistent legal framework for addressing postpartum mental illness. Despite a documented history of severe postpartum psychosis, Yates was charged with capital murder and found guilty after a brief trial, receiving a life sentence rather than psychiatric care. The case provoked national concern, prompting organizations such as Postpartum Support International to call for clearer diagnostic criteria, better medical education, and legislative reform. The American Psychiatric Association also emphasized the urgent need for courts to align with modern neuroscience and recognize that mentally ill defendants require treatment, not punishment. This case underscored critical gaps in the legal system's handling of postpartum psychiatric disorders and the application of the insanity defense (Spinelli, 2004).

In the United States, insanity defense is a common avenue in cases of postpartum psychosis, where mental illness is used to argue for a reduction in charges (e.g., from murder to manslaughter). However, the application of this defense varies as per different state laws and public understanding of mental illness, leading to inconsistent rulings (Spinelli, 2004).

3.2 United Kingdom

In contrast, the United Kingdom has a more formalized approach to postpartum disorders within its legal framework. Under English law, infanticide is recognized as a distinct offense (Section 1 of the Infanticide Act 1938), and a mother can be charged with infanticide rather than murder if it is shown that her actions were due to a mental disorder related to childbirth (e.g., postpartum depression or psychosis). The UK legal system provides more explicit criteria for considering postpartum mental health in cases involving maternal child death, and there is a stronger emphasis on medical testimony regarding the mother's state of mind during the crime (Martinez et al., 2003).

4 Evaluation of Perinatal Psychiatry Cases in South Asia

4.1 Criminal Responsibility Laws Across South Asia

In South Asia, there is no uniform or systematic approach to forensic psychiatric evaluation during the perinatal period, as seen in the West. While some South Asian countries have provisions in their penal codes for dealing with mental illness, there is a lack of clear guidelines or standardized procedures for evaluating perinatal psychiatric disorders (Table 16.1). Even criminal responsibility laws vary significantly across countries (De Alwis, 2019, Munir & Wright, 2023). These differences impact how cases involving mental illness during the perinatal period are treated in the legal system. Some countries have laws that recognize diminished responsibility due to mental illness, while others do not.

4.2 Status of Specialized Prison Mental Health Services or Forensic Psychiatry Services in South Asia

Prison mental health services in South Asia are generally underdeveloped, with limited access to mental healthcare for incarcerated women, especially those with perinatal psychiatric disorders (United Nations Office on Drugs and Crime, 2008). Prisons in the region lack specialized services for women, and mental healthcare is often not integrated into the overall prison health services (Table 16.2). In South Asian countries, the legal system often relies on inconsistent expert testimony, without comprehensive psychiatric evaluation procedures. For instance, the concept of "unsoundness of mind" is recognized, but the lack of trained forensic psychiatrists means that these evaluations are either insufficient or based on limited understanding of perinatal psychiatric conditions.

Table 16.1 Criminal responsibility laws in South Asia

Country	Criminal responsibility law	Lacunae in law
Bangladesh	Bangladesh penal code, Section 84—Insanity Defense	Lack of mental health professionals in the criminal justice system and delayed psychiatric evaluations (Nahin, 2022)
India	Section 23-Bhartiya Nyaya Sanhita	Mental illness is often not adequately considered in cases involving perinatal issues, such as postpartum depression (Behl et al., 2025)
Pakistan	Pakistan penal code, Section 84—Insanity Defense	Lack of clear guidelines on how to treat mental illness in perinatal cases, leading to inconsistencies in rulings (Munir & Wright, 2023)
Sri Lanka	Penal code, Section 86—Insanity Defense	Insufficient consideration of perinatal psychiatric conditions such as postpartum psychosis (De Alwis, 2019)

Table 16.2 Status of prison mental health services in South Asia

Country	Prison mental health services available	Forensic psychiatrist available	Status of mental health services for women in conflict with law during perinatal period in prisons
Bangladesh	Minimal; mental health services are basic (Arafat et al., 2024)	No forensic psychiatrists available	Women's mental healthcare is inadequately funded, and prison systems lack designated provisions for perinatal psychiatric care
India	Limited; basic mental health services available (Arafat et al., 2024)	Rarely available	Women often lack access to specialized psychiatric care. Mental health issues, especially perinatal disorders, are not adequately addressed
Nepal	Limited; mental health care is provided in some prisons (Arafat et al., 2024)	Limited forensic psychiatric services	Women face inadequate mental healthcare, and perinatal psychiatric conditions are not prioritized
Pakistan	Limited; some basic mental healthcare services	Rarely available	Women's mental health is underfunded, and there are no specific provisions for perinatal psychiatric care in prisons
Sri Lanka	Limited mental health services; some rehabilitation programs (Arafat et al., 2024)	Limited availability	Prisons provide minimal psychiatric care, with insufficient focus on perinatal mental health

4.3 Mothers in Conflict with the Law During the Perinatal Period in South Asia

Forensic issues during the perinatal period has not been an area of priority in the South Asian context, so data available on the exact magnitude of cases is scarce. However, research indicates that women charged with crimes like infanticide or child abandonment may often be suffering from untreated perinatal psychiatric disorders (Jefferies et al., 2016). In India, for example, a significant number of women incarcerated for infanticide or child neglect were found to be suffering from untreated postpartum depression or psychosis (Gowda et al., 2018). These women often lack access to psychiatric assessments and are imprisoned without consideration of their mental state at the time of the offense (Bera & Sarkar, 2015).

Shoib et al. (2023) provide a comprehensive overview of filicide cases in South Asia, focusing on India and Pakistan. The study identified 13 reports of filicide between 2000 and 2020, with 12 cases from India and 1 from Pakistan. Mental illness played a significant role, with depression identified in seven cases and schizophrenia in one case as contributing psychiatric conditions. Most victims were young female children under the age of six, and the majority of perpetrators were mothers. From a legal standpoint, outcomes varied. In India, several women were arrested and imprisoned, with little consistency in the evaluation of fitness to stand trial. This highlights glaring issue that in the absence of standardized assessment tools many cases proceeded without formal mental health evaluations, despite the clear role of psychiatric illness highlighting need for broader regional investigation and legal reform. The narrow interpretation of insanity defenses and lack of mandatory psychiatric evaluations frequently lead to convictions without fully considering the mother's compromised mental state. This gap highlights a critical need for reforms that integrate mental health expertise into legal proceedings, ensuring compassionate and just treatment for affected women. Table 16.3 summarizes key Indian case laws where maternal mental illness was a significant factor in infanticide trials.

4.4 Dilemmas and Challenges

The South Asian context presents several dilemmas and challenges in addressing forensic psychiatry issues in the perinatal period.

- **Stigma and Cultural Barriers**: Mental illness is often stigmatized in South Asian societies, particularly in women, making it difficult for these women to

Table 16.3 Notable case laws on maternal mental illness leading to infanticide in India

Case	Jurisdiction	Mental health condition	Outcome
Shanti Devi v. State (1967)	Delhi high Court	Schizophrenic psychosis	Acquitted under Section 84 IPC due to lack of motive and evidence of mental illness at the time of the act
Pappathi Ammal (1958)	Madras high Court	Suspected puerperal psychosis	Convicted; court acknowledged possible postpartum disorder but denied insanity defense due to lack of expert evidence
Kumari Chandra v. State (2018)	Rajasthan high Court	Premenstrual syndrome (PMS)	Acquitted under Section 84 IPC; supported by medical testimony from three doctors
Siddheswari Bora (1981)	Assam high Court	Claimed mental derangement	Convicted; court noted possible "impulsive insanity" but denied defense due to insufficient evidence
Savita Manish Chaudhari vs The State of Maharashtra 2017	Mumbai High Court	Postpartum depression	Convicted; insanity plea rejected due to absence of diagnosis or treatment at the time of the crime
Case Report: Rural India (Saha et al., 2015*)*	Unspecified	Schizophrenia	Convicted; lack of prior treatment and awareness led to infanticide under command hallucinations
Chunni Bai v. State of Chhattisgarh (2025)	Supreme Court of India	Temporary mental disorder influenced by superstition	Conviction reduced from murder to culpable homicide not amounting to murder under Section 304 part II IPC; released based on time served

seek help. This stigma extends to the criminal justice system, where psychiatric disorders are often overlooked.
- **Inadequate Legal Protections**: Although some South Asian countries have legal mechanisms in place to safeguard women with mental illnesses, these provisions are often poorly enforced, and the legal system does not adequately address perinatal psychiatric conditions.
- **Underdeveloped Prison Mental Health Services**: The lack of specialized mental health services in South Asian prisons means that women with mental illnesses, particularly those with perinatal conditions, are often left untreated, exacerbating their conditions.
- **Lack of Forensic Psychiatrists**: Many South Asian countries lack forensic psychiatrists trained to assess and address the complex psychiatric conditions of mothers during the perinatal period, leading to inconsistent and inadequate evaluations.

5 The Way Forward

Addressing the forensic psychiatry issues related to the perinatal period in South Asia requires several key reforms:

- **Improved Legal Frameworks**: South Asian countries need to revise their criminal responsibility laws to include specific provisions for mental health conditions during the perinatal period.
- **Development of Mother-Baby Units**: Establishing mother-baby units within prisons could provide an environment where incarcerated mothers can remain with their children while receiving the necessary psychiatric care.
- **Increased Training for Legal and Medical Professionals**: Forensic psychiatrists, judges, and lawyers should receive training on perinatal psychiatric conditions to ensure better outcomes for mothers with mental illness.
- **Strengthening Prison Mental Health Services**: Prisons should invest in specialized mental healthcare for incarcerated women, particularly those with perinatal mental health issues.

6 Conclusion

The perinatal period presents unique forensic psychiatry challenges, particularly in South Asia, where cultural, legal, and healthcare systems are often ill-equipped to address the complex needs of women with mental illness during this period. Despite some legal provisions, gaps in the understanding and application of mental health laws in the perinatal period persist. There is a need to develop structured legal frameworks sensitive to needs of women with perinatal mental disorders.

References

Anand, S. (2010). Rationalizing infanticide: A medico-legal assessment of the criminal code's child homicide offence. *Alberta Law Review, 47*(3), 705–725. https://doi.org/10.29173/alr184

Arafat, S. M. Y., Kar, S. K., Abhayanayake, C., Sharma, P., & Marthoenis, M. (2024). Prison mental health in South-East Asia: A narrative review. *Brain and Behavior, 14*(8), e70004. https://doi.org/10.1002/brb3.70004

Arafat, S. M. Y., Kar, S. K., & Kabir, R. (2022). Reproductive health care challenges for married female university students in Bangladesh. *The Lancet Regional Health Southeast Asia, 1*, 100001. https://doi.org/10.1016/j.lansea.2022.03.001

Behl, R., Nemane, V., & Gurpur, S. (2025). Legal interventions for perinatal depression in India: A qualitative study with clinical specialists having expertise in perinatal mental health. *BMJ Open, 15*(4), e059123. https://doi.org/10.1136/bmjopen-2021-059123

Bera, S. C., & Sarkar, S. (2015). Delusion of pregnancy: A systematic review of 84 cases in the literature. *Indian Journal of Psychological Medicine, 37*(2), 131–137. https://doi.org/10.4103/0253-7176.155609

Chunni Bai v. State of Chhattisgarh, Supreme Court of India. (2025). Retrieved from https://indiankanoon.org/doc/8644145/

D'Orbán, P. T. (1982). Child stealing and pseudocyesis. *The British Journal of Psychiatry, 141*(2), 196–198. https://doi.org/10.1192/bjp.141.2.196

De Alwis, L. (2019). Historical origins of the insanity defense in Sri Lanka and India. *Sri Lanka Journal of Psychiatry, 10*(2), 4–10. https://doi.org/10.4038/sljpsyc.v10i2.8211

Dolan, R. (2018). *Pregnant women in prison: Mental health, admission to prison mother and baby units and initial outcomes for mother and child (doctoral dissertation, University of Manchester).* University of Manchester. https://research.manchester.ac.uk/en/studentTheses/pregnant-women-in-prison-mental-health-admission-to-prison-mother

Friedman, S. H., Sorrentino, R., Kaempf, A., Price, M., Landess, J., Glezer, A., Penn, J., Westmoreland, P., Lewis, C., Cerny, C., & Janofsky, J. (2024). AAPL practice resource: Reproductive psychiatry/women's mental health in forensic psychiatry practice. *Journal of the American Academy of Psychiatry and the Law, 52*(1), 3–12. https://doi.org/10.1176/appi.focus.17401

Government of India. (2015). *The juvenile justice (care and protection of children) act, 2015.* Ministry of Law and Justice. https://www.indiacode.nic.in/handle/123456789/2148

Government of India. (2017). *The Mental Healthcare Act, 2017 (Act No. 10 of 2017).* Ministry of Health and Family Welfare. https://www.indiacode.nic.in/handle/123456789/2249

Gowda, G. S., Kumar, C. N., Mishra, S., Malathesh, B. C., Komal, S., Math, S. B., & Chandra, P. S. (2018). Maternal filicide: A case series from a medico-legal psychiatry unit in India. *Asian Journal of Psychiatry, 36*, 42–45. https://doi.org/10.1016/j.ajp.2018.06.004

Goyal, S., Gupta, B., Sharma, E., Dalal, P. K., & Pradeep, Y. (2020). Psychiatric morbidity, cultural factors, and health-seeking behaviour in perinatal women: A cross-sectional study from a tertiary care Centre of North India. *Indian Journal of Psychological Medicine, 42*(1), 52–57. https://doi.org/10.4103/IJPSYM.IJPSYM_96_19

Insan, N., Weke, A., Rankin, J., et al. (2022). Perceptions and attitudes around perinatal mental health in Bangladesh, India and Pakistan: A systematic review of qualitative data. *BMC Pregnancy and Childbirth, 22*, 293. https://doi.org/10.1186/s12884-022-04642-x

Jefferies, D., Horsfall, D., & Schmied, V. (2016). Blurring reality with fiction: Exploring the stories of women, madness, and infanticide. *Women and Birth, 30*(1), e24–e31. https://doi.org/10.1016/j.wombi.2016.07.001

Jenkins, A., Millar, S., & Robins, J. (2011). Denial of pregnancy: A literature review and discussion of ethical and legal issues. *Journal of the Royal Society of Medicine, 104*(7), 286–291. https://doi.org/10.1258/jrsm.2011.100376

Kenny, K. S. (2018). Mental health harm to mothers when a child is taken by child protective services: Health equity considerations. *Canadian Journal of Psychiatry, 63*(5), 304–307. https://doi.org/10.1177/0706743717748885
Kumari Chandra v. State, Rajasthan High Court. (2018). Retrieved from https://indiankanoon.org/doc/197692173/
Martinez, M., et al. (2003). Infanticide: Psychosocial and legal perspectives on mothers who kill. *Journal of the American Academy of Child & Adolescent Psychiatry, 42*(12), 1531–1532. https://doi.org/10.1097/01.CHI.0000089880.32852.63
Munir, M. A., & Wright, B. (2023). Reshaping insanity in Pakistani law: The case of Safia Bano. *American Journal of Law & Medicine, 49*(2–3), 301–313. https://doi.org/10.1017/amj.2023.33
Nahin, S. I. (2022). *Insanity plea in criminal and civil litigation in Bangladesh*. Jahangirnagar University. https://www.researchgate.net/publication/375698130_INSANITY_PLEA_IN_CRIMINAL_AND_CIVIL_LITIGATION_IN_BANGLADESH
O'Hara, M. W., & Wisner, K. L. (2014). Perinatal mental illness: Definition, description and aetiology. *Best Practice & Research Clinical Obstetrics & Gynaecology, 28*(1), 3–12. https://doi.org/10.1016/j.bpobgyn.2013.09.002
Pappathi Ammal, Madras High Court. (1958). Retrieved from https://indiankanoon.org/doc/1516345/
Rogers, R., & Shuman, D. W. (2000). The mental state at the time of the offense measure: Its validation and admissibility under Daubert. *The Journal of the American Academy of Psychiatry and the Law, 28*(1), 23–32.
Saha, R., Singh, S. M., & Nischal, A. (2015). Infanticide by a mother with untreated schizophrenia. *Shanghai Archives of Psychiatry, 27*(5), 311–314. https://doi.org/10.11919/j.issn.1002-0829.215058
Sapkota, D., Dennison, S., & Thompson, C. (2024). Mental disorders among mothers in contact with the criminal justice system: A scoping review and meta-analysis. *Community Mental Health Journal, 60*(4), 699–712. https://doi.org/10.1007/s10597-023-01222-x
Saravanan, S. (2002). Female infanticide in India: A review of literature. *Social Change, 32*(2), 58–66. https://doi.org/10.1177/004908570203200205
Savita Manish Chaudhari v. State of Maharashtra & Anr., Criminal Application No. 117 of 2016, Bombay High Court. (2017, March 27). Retrieved from https://indiankanoon.org/doc/11594484/
Seeman, M. V. (2014). Pseudocyesis, delusional pregnancy, and psychosis: The birth of a delusion. *World Journal of Clinical Cases, 2*(8), 338–344. https://doi.org/10.12998/wjcc.v2.i8.328
Shanti Devi v. State, Delhi High Court. (1967). Retrieved from https://indiankanoon.org/doc/481181/
Sher, L. (2015). Forensic psychiatric evaluations: An overview of methods, ethical issues, and criminal and civil assessments. *International Journal of Adolescent Medicine and Health, 27*(2), 109–115. https://doi.org/10.1515/ijamh-2015-5001
Shoib, S., Saleem, T., Menon, V., Ali, S. A., & Arafat, S. M. Y. (2023). Filicide in South Asia: Demography, risk factors, psychiatric, and legal aspects. *Medicine, Science, and the Law, 63*(2), 159–167. https://doi.org/10.1177/00258024221122248
Siddheswari Bora, Assam High Court. (1981). Cited in Vashist, L. (2023). Infanticide and the Indian legal response. Seminar India. Retrieved from https://www.india-seminar.com/2023/764/764-07%20LATIKA%20VASHIST.htm
Spinelli, M. G. (2004). Maternal infanticide associated with mental illness: Prevention and the promise of saved lives. *American Journal of Psychiatry, 161*(9), 1548–1557. https://doi.org/10.1176/appi.ajp.161.9.1548
Srivastava, S. P. (2001). The perils of pre-birth murder: A sociological analysis of female foeticide. *Journal of Social Welfare, 47*(10), 7–12.
United Nations Office on Drugs and Crime. (2008). *Handbook for prison managers and policymakers on women and imprisonment*. United Nations. https://www.un.org/ruleoflaw/blog/document/handbook-for-prison-managers-and-policymakers-on-women-and-imprisonment/
Yadav, T., Balhara, Y. P., & Kataria, D. K. (2012). Pseudocyesis versus delusion of pregnancy: Differential diagnoses to be kept in mind. *Indian Journal of Psychological Medicine, 34*(1), 82–84. https://doi.org/10.4103/0253-7176.96167

Index

P. Kukreti et al. (eds.), *Women's Reproductive Mental Health in South Asia*, South Asian Perspectives in Mental Health and Psychology,
https://doi.org/10.1007/978-981-96-9219-4

MIX
Papier aus verantwortungsvollen Quellen
Paper from responsible sources
FSC® C105338

If you have any concerns about our products,
you can contact us on
ProductSafety@springernature.com

In case Publisher is established outside the EU,
the EU authorized representative is:
Springer Nature Customer Service Center GmbH
Europaplatz 3, 69115 Heidelberg, Germany

Printed by Libri Plureos GmbH
in Hamburg, Germany